TRISOMY 21
(DOWN SYNDROME)

Proceedings of the conference, Trisomy 21 (Down Syndrome):
Research Perspectives, held in Boston, Massachusetts.

Sponsored by the National Institute of Child Health and
Human Development of the National Institutes of Health,
Bethesda, Maryland.

Organizing committee:
Park S. Gerald, M.D., Chairman
Felix F. de la Cruz, M.D., M.P.H.
Allen Gates, Ph.D.
Georgiana Jagiello, M.D.
Pamela Pierce, M.S., Genetics Associate
Siegfried Pueschel, M.D., M.P.H.

TRISOMY 21 (CHRISTA MACK)
(DOWN SYNDROME)

Research Perspectives

Edited by
Felix F. de la Cruz, M.D., M.P.H.
Special Assistant for Pediatrics
Mental Retardation and Developmental Disabilities Branch
National Institute of Child Health and Human Development
National Institutes of Health
and
Clinical Associate Professor
Georgetown University School of Medicine

and

Park S. Gerald, M.D.
Chief, Clinical Genetics Division
Children's Hospital Medical Center
and
Professor
Harvard Medical School

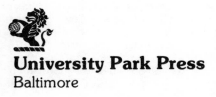

University Park Press
Baltimore

UNIVERSITY PARK PRESS
International Publishers in Science, Medicine, and Education
233 East Redwood Street
Baltimore, Maryland 21202

Composed by University Park Press, Typesetting Division.
Manufactured in the United States of America by
Universal Lithographers, Inc.,
and The Maple Press Company.

Library of Congress Cataloging in Publication Data
Main entry under title:
Trisomy 21 (Down syndrome)
(NICHD—Mental retardation research centers series)
"Proceedings of the conference . . . held in Boston,
Massachusetts, September 18-19, 1978. Sponsored by the
National Institute of Child Health and Human Development
of the National Institutes of Health, Bethesda, Maryland."
Includes indexes.
1. Down syndrome—Genetic aspects—Congresses.
I. de la Cruz, Felix F. II. Gerald, Park S.
III. United States. National Institute of Child
Health and Human Development. IV. Series: United
States. National Institute of Child Health and Human
Development. NICHD—Mental retardation research
centers series. [DNLM: 1. Down syndrome—Etiology
—Congresses. 2. Down syndrome—Congresses. WS107
T837 1978]
RC571.T74   616.85'8842'042   80-14035
ISBN 0-8391-1588-1

Contents

The Trisomy State

Animal Models

Contributors and Conference Participants

Eva D. Alberman, M.D., M.F.C.M.
London Hospital Medical College
University of London
Turner Street
London E12AD, England

Charles F. Barlow, M.D.
Department of Neurology
Children's Hospital Medical Center
300 Longwood Avenue
Boston, Massachusetts 02115

W. Roy Breg, M.D.
Department of Human Genetics
Yale University
333 Cedar Street
New Haven, Connecticut 06520

Thomas G. Brewster, M.D.
Foundation for Blood Research
Route 1
Scarborough, Maine 04074

Jan Chamberlin, B.A.
Crippled Children's Division
Division of Medical Genetics
University of Oregon Health
  Sciences Center
Portland, Oregon 97201

Thomas E. Cone, Jr., M.D.
Division of Clinical Genetics
Children's Hospital Medical Center
300 Longwood Avenue
Boston, Massachusetts 02115

Bruce Cushna, Ph.D.
Developmental Evaluation Clinic
Children's Hospital Medical Center
300 Longwood Avenue
Boston, Massachusetts 02115

Richard L. Davidson, Ph.D.
Division of Clinical Genetics
Children's Hospital Medical Center
300 Longwood Avenue
Boston, Massachusetts 02115

Felix F. de la Cruz, M.D., M.P.H.
NICHD, National Institutes of Health
Landow Building
7910 Woodmont Avenue
Bethesda, Maryland 20205

Peter Dignan, M.D.
Director, Institute for Developmental
  Research
Children's Hospital Research Foundation
Department of Pediatrics
Elland and Bethesda Avenue
Cincinatti, Ohio 45229

Irvin Emanuel, M.D.
Director, Child Development and MR
  Center
University of Washington
Seattle, Washington 98195

Charles J. Epstein, M.D.
Department of Pediatrics
Department of Biochemistry and
  Biophysics
University of California
San Francisco, California 94143

Lois B. Epstein, M.D.
Department of Pediatrics
The Cancer Research Institute
University of California
San Francisco, California 94143

Robert M. Fineman, M.D., Ph.D.
Department of Pediatrics
University of Utah College of Medicine
50 Medical Drive
Salt Lake City, Utah 84132

Ellen Fleischnick, M.D.
Division of Clinical Genetics
Children's Hospital Medical Center
300 Longwood Avenue
Boston, Massachusetts 02115

Uta Francke, M.D.
Departments of Human Genetics and
    Pediatrics
Yale Medical School
333 Cedar Street
New Haven, Connecticut 06520

Allen H. Gates, Ph.D.
Division of Genetics
Box 461
University of Rochester Medical Center
Rochester, New York 14642

Park S. Gerald, M.D.
Chief, Division of Clinical Genetics
Children's Hospital Medical Center
300 Longwood Avenue
Boston, Massachusetts 02115

John L. Hamerton, D.Sc., F.C.C.M.G.
Division of Genetics
University of Manitoba Children's Center
Winnipeg, Manitoba
Canada R3E 0Z3

Ernest B. Hook, M.D.
Birth Defects Institute
Division of Laboratories and Research
New York State Department of Health
Albany, New York 12237
and
Department of Pediatrics
Albany Medical College
Albany, New York 12208

Georgiana Jagiello, M.D., D.Sc.
Virgil Damon Professor of Obstetrics and
    Gynecology and of Human Genetics
    and Development
Director, Center for Reproductive Studies
Columbia University College of Physicians
    and Surgeons
630 West 168th Street
New York, New York 10032

A. Myron Johnson, M.D.
Department of Pediatrics
School of Medicine
University of North Carolina
Chapel Hill, North Carolina 27514

Kenneth K. Kidd, Ph.D.
Department of Human Genetics
Yale University School of Medicine
333 Cedar Street
New Haven, Connecticut 06510

David Kram, Ph.D.
Gerontology Research Center
National Institute on Aging
Baltimore, Maryland 21224

Samuel A. Latt, M.D., Ph.D.
Division of Clinical Genetics
Children's Hospital Medical Center
300 Longwood Avenue
Boston, Massachusetts 02115

R. Ellen Magenis, M.D.
Division of Medical Genetics
Crippled Children's Division
University of Oregon Health Sciences
    Center
Portland, Oregon 97201

Orlando J. Miller, M.D.
Departments of Human Genetics and
    Development and Obstetrics and
    Gynecology
Health Science Center
Columbia University
701 W. 168th Street
New York, New York 10032

Montrose J. Moses, Ph.D.
Department of Anatomy
Duke University Medical Center
Durham, North Carolina 27710

Harold Nitowsky, M.D.
Department of Pediatrics and Genetics
Genetic Counseling Program
Albert Einstein College of Medicine
Bronx Municipal Hospital Center
Bronx, New York 10461

Paul E. Polani, M.D., F.R.C.P.,
    F.R.C.O.G., D.C.H., F.R.S.
Pediatric Research Unit
The Prince Philip Research Laboratories
Guy's Tower
Guy's Hospital Medical School
London SE1 9RT, England

Siegfried M. Pueschel, M.D., M.P.H.
Child Development Center
Rhode Island Hospital
593 Eddy Street
Providence, Rhode Island 02902

L. Sandler, Ph.D.
Professor of Genetics
Department of Genetics
University of Washington
Seattle, Washington 98195

Roy Schmickel, M.D.
K2015 Holden Building
University of Michigan Medical Center
Ann Arbor, Michigan 48109

Edward L. Schneider, M.D.
Gerontology Research Center
National Institute on Aging
Baltimore, Maryland 21224

Margaret Siber, M.D.
Developmental Evaluation Center
Children's Hospital Medical Center
300 Longwood Avenue
Boston, Massachusetts 02115

Richard L. Sidman, M.D.
Division of Neuroscience
Children's Hospital Medical Center
300 Longwood Avenue
Boston, Massachusetts 02115

Shirley Soukup, Ph.D.
Children's Hospital Research Foundation
Elland and Bethesda Avenue
Cincinnati, Ohio 45229

Robert L. Summitt, M.D.
Departments of Pediatrics and Anatomy
   and Child Development Center
University of Tennessee
Center for the Health Sciences
Memphis, Tennessee 38163

John A. Sved, Ph.D.
School of Biological Sciences
Sydney University
N.S.W. 2006, Australia

Irene A. Uchida, Ph.D.
Department of Pediatrics
McMaster University
Hamilton, Ontario
Canada L8N 3Z5

Golder Wilson, M.D., Ph.D.
K2015 Holden Building
University of Michigan Medical Center
Ann Arbor, Michigan 48109

John W. Wood, M.D.
Division of Clinical Genetics
Children's Hospital Medical Center
300 Longwood Avenue
Boston, Massachusetts 02115

Foreword

The most important process underlying the more severe grades of mental deficiency is cerebral dysgenesis, that is, fault in the formation and early development of the central nervous system during gestation. This accounts for at least 50% of people with mental retardation, and it is the hard core of the problem. Cerebral dysgenesis is a major point of emphasis at the Children's Hospital Medical Center Mental Retardation Research Program, in particular, the Genetics Program, directed by Dr. Park S. Gerald, and the Neuroscience Program, under Dr. Richard L. Sidman. Cerebral dysgenesis refers to a heterogeneous group of patients. However, with reasonable frequency, somatic markers identify specific syndromes, and of these the most common is Down syndrome, an abnormality of chromosome 21. Recently, amniocentesis has been used to identify an affected fetus early enough to decide whether to interrupt pregnancy.

The problem is hardly solved, however, and that is why this conference was convened. We need to know more of the basic causes of perturbation of chromosome 21 and other chromosomes, and how this leads to false signals to the developing brain. When the process is better understood, where, when, and how may it be interrupted?

There have been two truly major developments in the diagnosis of Down syndrome: its identification as an abnormality of chromosome 21, and the application of this knowledge through amniocentesis to assist in genetics counseling. I am hopeful that there will soon be others.

Charles F. Barlow, M.D.

TRISOMY 21
(DOWN SYNDROME)

EPIDEMIOLOGY OF TRISOMY 21

Down Syndrome
Frequency in Human Populations and Factors Pertinent to Variation in Rates

Ernest B. Hook

There are at least four reasons for interest in the epidemiology of Down syndrome. These are related to:

1. Understanding of factors in the causal chain that result in affected persons and the possible implications of this information upon prevention, either directly, through intervention programs involving amniocentesis and prenatal diagnosis, or indirectly, through changes resulting from an understanding of empirical risks and putative "causal" factors
2. Greater precision of genetic counseling
3. Prediction of the numbers of affected people so that the magnitude of their needs for special educational, rehabilitative, and therapeutic services may be anticipated
4. Understanding that may be gained concerning related cytogenetic disorders, such as other trisomies, as well as defects that occur in high frequency in those affected, such as acute leukemia.

In this review I consider data on the frequency of Down syndrome in various populations, and some associated factors, most of them putative, not established. I focus upon observations, trends, and developments that have been reported recently, i.e., in the past 5 to 10 years, as well as on some observations of interest from the earlier literature that are pertinent, particularly if additional comment appears of

With the permission of editors and publishers, most of this chapter also appears in the volume *Down Syndrome: Advances in Biomedicine and the Behavioral Sciences,* edited by S. M. Pueschel, Garland SPPM Press, New York.

value. I have been surprised in reviewing much of the earlier work, that matters that I had considered established, such as the recurrence risk for 47,trisomy 21, or the putative association of trisomy 21 and extra X chromosomes, are far from certain. I have therefore also reviewed critically and in some detail some other issues, even though no recent data have been available.

SOURCES

Anyone attempting such a review is indebted to two major sources. One is the book by Penrose and Smith on Down's anomaly (1966), the second edition of which, by Smith and Berg (1977), appeared after Penrose's death. The second major source is that of Lilienfeld, who reviewed the epidemiology of Down syndrome in 1969.

Three other sources have also been very helpful: Hamerton's volume (1971) on clinical cytogenetics, an extensive bibliography and review provided by Cohen et al. (1977) in their summary of their second Baltimore case-control study, and a symposium of the New York Academy of Sciences in 1970 (Apgar, 1970).

PHENOTYPE AND GENOTYPE

Until the advent of the chromosomal era, Down syndrome could only be a clinical diagnosis. After discovery of the significance of extra chromosome material on chromosome 21, more precise delineation became possible. The terms *trisomy 21* and *Down syndrome* are often used interchangeably now, but they should be clearly understood as applying "operationally" to genotype and phenotypic diagnosis, respectively. The approximate distribution of cytogenetic findings in persons with the phenotypic diagnosis Down syndrome are given in Tables 1 and 2. (Precise data on the specific chromosomes involved in translocations are not yet available.) These proportions vary between populations, in that the higher the proportion of older parents having live births, the higher the proportion of individuals with 47,trisomy 21 and probably 47,trisomy 21 mosaics. (See Table 3, illustrating change with age.)

Table 1.   Estimated distribution of genotypes in live births associated with Down syndrome

47,trisomy 21 (presumably nonmosaic)	93%–96%
47,trisomy 21 mosaic	2%–4%
46,interchange trisomy (Robertsonian translocations)[a]	2%–5%
Other aberrations	<1%
Apparently normal karyotype	<1%

These estimates are derived from reports in the literature but are corrected for a bias in such surveys toward selection inclusion of Down infants born to younger mothers in cytogenetic surveys (see text). The proportion also depends upon the maternal age structure of the populations involved and the relative use of prenatal diagnosis. The estimates are meant to apply to the proportions in those populations on which cytogenetic studies are reported in Table 2.

[a]Includes mosaic translocations.

Table 2. Proportion of cytogenetic abnormalities among those with Down syndrome in several studies in which 300 or more persons have been studied[a]

Abnormality	Sutherland et al. (1979)	Papp et al. (1977)	Fabia (1970)[c]	Higurashi et al. (1969)	Gardner et al. (1973)	Aula, Leisti, & von Koskull (1973)
47,+21	94.0%	91.7%[b]	92.4%[d]	93.5%	91.8%[e]	91.5%[h]
47,+21 mosaicism (i.e., with 46 normal line)	2.1%	4.4%	3.0%	2.2%	4.4%	1.6%
Translocation	3.1%	3.9%	4.6%	4.4%	3.7%	5.6%
D/21		2.5%	1.9%	3.4%	2.4%[f]	2.8%
G/21		1.4%	2.8%	0.9%	1.3%[g]	2.8%
Other	0.8%					1.2%[i]
Total N	774	362	471	321	972	425

[a]Proportions will vary with maternal age composition of population. See text.

[b]One with XXY, two with XXX.

[c]Data on other cases are summarized in text. (Mean maternal age of karyotyped cases = 32.0; of others = 34.4).

[d]Two with C/C balanced translocation, one with D/D balanced translocation, one with XXY.

[e]Three with reciprocal translocation, two with XXY, two with XXY mosaicism, two with XXX mosaicism, two with 46-D,t (Dq21q) (mosaicism) are among those with trisomy 21 included here.

[f]Of 23 cases, 5 were familial, 2 were of unknown status.

[g]Of 13 cases, 3 were familial.

[h]Includes one balanced D/D carrier and one case with two fragments.

[i]Includes three cases with 47,+21q− genotypes in whole or in part and one 46,XY,15p+ with typical Down features and clinical interpretation that the 15p+ region includes 21q maternal. Also includes one 46,21 qi mosaic.

Table 3. Proportion of major etiologies of Down syndrome by maternal age

Maternal age (years)	47, +21	47, +21 mosaicism	21/D interchange trisomy	21/G interchange trisomy	Total N	
15–19	84.9%	5.0%	4.2%	5.9%	119	(100.1%)
20–24	89.8%	1.2%	5.9%	3.1%	323	(100.0%)
25–29	91.1%	2.1%	3.0%	3.9%	438	(100.1%)
30–34	92.7%	2.7%	2.0%	2.5%	441	(99.9%)
35–39	97.2%	1.4%	1.1%	0.4%	566	(100.1%)
40–44	97.1%	2.0%	0.0%	0.8%	491	(99.9%)
≥45	96.6%	2.3%	0.0%	1.1%	88	(100.0%)
All	93.7%	2.1%	2.1%	2.1%		
N	2311	52	52	51	2466	(100.0%)

Recalculated from data of Richards (1969) in data from 20 studies. The 51 mosaics include three with structural change (2 G/21 mosaics) and one triple line mosaic. Note the increasing proportion of 47, +21 cases with increasing age and the decreasing proportion of those with interchange trisomy.

In considering epidemiological investigations of Down syndrome, one must distinguish the preponderance of studies based on phenotypic evaluation only from those relatively few studies in which cytogenetic evaluation has been done on all diagnosed persons. Since about 95% of cases of Down syndrome phenotype are associated with 47,trisomy 21 (and more if we include 46/47, + 21 mosaics), epidemiological investigations of the phenotype are predominantly studies of the epidemiology of the 47, + 21 genotype. The inclusion of translocation cases in phenotypic surveys contributes a small amount of "noise," which for the most part will not seriously distort inferences concerning 47, + 21 that may be drawn from these studies. The main sections of this review consider primarily, but not exclusively, the epidemiology of 47, + 21 Down syndrome and some of the problems raised by mosaicism. The last section considers specifically the epidemiology of translocation Down syndrome, which is different in that, among other factors, there is a much higher proportion of familial cases and a much less marked parental age effect, if any.

THE FREQUENCY OF DOWN SYNDROME IN LIVE BIRTHS

It is most useful to consider the "incidence" rate, which for birth defects is best understood to mean, formally, the *prevalence* rate in *live births*.

There is clear evidence from many different studies that the crude rate has dropped recently in many different jurisdictions. With the widespread availability of birth control, a dramatic worldwide drop in the relative fertility of older mothers has occurred, along with a drop of the absolute fertility in the entire childbearing population, which may be defined for these purposes as women ages 15–49 (Figure 1). In view of the marked increase of rate of Down syndrome with maternal age, it is not unexpected that the ubiquitous drop in the proportion of older women among those having live births is also associated with a drop in the crude incidence rate in many different areas. The rates in many studies of European and U.S. live births have gone from about 1.5 per 1000 in the 1950s to close to about 1.0–1.2 per 1000 in the 1970s (Holmes, 1978a; Hook and Porter, 1977; Lowry et al., 1976; Stein et al., 1977).

A decreased proportion of older mothers in the population not only results in a declining crude rate of Down syndrome in live births but also should be expected to result in a lower average maternal age of those born with Down syndrome. This trend has also been noted in many studies (e.g., Gardner et al., 1973; Kuroki et al., 1977; Shiono, Kadowaki, and Nakao, 1975). Shiono et al. provided evidence that the same demographic trends in Europe and the U.S. have occurred also in Japan. Some apparent misunderstandings of this trend in mean maternal age may be fostered by a review by Holmes (1978a) in which the change in the *proportion* of Down syndrome infants born to older mothers was ambiguously discussed in the context of genetic counseling concerning the rates of infants with Down syndrome born to older mothers (see also Hook, 1978e; Holmes, 1978b). This has led to the misunderstanding by some that maternal age is no longer of significance (see Holmes, 1978b). There seems to be no clinical or epidemiological utility in considering a proportional analysis such as that discussed by Holmes (1978a) once one realizes that the changes in rates are exactly what would be expected of the demographic changes resulting from

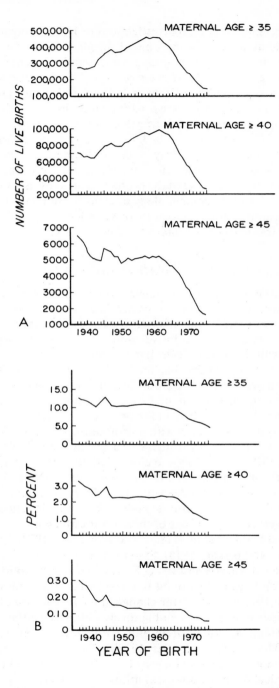

Figure 1. A, Changes in numbers of live births to older mothers in the United States, 1937–1975. B, Changes in proportions of live births to older mothers in the U.S., 1937–1975.

Table 4.   Regression equations for Down syndrome rate and maternal age

Study	20–31 years		33–49 years	
	b_1	b_0	b_1	b_0
New York[a] (Hook and Chambers, 1977)	0.066	−1.874	0.242	−7.466
Sweden (Hook and Lindsjo, 1978)	0.053	−1.511	0.268	−8.460
Massachusetts (Hook and Fabia, 1978)	0.045	−1.458	0.243	−7.578

[a]The equation for New York was re-derived from the Hook and Chambers data because a linear—not exponential—model was used in the younger age interval of that study. The rates in Table 5 are those of the original study.

the relatively fewer number of older women having live births. Proportional analysis was used by earlier workers, particularly Penrose (e.g., Penrose and Smith, 1966), in comparing trends from different countries whose data sources were known to be incomplete. This is different than estimating risks or rates, however. (See further discussion in Hook and Porter, 1977).

There have been several recent detailed studies on maternal age-specific rates (Hook and Chambers, 1977; Hook and Fabia, 1978; Hook and Lindsjo, 1978; Trimble and Baird, 1978). The data from these studies indicated that after age 30 the incidence rate can be approximated well by a first-degree exponential equation of the form $y = e^{(b_1x + b_0)}$ (which may also be written $y = \exp(b_1x + b_0)$ or $\ln y = b_1x + b_0$), where $x =$ maternal age at birth of child and $y =$ rate per 1000 live births); these equations all suggest an increase in incidence of about 30% per year over age 30—a convenient mnemonic. Between ages 20 and 30, the rates exhibit a much flatter change with increasing age and can be fit well to a linear equation: $y = b_1x + b_0$. They can also be fit well in this interval to a first-degree exponential equation, but to one different from that for the 33–49 interval. This is because when the rate of increase is very small, as in the 20–30 interval, there is little difference between a first-degree linear or exponential increase. Another way of putting this condition is that when x is very small, $e^x \doteq 1 + x$, so $\ln (1 + x) \doteq x$.[1]

Equations and rates by 1-year intervals appear in Tables 4 and 5, and Table 6 gives cumulative rates by 5-year intervals for the older ages.

What is striking is the apparent, very abrupt change in rates that occurs at about age 30 when the observed rates are plotted on semilogarithmic paper against maternal age by single-year interval (see Figure 2). This observation had been noted earlier by others, when data by 5-year intervals were analyzed (e.g., Lilienfeld, 1969; Penrose and Smith, 1966), although this latter approach has produced at least one statistical artifact at the upper extreme of age. This abrupt increase suggests that there is some "basic" biological change that occurs at this point. Sharp changes of this type may be

---

[1]Since this has been written, it has been discovered that a simple single equation fits about as well over the entire age range as do two separate first-order differential equations (Lamson and Hook, in press). This equation is of the type $\ln (y − a) = b_1x + b_0$ or $y = a + \exp (b_1x + b_0)$. In this formulation the constant a represents a constant factor independent of age and the expression b_1x represents an age-related factor.

Table 5.   Estimates of rates of Down syndrome per 1000 live births by single-year maternal age interval in three studies

Maternal age (years)	Massachusetts study[a]	New York study[b]	Swedish study[c]
20	0.57	0.52	0.64
21	0.60	0.59	0.67
22	0.64	0.65	0.71
23	0.67	0.71	0.75
24	0.70	0.77	0.79
25	0.74	0.83	0.83
26	0.77	0.89	0.87
27	0.80	0.95	0.92
28	0.84	1.01	0.97
29	0.87	1.07	1.02
30	0.90	1.13	1.08
31	0.93	1.21	1.14
32	1.15	1.38	1.25
33	1.55	1.69	1.47
34	1.98	2.15	1.92
35	2.53	2.74	2.51
36	3.22	3.49	3.28
37	4.11	4.45	4.28
38	5.24	5.66	5.60
39	6.68	7.21	7.32
40	8.52	9.19	9.57
41	10.86	11.71	12.51
42	13.85	14.91	16.36
43	17.66	19.00	21.39
44	22.51	24.20	27.96
45	28.71	30.84	36.55
46	36.61	39.28	47.79
47	46.68	50.04	62.47
48	59.52	63.75	81.67
49	75.89	81.21	106.76

[a]Hook and Fabia (1978).
[b]Hook and Chambers (1977); see footnote to Table 4.
[c]Hook and Lindsjo (1978).

Table 6.   Cumulative rates of Down syndrome per 1000 live births for older mothers from three studies

Maternal age (years)	New York[a]	Sweden[b]	Massachusetts[c]
All ≥ 30	3.39	3.19	3.15
All ≥ 35	6.61	6.68	5.96
All ≥ 40	14.48	17.70	14.20
All ≥ 45	38.40	62.09	35.25

[a]Hook and Chambers (1977).
[b]Hook and Lindsjo (1978).
[c]Hook and Fabia (1978).

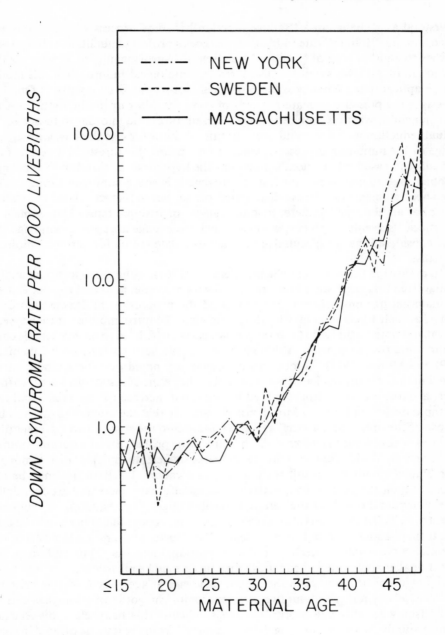

Figure 2.   Rates of Down syndrome by single-year maternal age interval in three studies. The rates for the New York study are corrected for underreporting (see Hook and Chambers, 1977). Other references are: Sweden, Hook and Lindsjo (1978); and Massachusetts, Hook and Fabia (1978).

understood as a change in a "failure function" if some process with a certain expected baseline "failure" rate suddenly undergoes a profound qualitative change and switches to another type of "failure" function of higher magnitude. If we view the production of a Down syndrome live birth as a biological failure, then this model may be appropriate. What possible biological factors could be involved? One hypothesis is the presence in maternal cells of some inhibitor or inhibiting process of nondisjunction, which is required above a certain threshold in order to be active. A gradual reduction with age could occur in this inhibitor (or else there is, with age, a change of the inhibiting processes); when it falls below this threshold it results in a markedly increased rate of nondisjunction. The hypothesis of threshold for change just above age 30 may apply not just to cytogenetic events resulting in formation of unbalanced gametes, i.e., in nondisjunction per se, but in factors related to relative survival of an abnormal gamete, trisomic zygote, or trisomic fetus. Thus it may be the natural "screening" processes whose functions change abruptly around age 30. These considerations are speculative but may stimulate search for pertinent biological factors.

In discussing this apparent change, Penrose (1961), using a proportional analysis, suggested that there were two types of Down syndrome: maternal age-dependent and maternal age-independent. He compared the proportion of Down syndrome mothers at each 5-year interval with the proportion of control mothers at each 5-year interval and noted a biphasic (or bitangential) curve, which led to his hypothesis concerning these two categories. Although he may have been correct, both Lilienfeld (1969) and Moran (1974), in more detailed analyses, noted that the bimodal curve derived in the proportional analysis is probably the result of a statistical artifact (or, better, a statistical coincidence) caused by the rapid increase of risk in age and the very rapid decline in fertility. Moran noted explicitly that the attempted division by Penrose of the observed maternal age distribution into the sum of two different distributions is not "logically necessary," because if the probability of a normal mother producing a child with Down syndrome increases sufficiently quickly, then bimodality or bitangentiality can result without separate causes. I believe this may be rephrased as indicating that even if maternal age-specific rates increased exponentially at the same rate throughout the period of fertility (e.g., if one equation of the form $y = \exp(b_1 x + b_0)$ fit the observations over all maternal ages so that there would be evidence from this source for only one "category" of Down syndrome), a bimodal or bitangential curve would be derived in the proportional analysis. Thus, although the proportional analysis can be heuristically useful, it may be misleading.

In any event, the change in the rate of incidence at age 30 is at least consistent with Penrose's hypothesis about two different major categories of etiological events for 47,trisomy 21, although Moran's analysis indicates that he reached this conclusion on grounds that were not "logically necessary" from the data he offered in support. (The translocation Down syndrome infants born to mosaic parents are of course maternal age-independent in Penrose's sense, but these do not exhaust what he implied by the age-independent category. There must also be 47,trisomy 21 cases in this as well.) Penrose suggested class "A" events, the maternal age-independent group, to be 40% of all cases and the class "B" maternal age-independent group to be 60% of all cases of Down syndrome.

These figures must depend upon the proportion of older mothers in the child-bearing population. One way of roughly estimating what these proportions are in any population in which maternal age-specific rates are available is as follows. If the rate in those of maternal age under 30 is assumed to be roughly constant, then multiply the best estimate of this rate by the total number of live births in this population. This is presumably the proportion of cases that are age-independent. (Note that some of them will be born to older mothers.) The residue is the maternal age-dependent class. For the Swedish, New York, and Massachusetts data sources (see Tables 4, 5, 6), the proportions of maternal age-independent cases are 62.7%, 57.5%, and 49.3%, respectively. The differences between them are because of differences in the proportion of older mothers in each of the three populations (7.5%, 9.0%, and 12.9%, respectively, are ≥ 35).

Penrose (Penrose and Smith, 1966) discussed three mathematical models for the age-dependent cases: 1) an exponential increase with age of the type discussed previously; 2) an increase with the 10th power of age, i.e., a rate proportional to x^{10}, where x is maternal age in years; and 3) a complex model in which: a) there is apparently a mean frequency of 0.19565 "events" at either of two sites per person per year from age 17 on that have a Poisson distribution and b) a Down syndrome live birth occurs after 17 "events" have taken place. Analysis of one incomplete data set led him to conclude that the models are in ascending order of agreement with "observation" and that the third model produces an excellent "fit." (Recent analyses indicate that these conclusions do not apply to some more complete data sets available recently and that the exponential increase fits better than does a Poisson model (Hook and Lamson, 1980; Lamson and Hook, in press).)

Three different types of etiological hypotheses are discussed by Penrose to accord with his three models: 1) an exponential rise is consistent with some slowly growing infective factor gradually disturbing more and more cells or, alternatively, involving failure of nucleolus breakdown in the meiotic prophase with age; 2) a rise with the power of age is interpreted as indicating that the error in the ovum leading to nondisjunction depends upon a "succession of independent accidents"; 3) a theory postulating 17 deleterious events of chance occurrence (affecting a centromere of one of the chromosomes involved) is consistent with a "progressive deterioration by accidental occurrences," which is "equivalent to postulating a natural aging of the nucleus of the ovum." The latter is the preferable hypothesis to Penrose, because of the fit.

Penrose's rejection of the exponential model and preference of a Poisson model depends on his interpretation that maternal age-specific rates "level off" (when plotted on a logarithmic scale for rate and linear scale for age). This inference based on one data set is not borne out by recent analyses (Hook and Lamson, 1980). (See also below.)

Two other factors concerning maternal age effects are pertinent to this discussion.

First, under age 20 there has been persistent evidence from several studies for a slight rise in rate with falling age. Some studies that present data by 5-year intervals have not found this effect (e.g., see Figure 2.1 and p. 109 in Lilienfeld, 1969).

Such an effect may be missed because of pooling of data. Because there are many more mothers ages 18 and 19 than ages 17, 16, or 15, pooling all data in the under-20 group may obscure the higher rates in those at the lower extreme, if only the entire group under 20 is compared with those 20–24. Reports by 1-year intervals are more likely to reveal an effect. A suggestive trend is particularly notable in data of Erickson (1978) and Zellweger and Simpson (1973). A suggestion of such an effect also appears in the New York (Hook and Chambers, 1977) and Massachusetts (Hook and Fabia, 1978) studies, but it is not notable in the Swedish study (Hook and Lindsjo, 1978) (see Table 7). In a few studies (e.g., Mikkelsen et al., 1976), even rates by 5-year intervals show an increase in mothers ages 15–19 compared to mothers ages 20–24.

What could account for this effect? It may be due to a combination of higher fertility rate among slightly retarded teenagers and the association of cryptic trisomy 21 mosaicism with diminished intelligence. If so, the rates of Down syndrome live births at the very young maternal ages would be expected to vary with social and cultural factors. This might explain why an effect was not striking in the Swedish data when analyzed by 1-year interval, but is noted in data of others. Alternatively, it may be due to differential survival of Down syndrome fetuses in very young mothers.

Second, it has been suggested that among women age 45 or older, the increase in incidence with maternal age begins to level off when plotted on a semilogarithmic graph (see Lilienfeld, 1969, Figure 2.1 and p. 27). In fact, Penrose (Penrose and Smith, 1966) stated without citation that the increase with age tends to slow down after 40 years. This leveling is not evident in data from more recent studies, whether plotted by 5-year intervals or, as is optimal, by 1-year intervals (Hook and Lamson, 1980). There is, moreover, a statistical artifact that tends to contribute to the impres-

Table 7.   Down syndrome rates per 1000 live births from four studies on observations at younger ages

Maternal age (years)	Iowa[a]	Sweden[b]	New York[c]	U.S.[d]
< 15			0.19	0.68
15	1.15	0		0.33
16	0.78	0.51	0.32	0.22
17	0.86	0.57	0.25	0.23
18	0.80	1.09	0.27	0.20
19	0.52	0.30	0.20	0.19
20	0.67	0.60	0.18	0.17
20–24	0.67	0.74	0.24	0.22

[a]Zellweger and Simpson (1973).
[b]Hook and Lindsjo (1978).
[c]Hook and Chambers (1977).
[d]Erickson (1978). Erickson's numerator data were all birth certificate reports of Down syndrome live births. His denominator data were at 1% systematic sample of all live births reported on birth certificates. The proportions he reported at each maternal age have been multiplied by 10 (divided by 100, multiplied by 1000) to provide the best estimate of what the rate per 1000 live births in the original data base would be.

sion of a leveling effect at the oldest ages that arises from pooling data by 5-year intervals. In the 45–49 age group the average age of mothers is much closer to 45 than 49, but the pooled rate is usually plotted at the midpoint of the quinquennium in these graphs. This also occurs to a lesser extent in the 40–44 age group and tends to result in at least some "leveling." Analyses of rates by 5-year intervals when plotted also result in graphical underestimates of rates at single-year intervals by 20% to 30% in the older ages for similar reasons. For further discussion of other methodological artifacts that would result in a spurious leveling effect at the oldest ages, see discussion in Hook and Lamson (1980).

PROBLEMS CONCERNING THE ACCURACY OF REPORTED RATES

A major concern in evaluation of the data on crude and maternal age-specific rates is the accuracy and completeness of the data sources. Most phenotypic surveys have involved collection of data from a wide variety of medical sources some time after birth, and incomplete ascertainment is quite possible. Collman and Stoller's (1962) Australian study—which Christianson (1976) indicated was generally regarded as most complete—may have had some underascertainment of cases. Compare the maternal age-specific rates in this study with those of Lindsjo (1974) (Table 8). Note that although the crude rate is higher in the Australian study, the maternal age-specific rates are all lower than in the Swedish study. This discrepancy reflects the fact that there are proportionally fewer older mothers in the Swedish group than in Australia, but it is likely that there was better ascertainment in the Swedish study. (It is possible that temporal and/or geographical differences rather than differential ascertainment account for these and other differences between surveys, but this seems implausible.)

For this reason the best data are from those surveys that involved complete systematic evaluation of all newborns at birth using the same protocol as the U.S. collaborative study (Marmol, Scriggins, and Vollman, 1969; Sever et al., 1970), the Oakland study (Christianson, 1976), or those studies involving cytogenetic evaluation of consecutive newborns (e.g., Jacobs et al., 1974). There are relatively few persons evaluated in such intensive studies, but the rates from the available data (Table 9) are consistent with those from the large-scale phenotypic surveys. The data from

Table 8. Comparison of rates of Down syndrome in two studies

Maternal age (years)	Australia[a]	Sweden[b]	Ratio
≤20	0.42	0.59	0.71
20–24	0.02	0.74	0.84
25–29	0.82	0.88	0.93
30–34	1.13	1.45	0.78
35–39	3.45	3.74	0.92
40–44	9.80	14.96	0.66
45–49	21.68	62.09	0.35
Total crude rate	1.45	1.32	1.13

[a]Collman and Stoller (1962).
[b]Lindsjo (1974).

Table 9.   Comparison of maternal age-specific rates of Down syndrome by 5-year intervals

Maternal age (years)	Intensive surveys[a]	Swedish study	Ratio
<20	0.66	0.59	1.12
20–24	0.68	0.74	0.92
25–29	0.81	0.88	0.92
30–34	1.74	1.45	1.20
35–39	3.38	3.74	0.90
40–44	15.19	14.96	1.02
45–49	52.63	62.09	0.85

[a]These are pooled data from studies by Jacobs et al. (1974) in Edinburgh, Christianson (1976) in Oakland, Erickson (personal communication) in Atlanta on white live births, and the U.S. collaborative study (Rosenberg, personal communication) on white live births.

the intensive surveys are not sufficient to construct regression estimates by 1-year intervals but at least provide some reassurance that the larger surveys in which the 1-year estimates are derived have not grossly underestimated or overestimated rates (see Figure 3).

THE PROBLEM OF VARIABLE ASCERTAINMENT

The possibility of variable ascertainment is worth considering in further detail because it also enters into the evaluation of possible temporal, ethnic, or geographical variation.

The crude rates in the intensive surveys provide a type of benchmark with which to compare the results of large-scale phenotype surveys. With one exception (in non-European Israelis), crude rates in these intensive surveys are consistent with each other. Differences in maternal age distributions may contribute to some variability among the rates in the intensive surveys, but the crude rates are all between 1.0 and 1.3 per 1000 live births, with the exception of the small-scale study of Jacobs et al. (1974), in which the crude rate was 1.45 per 1000.

Now consider a large-scale phenotypic survey in which a crude rate has been observed that is higher than this range of 1.0 to 1.3 per 1000 in the intensive studies: perhaps 1.4 to 1.5 per 1000 or as high as 1.86 per 1000, as found by McDonald (1972b) in Quebec province. This may be attributable to a higher proportion of older mothers in the study population than in the intensive surveys, as would be expected for studies of live births in the 1940s, 1950s, and early 1960s. Logically, if maternal age is already "adjusted" for, it may also be attributable to: 1) higher maternal age-specific rates in the population studied, 2) a high rate because of sampling fluctuation (in a survey involving small numbers), or 3) false diagnoses of Down syndrome cases in the population. To my knowledge (with one exception, noted later), all studies in which crude rates higher than those of intensive surveys noted have been from populations involving proportionally more older women than in the intensive investigations and/or a population in which sampling fluctuation cannot be excluded with high confidence.

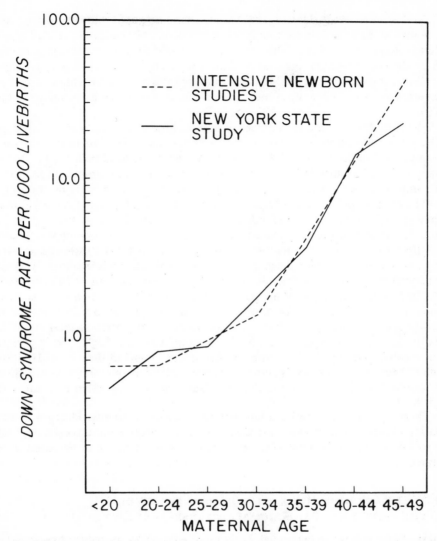

Figure 3.   Comparison of rates in intensive newborn studies (see text) and those in the New York State study by 5-year interval. The New York rates by 5-year interval (given in Hook, 1978b) are close approximations to those in the Swedish study of Lindsjo (1974).

Now consider the opposite outcome: large-scale phenotypic surveys in which rates lower than those of the intensive studies have been noted—e.g., under 1.0 per 1000, as in the Stark and Mantel (1967) survey—or studies from some years ago in which, despite a higher proportion of older mothers in the population, crude rates of 1.0 to 1.2 were observed. This may be due to incomplete ascertainment of cases, to sampling fluctuation in studies involving small numbers of cases, or to truly lower maternal age-specific rates in the population in question. It is of interest that the methods of these phenotypic studies that have found lower rates, such as those of

Stark and Mantel (1967), Halevi (1967), and others, do not exclude incomplete ascertainment with any confidence (see Hook and Porter, 1977). Even the Collman and Stoller (1962) survey falls into this category as somewhat suspect because, despite the high crude rate, the maternal age-specific rates are lower than in the intensive surveys. While it cannot be proved that these lower rates are attributable to incomplete ascertainment, this appears the most parsimonious explanation (compare Tables 8 and 9).

The complex interacting problem of ascertainment and the proportion of older mothers in a population may be illustrated well by considering data reported from the British Columbia Birth Defects Registry (Lowry et al., 1976). From 1952 to 1973 the apparent crude live birth rate in the population fell slightly from 1.38 to 1.18 per 1000, almost certainly because there were proportionally fewer older mothers (Table 10). (The proportion for ages 35 and over dropped from 11.1% to 4.8%.) Yet maternal age-specific rates rose in the second half of this interval, about 20%. Lowry et al. stated: "In 1964 and 1966, two new important sources of ascertainment were added to the Registry. . . . The first involved. . .death or stillbirth registrations and the second. . .a copy of the hospital discharge face-sheet from all children under 7 years. . . . The age adjusted incidence rate has increased in recent years and as a result the expected decline in crude rate has not materialized. *The possibility that* this has resulted from better ascertainment. . .cannot be excluded" (emphasis added). These authors have stressed the wrong point. Not only can the effects of better ascertainment upon age-adjusted rates not be excluded, but if anything it appears highly likely to explain all the trends, particularly the abrupt change in 1964–1967 in their data. Had ascertainment been consistent in this period, it seems very likely that maternal age-specific rates would have been stable and the crude rate would have fallen even more than it did.

There are very few studies that provide evidence of secular changes or ethnic variation in rates for which variable ascertainment, although hard to exclude, is difficult to invoke as an explanation for the differences. These are discussed in later sections.

THE ACCURACY OF DIAGNOSIS IN PHENOTYPIC STUDIES
AND THE PROBLEMS OF MOSAICISM AND "PSEUDO-DOWN SYNDROME" CASES

Even if all live births are examined, what are the effects of possible phenotypic misdiagnoses of Down syndrome and the consequences for estimated rates and other epidemiological inferences? This "simple" question has subleties that lead to deep questions concerning exactly what is meant by Down syndrome and whether it should be a

Table 10.   Rates of Down syndrome per 1000 live births by year of birth, in British Columbia

Rates	1952–1955	1956–1959	1960–1963	1964–1967[a]	1968–1971[a]	1972–1973[a]
Crude	1.38	1.22	1.23	1.41	1.25	1.18
Age-adjusted	1.24	1.13	1.14	1.39	1.50	1.51

Data from Lowry et al. (1976).
[a]Two ascertainment sources added.

phenotypic or genotypic diagnosis and the optimal method for evaluating cases where phenotype and genotype diagnoses conflict. This also overlaps with the question of the criteria for mosaicism.

Although there are exceptions, in most phenotypic studies not all cases are examined cytogenetically. This brings up the possibility of inclusion of those without extra 21q + material in such surveys, i.e. those with so-called pseudo-Down syndrome.

If such cases are "falsely" included in any series, then the maternal age effect inferred for the entire group studied would be biased downward, unless the confusion is with a rare condition like trisomy 18, which has a similar maternal age effect.

(Stene and Stene, 1978, have stated unequivocally, without citation, that the Down syndrome child is more likely to be diagnosed if the mother is of advanced age. In my clinical experience, however, there has never been a situation in which maternal age was considered in reaching a phenotypic diagnosis of either Down syndrome or questionable Down syndrome.)

In the past, a clinician's decision to seek cytogenetic diagnosis was probably selectively biased to those born to younger mothers, because of the greater likelihood of a translocation in such instances. A recent comparison of the maternal age distribution of Down syndrome cases reported to the New York State chromosome registry (which is limited only to cytogenetically confirmed cases) and the maternal age distribution of cases reported on birth certificates in New York State—which is unlikely to be highly biased in maternal age—indicates that approximately 17% fewer cases born to older mothers were reported to the registry than would be expected from the vital record data (Hook, Woodbury, and Albright, 1979). This is consistent with the explanation that for cases in this jurisdiction from 1968 to 1977, a Down syndrome infant born to an older mother had only a 0.83 likelihood of being studied as an infant born to a younger mother. (Until recently, cytogenetic investigation of Down syndrome was usually felt to be indicated only if the mother was under 35 (because of the possibility of a translocation), there were affected relatives, or there was uncertainty concerning the diagnosis.)

The results of a major study by Fabia (1970) in Massachusetts are of interest. She has kindly made her data available to me for further analysis. She investigated over 2400 cases and found data on 583 persons for whom the notation of Down syndrome (or mongolism) had been entered in some medical or school record and who had been studied cytogenetically in some laboratory. (Fabia's thesis, data from which are included in Table 2, reports fewer cases studied cytogenetically, but the totals analyzed here include all birth years and infants born outside Massachusetts or in Massachusetts to nonresidents.) Of these, 25 were found to have "normal" peripheral blood chromosomes. Three of these were felt, despite this, to be clinical cases of Down syndrome; three were possible or questionable cases; and the remaining 19 were classified phenotypically as "not Down." One of the latter cases had "6% trisomic cells," hydrocephalus, and Crouzon's disease, and was classified as a "doubtful mosaic." Another infant in the latter category had the phenotypic stigmata of Down syndrome, but his normal intelligence and karyotype led to the exclusion of this diagnosis. In addition to these 25, there were two infants with other chromosomal abnormalities: one trisomy 18 and one XO/XY. Thus, based on cytogenetic analysis,

$27/583 = 4.6\%$ of those suspected of having the disorder, based on entries in institutional records elsewhere, did not have Down syndrome. It is probable that among the over 2400 cases that Fabia investigated, those who had chromosome studies selectively included questionable cases. Therefore, 4.6% may be an upper limit of the proportion of cases phenotypically diagnosed as Down syndrome in some institutional source in this jurisdiction but who would have had "normal chromosomes" in laboratory investigation. However, many of these infants may well be cryptic mosaics—even those with minimal stigmata or with borderline low or normal intelligence.

In a series of 43 suspected mongoloid children reported by Hall (1964), 38 were found to be trisomic and 5 (11.6%) were not. Two of the latter had suggestive clinical signs leading to the diagnosis of pseudomongolism. The method of ascertainment used here may have increased the number of reports of pseudo and/or false cases. Gustavson (1964) reported results of cytogenetic investigation of 62 "clear-cut" cases of Down syndrome studied because of young maternal age or because of the presence of affected relatives, all of whom had trisomy 21. He also investigated 57 "questionable cases" to confirm the diagnosis. Of these 57, 16 had normal chromosomes, 1 had trisomy 21 mosaicism and normal intelligence, 1 had another undescribed chromosome abnormality, and the remainder had a Down syndrome genotype. At face value, these results suggest that a case diagnosed as questionable Down syndrome in Gustavson's jurisdiction in any event had a likelihood of 0.76 (40/57) of having confirmatory chromosomal findings. (See also results of Hamerton, Giannelli, and Polani, 1965, discussed in the next section.)

An interesting case seen at the Birth Defects Institute in Albany illustrates this possibility.[2] A child with some Down syndrome stigmata and an endocardial cushion defect—the heart defect very frequent in Down syndrome—was found in the 1960s to have 47 chromosomes and an extra acrocentric group G chromosome. Despite development being somewhat more advanced than for a Down syndrome infant, he was given this diagnosis. In the 1970s, however, banding studies revealed that he had the 47,XYY genotype, and the diagnosis was changed. It was assumed that the heart defect and stigmata were coincidental, although they appeared to be unusual coincidences. Subsequently, metaphase preparations from this person were used for New York State cytogenetic proficiency evaluation and sent to about 20 different laboratories, each of which counted at least 20 cells. None of the laboratories knew of the phenotypic diagnosis or had any reason to expect unusual findings. Two laboratories reported finding at least one cell, on separate slides, with a 48,XYY,+21 constitution. The metaphase plates indicated that these counts were unlikely to be artifacts. Thus the child is very probably a mosaic for trisomy 21, but a mosaic detected only because over several hundred cells were counted. Yet Down syndrome was excluded after the initial "definitive" cytogenetic findings using banding.

This and similar cases involving intermediate phenotypes raise some profound issues as to what exactly is meant by a Down syndrome case, and whether the pheno-

---

[2]I thank I. H. Porter for permission to cite the details of this case.

type or genotype should be the more significant in making the diagnosis. A precise definition of Down syndrome to which everyone will agree will probably never emerge. There will always be some intermediate cases and even phenotypically clear-cut cases with "negative" cytogenetic study who are probably 47,trisomy 21 mosaics or who have cryptic translocations.

Some of the difficulties posed by mosaicism are illustrated by clinically apparent Down syndrome cases with no detectable trisomy 21 cells in the blood and just a small proportion in fibroblasts (e.g., Warkany et al., 1964). Other perplexing cases are cited by Smith and Berg (1976). Mikkelsen (1970) found a phenotypically normal mother in whom the presence of a trisomy 21 line was missed after birth of the first affected child (in 30 cells counted in peripheral blood) but was detected after birth of the second child in 3% of 100 leukocytes and 13% of 100 fibroblasts. Similarly, Sutherland, Fitzgerald, and Danks (1972) reported a mother with some stigmata of Down syndrome with three affected children. In 59 cells of blood and marrow (studied on three occasions), only a normal karyotype was detected—but a further leukocyte culture revealed trisomy 21 in 5 of 70 cells (7.1%).

The observation of no extra trisomy 21 material whatsoever in any tissue studied from a clinically typical Down syndrome (as in Bowen et al., 1974; Day and Miles, 1965; Fabia, 1970; Sergovich et al., 1964) can, of course, be attributable not only to cryptic 46,trisomy 21 mosaicism but also to a cryptic translocation involving extra 21q material; it may not be detectable at the resolution of the methods employed. Such an interpretation appears particularly likely to explain the fascinating family studied by Day and Miles (1965), in which the presence of a cryptic translocation could be inferred in two persons with Down syndrome and normal genotype from its presence in other affected relatives and carrier parent. Two persons had Down syndrome with normal chromosomes, one had the syndrome with 46 chromosomes and a "minute," and the mother of two affected children had 45 chromosomes and a "minute." If there had been only one affected person in this family, a cryptic translocation probably would have been regarded as an unlikely deus ex machina and the case would have been dismissed as pseudo-Down syndrome.

Some observations on long-term cultures may be pertinent to the explanation for cryptic mosaicism. It is known that the proportion of mosaicism for trisomy 21 mosaicism is variable in tissue culture, in some cases the normal line tending to predominate and, in others, the abnormal line (Taylor, 1968, 1970; Taysi, Kohn, and Mellman, 1970; Richards, 1969). "Disappearing" mosaicism for chromosomal abnormalities has also been demonstrated in vivo, at least for peripheral blood studies (LaMarche, Heisler, and Kronemer, 1967). In Penrose's study of mosaics (cited by Smith and Berg, 1976), it was suggested that there is a higher frequency of trisomic cells in fibroblasts than in leukocytes of those with trisomy 21 mosaicism. He classified a mosaic as one with 10% to 90% of trisomy 21 cells, and appears to have overlooked an ascertainment bias here, since apparently nonmosaic cases based on leukocyte findings would not be as likely to have their fibroblasts investigated. (Most Down syndrome cases that undergo cytogenetic investigation only have fibroblasts studies, if at all, after peripheral blood studies.)

THE EPIDEMIOLOGY OF TRISOMY 21 MOSAICISM

As may be inferred from the previous discussion, the great difficulty in studying the epidemiology of trisomy 21 mosaicism is that it is hard to find a definition of cytogenetic mosaicism for which there would be universal agreement. If one observes all but one cell with an extra chromosome 21, the temptation may well be to dismiss the exception as artifact, although it may represent an in vivo cell line, and one with wide distribution in the body. It is always possible that in any presumed nonmosaic $47, +21$, in which all cells examined are affected, another line may be discovered if further cells or additional tissues are studied. Thus, any algorithms for deciding if mosaicism is present (e.g., those of Bochkov et al., 1974) are purely arbitrary.

They replace scientific judgment by rote and sometimes inaccurate formulae. About all we can hope to do is state at what confidence level some specific level of mosaicism has been excluded in the cells from the tissue line examined (Hook, 1977, 1978c). To do this, the number of cells evaluated in each person, the number of separate studies, and the criteria used (if any) for scoring exceptional results as artifacts should be specified.

Unfortunately, this is done rarely, even for series of persons with Down syndrome reported from a single laboratory. Most laboratories routinely count somewhere between 10 and 30 cells as part of a clinical study. This will exclude, with 95% confidence, levels of mosaicism equal to or greater than 26% and 10%, respectively, if all cells examined have the same genotype (Hook, 1977). Some occasionally count much less. Even two cells had been reported as used in some surveys (see review in Hook and Hamerton, 1977), although it is likely that additional cells would be evaluated if some abnormality were detected. However, the proportion of mosaicism (i.e., $47, +21/46$) in various series of cases of Down syndrome is a function not only of how many cells from each person are evaluated, how many tissues may be examined, and how many repeat samples may be obtained, but also of what proportion of cases studied cytogenetically includes those with clear-cut phenotypic Down syndrome and what proportion has questionable, uncertain, or intermediate Down syndrome phenotypes. The greater the proportion in the latter group, the higher the proportion of genotypic mosaics detected, other things being equal. For example, Hamerton et al. (1965) found four trisomy 21 mosaics in (a maximum of) 47 cases examined cytogenetically in which the clinical diagnosis of Down syndrome was in doubt (of these, a maximum of 28 had nonmosaic, cytogenetically confirmed Down syndrome) and one case of $47, +21/46$ mosaicism in (a minimum of) 126 apparently unequivocal cases with the genotype. There was also a tetrasomic-trisomic mosaic in their series. (Only maximum and minimum can be given for the denominators of the proportions for this study because although there were 260 persons referred for study, and this included 47 with uncertain diagnoses and 213 with apparently confirmed diagnoses, chromosome studies were done only upon 173 persons, and it is not clear how those studied were distributed in the two subcategories.) The criteria for mosaicism were unspecified in their report and it is possible the authors looked harder on the average at cases of uncertain phenotype than they did at those with definite phenotype. In any event, they suggested a frequency of mosaicism (of unspecified criteria) in 1% of those with unequivocal Down syndrome and 10% among those "in whom the diagnosis of Down syndrome is in doubt" (Hamerton et al., 1965).

Thus it is clear that precise estimates of the frequency of trisomy 21 mosaicism in the newborn population or among clinically typical cases of Down syndrome are impossible. In pooled data from various clinical surveys, the reported proportion of 47, + 21 mosaics among cases of Down syndrome ranges from about 2%, estimated by Richards (1969) from a review of about 20 clinical series, to about 4%–5% in the larger series (see Table 2). It is not clear why the results from the larger surveys indicate higher proportions than those summarized by Richards, but heterogeneous criteria of the type discussed previously may explain this difference.

Another question arises concerning the frequency of cryptic mosaics among ostensibly normal parents of Down syndrome children. Some interesting calculations are presented on this by Smith and Berg (1976). Based on dermatoglyphic findings in parents, they estimated that "some 10 percent of mothers of Down's syndrome children could be mosaics... [but] not more than 1 percent of fathers..." Citing Penrose's work on age of maternal grandmothers of cases, they suggested that "it may be argued...at least 10 percent of mothers of Down's syndrome cases are themselves mosaic." Assuming that only 50% of women affected this way have a Down syndrome birth, they estimated a frequency of 1/4000 of such women in the total population of childbearing women. Apparently their calculation is derived by assuming a 1/800 frequency of Down syndrome in live births, that 10% (1/8000 live births) of these have cryptic mosaic parents, and that an equal number of cryptic mosaic women exist who do not happen to have Down syndrome infants. (Presumably the same proportion of males would have cryptic mosaicism since there is no reason to expect a differential frequency of male and female mosaics. Apparently, Smith and Berg postulated that cryptic mosaic males are less likely to have children with Down syndrome than are cryptic mosaic females.) These suggestions are provocative but must await confirmation.

Either meiotic or mitotic nondisjunction may result in mosaics. On the assumptions that only mosaic cases in which meiotic nondisjunction was the initiating event have a maternal age effect and that the effect is the same for these as for nonmosaic cases of meiotic origin—plausible assumptions that must still be documented—Richards (1969) calculated the proportion attributable to either origin in 51 mosaic cases in 20 series. "If the mean maternal age of trisomics is z, of mosaics is x, and of controls n, then p (the proportion of mosaics that started as normal zygotes) = $(z - x)/(z - n)$. Richards used values of $z = 33.1$, $x = 32.0$, and $n = 27.6$ and calculated $p = 0.2$, that is, 20% of mosaics are of mitotic origin, 80% of meiotic origin. This calculation depends on the assumption that the value of n for controls in all 20 series is appropriate. Another implicit assumption is that mosaics of meiotic and mitotic origin do not differ significantly in the distribution of their phenotypic manifestations. But, if, for example, mosaics of mitotic origin tend to have milder phenotypes than those of meiotic origin, as is likely, then the evaluation would be very sensitive to methods of patient selection. Cytogenetic studies that selectively include clear-cut cases of the phenotype would have proportionally more mosaics of meiotic origin in this event.

More complex mosaics than simple 46/47, + 21 genotypes can occur of course. In his series of 51 mosaics collected from the literature, Richards (1969) found 1 triple-stem cell mosaic and 3 cases with structural change. He collected five more mosaic structural translocations from questionnaires. In the total of eight, the mean maternal age of 26.7 was not very different from his control value. Of the eight, three had a normal cell line, and in two of these, mosaicism was presented in one tissue only; three of the eight had three or more cell lines. Five of the eight with a structural change involved a translocation; four, a G/21, and one, a D/21. Two of those with a G/21 translocation had a 47, + 21 line also.

To conclude this discussion of mosaicism, it is worth reemphasizing that it will probably be impossible to establish a definition of Down syndrome that will coincide exactly with everyone's understanding of the term. Under some definitions, cryptic mosaics will be excluded; with other definitions, mosaics may be included. All we can do is establish an operational definition in any particular study and attempt to estimate the magnitude of false inferences that may be drawn because of the cases that may be inappropriately included or excluded. Most phenotypic surveys will include some cases that on initial cytogenetic study will be found to have "normal" chromosomes in peripheral lymphocytes. Although this may tend to lead to overestimates, it must be emphasized that a certain fraction of those with normal genotypes will be cryptic mosaics. Cytogenetic surveys that exclude those with "normal" chromosomes may result in a slight underestimate of rates.

THE FREQUENCY OF DOWN SYNDROME IN EMBRYOS AND FETUSES

The frequency of Down syndrome embryos and fetuses has been widely studied using material from spontaneous and induced pregnancy terminations (see review in Carr and Gedeon, 1977). From these data the frequency of all chromosome anomalies among clinically recognized abortuses (fetal deaths up to the 20th week) is estimated to be 50%, of which 52% are trisomic. Nine percent of these had trisomy 21. Therefore it may be estimated that $(0.09 \times 0.50 \times 0.52 = 0.023)$ or 2.3% of all spontaneous abortuses have trisomy 21. (About the same proportion, 2.8%, may be estimated to have trisomy 22.)

This estimate may be high, because the estimate of 50% as the frequency of chromosomally abnormal spontaneous abortuses may be too high. However, if we accept the figures of 2% Down syndrome in the group of spontaneous abortuses, and if the frequency of spontaneous abortion is 15% of all pregnancies, then about 75%–80% of all Down syndrome conceptuses do not survive gestation. (Creasy and Crolla, 1974, using data from three sources and assuming an abortion rate of 15%, have estimated a slightly lower prenatal mortality rate of 70%.)

If, however, as many as 50% of all pregnancies end in spontaneous abortion, as some (e.g., Abramson, 1971) have projected, then it may be calculated that about

90%–95% of all Down syndrome conceptuses do not survive gestation, assuming that the Down syndrome cases are of the same proportion among unrecognized early abortuses as among the later clinically detected ones.

At the 16th to 18th week of gestation—the usual time of amniocentesis—the maternal age-specific rates of Down syndrome are greater than the baseline live-birth rates. There have been several questions and controversies concerning this. First, the actual excess has varied from report to report. Some reports of a very high excess may be attributable to sampling fluctuation and the preferential publication of apparently extreme observations. For example, of member centers of the New York State Chromosome Registry, the center observing the highest rates reported its observations (Kardon et al., 1978), but none of the other centers, at which much lower rates have been observed, did so. A similar explanation, sampling fluctuation, may explain in part the very high rates noted by Ferguson-Smith (1976) and Polani et al. (1976), which may have also been examples of selective publication from the United Kingdom.

Another contributing factor is that some comparisons have examined rates by 5-year intervals, not 1-year intervals. Because fertility falls so dramatically and amniocentesis utilization tends to increase with advancing maternal age, comparisons of live-birth rates and amniocentesis by 5-year intervals are too crude and will inflate the apparent difference (Hook, 1978a, b). Selective publication and inappropriate age adjustment cannot explain all discrepancies, however.

There are at least three other types of explanations. The first is that women having amniocentesis only because of advanced age are at higher risk for other cryptic reasons, such as "subfertility" or radiation exposure (Polani et al., 1976). The second is that rates in live births have increased since those studies whose results were used as a base line in comparison with the results from amniocentesis were carried out (Ferguson-Smith, 1978) or, alternatively, that such studies were gross underestimates of the live-birth rate in the group they did investigate (Ferguson-Smith, 1976). The third is that a high fetal death rate of Down syndrome fetuses after the usual time of amniocentesis accounts for the difference (Hook, 1978a).

All three factors could contribute to the discrepancy.

With regard to the suggestion of a change in live-birth rates, the results of two studies, in which ascertainment was unfortunately incomplete, do provide some suggestive data concerning rate increases in some jurisdictions (Evans, Hunter, and Hamerton, 1978; Hook and Cross, in preparation). One study with better ascertainment does not suggest a marked increase (Erickson, personal communication). See further comment on this in discussion of temporal trends below.

One cannot exclude the possibility of additional cryptic putative risk factors, but the evidence for such effects remains conjectural. (For radiation, for example, there are some suggestive positive studies, some apparently definitive negative studies, and one study suggesting that the major effect occurs after 10 years of exposure.) It is likely that if this does account for the discrepancy, then as amniocentesis becomes more widely utilized and publicized, selective inclusion of women with putative risk factors other than maternal age will diminish. Thus this hypothesis would predict that the excess will diminish with expansion of utilization.

The author recently surveyed the outcome of pregnancies in which chromosome abnormalities had been diagnosed prenatally but the mother elected not to terminate her pregnancy. The observed fetal death rate was about 20%, with a 95% confidence interval of about 9% to 46% (Hook, 1978d) (see Table 11). This is consistent with the differential between the live-birth rates and rates at amniocentesis in many studies, but not in all of them. There was, incidentally, no evidence in this series for a higher fetal death rate in affected fetuses of mothers ages 40 or over in this study than in those ages 35–39 (Hook, personal observation), as suggested by Oakley (1978). It is clear that spontaneous fetal death accounts for some of the differential; it is still far from certain that it accounts for all of it.

Two factors of separate interest emerged in this survey. First, twin pregnancies were disproportionately represented among cases that did not involve elective termination. Second, in New York State, it was possible to estimate the proportion of women in whom a Down syndrome fetus had been diagnosed but who elected not to terminate. This figure was $2/47 = 4.3\%$ (Hook, 1978d).

If all discrepancy between live births and amniocentesis is attributable to fetal death, then what is the predicted rate of Down syndrome fetuses among all late fetal deaths? A formula has been given (Hook, 1978b; Hook et al., 1979) for this: $f = \Delta/a + L$ where Δ is the difference between expected live-birth and amniocentesis rates (where the live-birth rate is adjusted to the distribution of maternal age of women having amniocentesis), L is the rate of Down syndrome in live births, a is the fetal death rate in the population in the interval in question, and f is the rate of Down syndrome among fetal deaths that would have occurred spontaneously without intervention. This formula is applicable irrespective of whether fetal deaths are natural or induced (see derivation of formula in Table 12).

Although the formula results from an algebraic identity, in application L (the rate of Down syndrome in live births) can never be known for the study group in question but must be estimated from other sources. Using values for L from the New York State study (Hook and Chambers, 1977), values of f (assuming various values of a) are presented:

a	f
2%	0.219
3%	0.134
4%	0.109
5%	0.081
7%	0.066
10%	0.049

In the data of the U.S. collaborative study, the Canadian collaborative study, and the New York State chromosome registry (as of Volume 19), the pooled rate of Down syndrome diagnosed at amniocentesis was 29 in 2238 cases, or 13/1000. The predicted rate in live births to mothers with the same maternal age distribution as those having amniocentesis was about 9/1000. Assuming various value of a, the projected value of f is given. These calculations suggest that (in the absence of prenatal diagnosis and termination) Down syndrome is likely to constitute a significant fraction of late fetal deaths to older mothers. The estimates depend, of course, upon the appro-

Table 11. Spontaneous fetal death rate after amniocentesis

Rates	Cases	Confidence interval
In all cases		
47, +21	5/21 = 23.8%	(8.2%–42.2%)
47, +18	3/4 = 75.0%	(19.4%–66.4%)
Milder or		
normal genotypes	2/73 = 2.7%	(0.3%–11.5%)
Collaborative studies		
U.S.	3.5%	
Canada	3.3%	
In singletons only		
47, +21	4/19 = 21.1%	(6.1%–45.0%)
47, +18	2/3 = 67.7%	(9.4%–99.1%)

Data from Hook (1978d).

Table 12. Derivation of formula $f = \Delta/a + L$*

	Total at amniocentesis =	Fetal deaths +	Live births
Affected	P	P_b	P_b
Unaffected	Q	q_d	q_b
Total	N	n_d	n_b

given: 1) $A = \dfrac{P}{N}$; 2) $L = \dfrac{P_b}{n_b}$; 3) $\Delta = A - L$; 4) $a = \dfrac{n_d}{N}$; 5) $f = \dfrac{P_d}{n_d}$;

then:

6)	$n_b = N - n_d = (1-a)N$	from 4)
7)	$P_b = LN(1-a)$	from 2), 6)
8)	$P = AN$	from 1)
9)	$P_d = P - P_b = AN - LN(1-a)$	from 7), 8)
10)	$n_d = aN$	from 4)
11)	$f = \dfrac{P_d}{n_d} = \dfrac{AN - LN(1-a)}{aN}$	from 5), 9), 10)
12)	$f = \dfrac{A - L(1-a)}{a} = \dfrac{A - L + aL}{a}$	from 11)
13)	$f = \dfrac{\Delta}{a} + L$	from 12)

*The rate of affected cases among the fetal deaths (f) is equal to the rate in live births (L) plus the difference between the rate at amniocentesis and in live births, divided by a rate of fetal loss in all those having amniocentesis (Δ/a). The equation applies whether fetal deaths are spontaneous or include induced terminations, although if affected cases are selectively terminated then the value of L must be adjusted accordingly. If L is the expected rate in live births and A is the observed rate at amniocentesis, and if all of the difference is due to fetal death, then the formula indicates what the fetal death rate of Down syndrome fetuses should be.

priateness of values used for A and L in any population analyzed. These are consistent with a high rate of late fetal loss for Down syndrome in women of all ages, although there are not sufficient data to document an effect with high precision (see next section). See also Table 12 for the formula used in calculation and further comments in Hook (1978b) and Hook et al. (1979).

There is one additional point with regard to the discrepancy. Spielman, Mellman, and Zackai (1975) suggested that the "excess" rate at amniocentesis is only in those ages 40 or over, not in those ages 35–39. On the whole, there does appear to be a trend to a greater excess at the older ages, i.e., at 40 or over, but there is an excess in the 35–39 group in at least some studies, according to this author's observations.

MORTALITY EXPERIENCE INCLUDING STILLBIRTHS

There have been only four studies of rates of stillbirths and early neonatal death rates for Down syndrome summarized in Table 13. The rate in all stillbirths studied to date is $4/452 = 0.9\%$ (95% confidence interval about 0.2%–2.3%) and in early neonatal deaths is $6/858 = 0.7\%$ (95% confidence interval about 0.3%–1.5%), which excludes the crude rate in live births (0.1%) found in most studies. These rates are about seven to nine times greater than the live-birth rates. (It should be noted, however, that fetal deaths are more likely to occur to older mothers and the rates in this group have not been age-corrected in comparison with the live births.)

The prevalence of Down syndrome after birth diminishes steadily because of the higher mortality of Down cases. Life tables have been published for the group studied by Fabia and Drolette (1970). The main difficulty in using these or other historical tables for prediction, however, is that variation in social and medical factors, not in intrinsic biological factors, will probably make the largest contribution to the variation in mortality. For example, whether corrective heart surgery is performed routinely on affected Down syndrome cases, or withheld routinely, or deferred until after extensive consultation with the parents, who realize the implications of their decision (the course this author prefers), will obviously markedly influence longevity, mortality, and prevalence after birth. There are strikingly different patterns at different medical centers and, moreover, striking differences between parents in their own decisions on whether to elect lifesaving heroic measures for children with Down syndrome. Although there probably always will be a higher mortality among those with Down syndrome than those with normal genotype, the magnitude of this difference and the long-range trends in longevity are extremely hard to predict.

Tarjan, Eyman, and Miller (1969) provided an example of the temporal trend in mortality in comparing death rates among retarded persons admitted to an institution between 1948 and 1952 and admitted between 1958 and 1962. There was a strik-

Table 13. Down syndrome in stillbirths (SB) and early neonatal deaths (NND)

Study	Macerated SB	Fresh SB	Early NND
Kuleshov et al. (1975)	0/22	1/61	1/92
Machin and Crolla (1974)	0/34	1/122	3/344[a]
Sutherland et al. (1978)			
Edinburgh study[b]	2/49	0/146	2/371
Adelaide study	0/7	0/11	0/48
Total	2/112 = 1.8%	2/340 = 0.6%	6/858 = 0.7%
	4/452 = 0.9%		

[a]Includes one 46, − 13t (13q 21q) but excludes one tetrasomic 21 (!), 47, + t(21q 21q).
[b]Also 27 spontaneous abortuses over 20 weeks of age with no Down syndrome cases noted.

ing improvement in mortality rate (within 4 years after admission) for all retarded persons in this period, but this was most marked for Down syndrome, with the mortality of the second cohort being only $1/16 = 6\%$ of that of the first—over a 90% improvement. The diminished mortality was probably attributable to more intensive therapy for infectious disorders and, perhaps, congenital heart defect (see Table 14).

Singer and Levinson (1976), in analyzing some older published mortality data, suggested that the mortality rate of those institutionalized with Down syndrome ages 50 or over may be considerably greater than the rate of others institutionalized with mental deficiency (although between ages 20 and 40 this gradient may be reversed). This may be due to the high frequency of presenile dementia in those with Down syndrome (Heston, 1977; Jervis, 1970).

In the U.S. collaborative study, 16 of 63 persons with Down syndrome died in the first year, and 3 more died in the next 3 to 5 years, although follow-up was not complete (Sever et al., 1970). Wahrman and Fried (1970), analyzing live births in Jerusalem from 1965 to 1969, found that only 60.8% of 53 cases reached age 6 months and 55.3% reached age 1 year compared to the first year death rate in Jerusalem of 21.1/1000 for all live births. And 5% of infants dying before 1 year of age in Jerusalem had Down syndrome. The mortality rate was higher among females than males in this period, but the numbers are too small to be conclusive.

Fabia and Drolette (1970) (Table 15) noted that among Down syndrome infants born to Massachusetts residents during 1950–1967, the survival to age 10 years was, in those without heart defects, about 75% in both sexes. In those with heart defects however, survival was 44.9% in males and 32.0% in females. This interaction of sex and congenital heart lesion with mortality remains unexplained. It does not seem to be consistent with mortality data in those with congenital heart defects without Down syndrome. It is consistent with some earlier data on mortality experience in Down syndrome unstratified by the presence of congenital heart defect, in which a higher death rate was noted in females (Record and Smith, 1955), although not all studies have found this (Forssman and Akesson, 1965, 1967b).

Table 14.   Death rate of Down syndrome in California institutions to 2.5 years of age

	Age (years)				
	0.5	1.0	1.5	2.0	2.5
1948–1952 cohort					
Death rate	17.7%	1.7%	1.8%	1.8%	5.5%
(Cohort size)	(70)	(59)	(58)	(57)	(56)
1958–1962 cohort					
Death rate	1.1%	2.2%	0.6%	0.0%	0.0%
(Cohort size)	(187)	(184)	(180)	(179)	(179)

Abstracted from Table 5 of Tarjan et al. (1969). The death rates given per 6-month interval are apparently in the cohort whose size appears immediately below the rate. Because admissions could occur at all ages, it cannot be assumed that the number in the next cohort can be predicted from the number in the previous cohort and the death rate. Thus, for example, although 17.7% of 70 cases = 12.3, the number at age 1 in the 1948–1952 cohort is not $70-12=58$, but 59. Apparently one subject entered between ages 0.5 and 1.0 in the 1948–1952 group.

Table 15.   Down syndrome survival rate to 10 years

Category	Males	Females
All cases	0.67	0.61
With congenital heart defects	0.45	0.32
Without congenital heart defects	0.76	0.77

Data from Fabia and Drolette (1970).

Differences in mortality rates between the U.S. studies and that in Israel may reflect differences in the treatment of infections or other disorders in Down syndrome persons.

ETHNIC AND RACIAL DIFFERENCES

Until now the discussion has implicitly assumed that although crude incidence rates may vary for reasons already discussed, maternal age-specific rates in live births are stable over time and between populations. Of course, intervention resulting from prenatal diagnosis will have an effect in the future upon maternal age-specific rates in live births, as well as upon the crude incidence, particularly in older mothers; but ignoring this factor, it is important to consider evidence bearing on the possibility of temporal and/or geographical, ethnic, and racial differences in maternal age-specific rates related to other factors.

With regard to racial differences in the U.S., a nearly 60% higher rate in older white than older black mothers was reported in one study, but no difference was found in those under age 30 (Stark and White, 1977). Unfortunately, this study had at least 20% underascertainment of cases and may have selectively detected older black compared to older white and/or younger black mothers of affected infants (Hook and Porter, 1977). In the U.S. collaborative study, there was actually an increased rate of Down syndrome in older black mothers compared to older white mothers, of borderline significance (Sever et al., 1970). Data from Atlanta collected by the Center for Disease Control (CDC) (Erickson, personal communication) indicate no evidence for any marked racial difference in rates, although there may be a trend to slightly higher (perhaps 20% greater) rates in whites than blacks, but the difference is not significant (see Table 16). This does not appear to be due to racial differences in ascertainment, judging by the distribution of length of time to diagnosis in the first year of life.

There have been reports of unexpectedly low rates of Down syndrome in several ethnic groups. For example, Morris (1971) found lower rates in the Maoris than in the Europeans in New Zealand, but her study for some reason excluded from the comparisons of maternal age-specific rates all persons who died, about 40% in both groups, so differential mortality by race may have contributed to her observation. In this study and almost all other studies in which ethnic, racial, or geographical differences have been noted, differential ascertainment has not been excluded (see Hook and Porter, 1977, for review). The variation in crude rates between countries reported by Stevenson et al. (1966) may be explained by sampling variation as well as by

Table 16.   Atlanta birth rates in whites and nonwhites (99% black)

Maternal age (years)	Whites	Nonwhites	Ratio	
< 20	0.83	0.70	1.19	
20–24	0.69	0.60	1.15	
25–29	0.86	1.09	0.79	
30–34	1.71	0.73	2.34	
35–39	2.98	2.46	1.21	
40–44	13.64	11.60	1.18	
≥ 45	56.60	0.00		
All ages	1.10	0.89	1.24	(crude)
			1.19	(Mantel-Haenszel–adjusted relative odds)
			$p \cong 0.33$	

Analyzed from data provided by Erickson (personal communication) from CDC survey of Atlanta births during 1969–1974.

differential ascertainment because of the relatively small numbers of births involved in each jurisdiction.

There is, however, one interesting exception to this.

Harlap conducted a West Jerusalem perinatal study on Down syndrome and has made her data available for analysis by single-year maternal age intervals and by ethnic group. These data indicate that the maternal age-specific rates in Jewish mothers of European origin are about the same as those in North America or Europe, already cited. The rates in non-Europeans (those from North Africa and the Middle East), however, are about 60% higher at all maternal ages, with the possible exception of those under 25 (see Table 17) (Hook and Harlap, 1979). The non-Europeans have lower socioeconomic background, different cultural traditions, and differ genetically within their own groups as well as from the Europeans. The maternal age-specific rates in the non-Europeans are among the highest in the world, and indeed the crude incidence rate in this group, over 2/1000 live births, is among the highest known to this author in studies involving substantial numbers of live births. It is hard to see how the observed difference from the European rate could be an artifact. The only conceivable artifacts are systematic overdiagnoses of Down syndrome in non-European births compared to European births in the same hospital in West Jerusalem, or errors in the average maternal age of the non-Europeans of 10 years or so in their documents, so that these women are much older than their official ages. Such effects both appear unlikely.

It would be of interest to see if these observations could be confirmed in other areas in Israel or in other Near-Eastern populations, but at present it is difficult to know how to interpret them.

In an earlier study from Israel, Halevi (1967), from data on 90,793 births (including 1213 stillbirths), found a rate of 1.21/1000 in (primarily Eastern European) Jews and 0.91/1000 in non-Ashkenazi Jews, predominantly those of Asian and North African origin. (Of 96 cases total, 37 were Ashkenazi, 59 were not). Halevi's analysis was based on hospital reports and records after birth and may have involved selectively greater ascertainment in the Ashkenazi group. His study involved primar-

Table 17. Down syndrome in Israeli Jewish births (rates per 1000 live births)

Maternal age (years)	Israeli Jewish births[a]			Rates elsewhere	
	Non-European	European	Ratio	Sweden[b]	Massachusetts[c]
<20	0.9 ⎫	0.0 ⎫	1.0	0.6 ⎫	0.7 ⎫
20–24	0.6 ⎭ 0.7	0.7 ⎭ 0.7		0.7 ⎭ 0.7	0.7 ⎭ 0.7
25–29	1.1	0.8	1.4	0.9	0.8
30–34	2.2	1.4	1.6	1.5	1.3
35–39	6.9	2.6	2.7	3.7	3.7
40–45	15.7 ⎫	12.8 ⎫	1.3	15.0 ⎫	13.2 ⎫
45–49	11.9 ⎭ 15.3	0.0 ⎭ 12.0		62.0 ⎭ 17.7	36.1 ⎭ 14.2

[a]Hook and Harlap (1979).
[b]Hook and Lindsjo (1978).
[c]Hook and Fabia (1978).

ily births in 1959 and 1960. The only other studies from the Near East seem to be one cited by Lilienfeld (1969) of Hashem and Sakr (1961), who found a rate of 1.25/1000 "total births" in one sector of Cairo, Egypt, and the report from Alexandria, Egypt, by Stevenson et al. (1966), who noted no cases in 9598 singleton births, but the latter report may have also involved underascertainment.

SEASONALITY AND OTHER ASPECTS OF TEMPORAL VARIATION

There are at least five separate components of possible temporal variation in rates that may be distinguished. Any deviation from "random" distribution over time may be understood as a temporal variation. In one sense this may also be understood as "clustering" since it means necessarily that cases must be concentrated in at least one or more subsection of the entire temporal interval. A temporal cluster per se usually is understood, however, as having a more restrictive meaning, namely, a nearly simultaneous occurrence of events consistent with and suggestive of a point outbreak in time with a common source.[3] It may be hard to distinguish formally the latter type of temporal clustering from simple, nonrandom occurrence in time by a suitable statistical definition. For example, seasonality could be understood formally as recurrent clusters with one type of cyclic pattern.

The term *secular trend* usually refers to a change in rates of an event over a period of years. Evidence for such effect for Down syndrome is discussed in the next section.

Seasonality usually refers to a consistent variation of rate with season (or sometimes, in a broader sense, month) over a period of some years. This is just one type of periodicity, which is a consistent temporal variation that is not necessarily seasonal. Patterns occurring in 5-month or 5-year "waves" would exhibit periodicity but not seasonality. Patterns in which cycles occur but in which the periods are irregular may exhibit cyclicity but not periodicity.

In this section, evidence primarily for seasonality is discussed. There have been numerous investigations of this variable for Down syndrome, in part because it is, superficially, easy to accumulate data, pool them by month, and search for variation. Any such analysis will find peaks in some months, troughs in others. Some authors report these peaks as apparent evidence for seasonality, others refrain unless there are consistent patterns in adjacent months. Some authors who report no evidence for seasonality often do not carry out detailed statistical tests of their data, so that the power of their observations to detect or exclude seasonality is uncertain. Moreover, in some cases the analysis is based on the post-hoc division of the temporal trend, e.g., an increase is observed in May–October and a statistical calculation is carried out as if that were the only period in which an increase could be observed.

What has been most impressive from the review of the data has been the inconsistency in the reported observations.

Lilienfeld (1969) summarized the conclusions of studies up to 1969, and these have been extended to include results of reports that have appeared since then (Table 18).

---

[3]The term *cluster* often implies a spatial as well as a temporal concentration.

Table 18.   Some reports bearing on seasonality of Down syndrome

Study	Outcome reported
Lunn (1959) (Glasgow, 1953–1958)	No seasonality
Collman and Stoller (1962) (Australia, 1942–1957)	No seasonality
Greenberg (1963) (England, 1953–1957)	> 35 years, no seasonality < 35 years, May, Aug., Oct. peaks
Slater, Watson, and McDonald (1964) (England and Wales, 1954–1960)	No seasonality
Lander, Forssman, and Akesson (1964) (Sweden, 1911–1958)	Sept. deficit
Leck (1966) (Birmingham, U.K., 1950–1968)	Deficit July to Dec.
Halevi (1967) (Israel 1959–1960)	Peaks Oct. to Dec.
Stark and Mantel (1967) (Michigan, 1950–1964)	No seasonality
Jongbloet (1971) (Netherlands, 1945–1968)	Peak deficit: Jan., Feb., March, ?Sept., April
Spielman et al. (1975) (Philadelphia, 1960–1975) (Indianapolis)	Peak deficit: July–Sept. April–June
Fabia (1970) (Massachusetts, 1954–1965)	Peak deficit: April–June, Aug., Jan.–March
McDonald (1972b) (Quebec, 1947–1967)	No seasonality
Harlap (1973) (Jerusalem)	Two peaks: Feb.–April, Aug.–Sept.
Goff et al. (1973) (Philadelphia, 1962–1975)	≥ 35 years, no effect < 35 years, peak Aug.–Oct.
Goad, Robinson, and Puck (1976) (Denver, 1964–1974)	≥ 35 years, no seasonality < 35 years, peak May–Oct.

Only some of the earlier studies receive comment here. Lander et al. (1964) in Sweden suggested that the trend to fewer cases in September may be regarded skeptically because of difficulty in getting suitable controls. Leck (1966), who found lower rates in July–December, suggested that this evidence for seasonality may have been due to lower ascertainment of infants born in those months because of early infant deaths, compared with those born in the rest of the years. The negative studies of Slater et al. (1964) and Stark and Mantel (1967) may, Lilienfeld (1969) suggested, be due to low ascertainment of cases which obscured a true temporal change. (This is in one sense the converse of Leck's suggestion.)

Some reports are of interest because they suggest etiological hypotheses. Jongbloet (1971) compared the month of birth of 441 infants born between 1945 and 1968 in the Netherlands with the distribution of live births and stillbirths between 1955 and

1959. He claimed for the control data a broad peak in February to May and a smaller peak in September, which he suggested is typical of Northwest European live-birth distributions. He claimed that the Down syndrome distribution (as well as the Klinefelter and Turner syndrome distributions) agrees with the control distribution but has greater amplitude. Of course, there are exceptions. Down syndrome has a decline in April (not a peak), a peak in January that the controls do not have, and only a questionable peak in September. Even more surprising is that the curves for parents of Down syndrome children, particularly for mothers, show a similar pattern: the same cycle as controls but a greater amplitude in peak months. The main difficulty is that no statistical tests are presented concerning his hypothesis and, moreover, it is not clear that the control data, which are limited to birth years 1955–1959, are at all appropriate for this study of infants born from 1945 to 1968.

Spielman et al. (1975), in a better study from Philadelphia, found an excess of Down syndrome live births from July through September and a deficit from April through June. The significance of this is not the actual months involved per se, but that the same pattern is found for all births in the U.S. but with an amplitude only one-quarter as great. The inference is that factors contributing to variation in frequency of all live births may contribute to variation in relative rates of Down syndrome in the U.S. Spielman et al. confirmed the variation in Down syndrome in a data source from Indianapolis. However, Hecht (1977), from Oregon, did not find evidence for this trend, nor apparently have other observers from the U.S.

The other interesting result with regard to seasonality is that of Harlap (1973), from Israel, who found an annual biphasic curve with peaks in February–April and August–October, with troughs in between. The trend was found among mothers of all ages, but was stronger among those under 35. (Ament, 1976, expressed some skepticism about the statistical conclusions for these data, but succeeded only in showing that the p value may be closer to 0.05 than the much lower value reported by Harlap, 1974. See also Rothman, 1976, who pointed out that the ratio of peak to low rates is 2.5 to 2.7, very suggestive of a strong variation.) It is not known if the trend was primarily in one of the ethnic subdivisions.

It has been suggested that seasonal variation of estradiol receptors in mammary tumors (in Germany) shows the same variation as that of the Down syndrome cases (in Israel) reported by Harlap (1973, 1974) (Janerich and Jacobson, 1977), but no statistical test of the concordance is presented. It also is not clear if the date associated with each tumor is the date of the first suspected diagnosis, of surgery, or of analysis of the tissue. In any event, these authors suggested that causal factors resulting in changes in estradiol receptors in tumors are the same as those that result in "changes in chromosome division during late states of meiosis."

An earlier study of Halevi (1967) on seasonality in Israel reported, for 92 cases of Down syndrome (about two-thirds non-Ashkenazi), proportions of 23.9%, 20.9%, 20.7%, and 34.8% in the four quarters of the year, compared to that for all live births of 24.9%, 24.2%, 26.4% and 24.5%. The peak in the last quarter is at variance with Harlap's observation. Nevertheless, the prevalence at birth in Harlap's study was about twice that in Halevi's study, so that underascertainment in the latter study can always be invoked. Harlap's study is noteworthy for several reasons other than the observations of biphasic seasonality: the high prevalence rates at birth, the high maternal age-specific rates in non-Europeans (non-Ashkenazis), and the trends of association with low socioeconomic status and diminished primogeniture (see next section). None of these seems to have been found in studies of populations of European origin. Perhaps the observations are all interrelated, and it is only in the non-Europeans in Harlap's study that all these exceptional patterns occur.

SECULAR CHANGES

The likely effect of amniocentesis and prenatal diagnosis upon the rates of Down syndrome in live births depends upon the use of these preventive measures. A search for evidence for an effect of this procedure upon the rates of Down syndrome noted in vital record reports in Upstate New York revealed only that the problems of sampling fluctuation and small numbers have obscured detection of an effect to date in this source, although the live-birth prevalence probably has fallen from what it would be because of this procedure. Use of amniocentesis and prenatal diagnosis is increasing so rapidly among pregnant women over 35, and even those of younger ages, that at this point it is probably premature to make any projections.

As to true long-term secular changes in maternal age-specific rates, there are two suggestive studies in which sampling fluctuation or differential ascertainment are difficult to invoke as explanations for the change.

Evans et al. (1978) reported a two-fold increase in Down syndrome in the 35–39 quinquennia ($19/7778 = 2.4 \times 10^{-3}$ versus $26/4567 = 5.7 \times 10^{-3}$) from 1965–1969 to 1970–1974. The published data indicated no evidence for a change in women ages 40 or over (11.5×10^{-3} in the first period versus 11.96×10^{-3} in the second). A Mantel-Haenszel test indicated that the summary trend in all women 35 or over was significant at the 0.02 level (see Table 19). There is not any evidence for change in those under age 35. These might be dismissed as simply a chance occurrence in one quinquennium; however, our New York State data, based on birth certificate reports, appear to show a similar effect. Comparing 1965–1969 with 1970–1974, there is no evidence for a rise in maternal age-specific rates of births to younger mothers, but there is for older mothers (see Table 20). The relative risk for those 35 or over to be born in the later period is 1.3, with $p < 0.05$.

Comparisons of direct age-standardized rates in the two time periods appear in Table 21. The search for a trend in New York State data by maternal age was stimulated by the Manitoba report. Earlier analyses of New York State trends had been confined to adjusted rates in births to mothers of all ages. The increase in the older mothers in Manitoba was 1.65-fold. Notice the lack of increase at younger ages. The increase in older mothers in New York State was about 1.30-fold. Again, note the lack of increase at the younger ages. The absolute rates were lower in New York State than in Manitoba because birth certificate reports of Down syndrome in New York State were only about 38% complete.

One of the difficulties with the New York State study is that it was based on birth certificate reports, and differential reporting by age of mother could have occurred. It is hard to understand why this should have happened for older mothers only in 1970 and later, but it cannot be excluded. A study of the completeness of birth certifi-

Table 19. Rates per 1000 of Down syndrome by maternal age quinquennia in Manitoba, 1965–1969 and 1970–1974[a]

Maternal age (years)	Rates			Frequencies	
	1965–1969	1970–1974	Relative change	1965–1969	1970–1974
Lt. 20	0.983	0.234	0.24	11/11,189	3/12,840
15	10.526	0		1/45	0/150
15–19	0.901	0.236		10/11,044	3/12,710
20–24	0.601	0.856	1.42	18/29,968	26/30,390
25–29	0.691	0.737	1.07	17/24,606	20/27,119
30–34	1.574	1.466	0.93	22/13,981	17/11,595
35–39	2.443	5.693	2.33	19/7,778	26/4,567
40–44	10.554	11.398	1.08	28/2,653	15/1,316
45–49	23.256	38.095	1.64	5/215	4/105
≥50	0	0		0/1	0/0
N.S.				1/5	1/14
All ages	1.339	1.274	0.95	121/90,396	112/87,946

Data from Evans et al. (1978) and Evans (personal communication).
[a] Summary Mantel-Haenszel relative odds for all ages = 1.20, $p = 16$, summary relative odds for ages ≥ 35 = 1.62, $p < 0.02$.

Table 20.   Rates of Down syndrome in Upstate New York (vital records)[a]—white live births[c]

Maternal age	Rates		Relative change	Frequency	
	1965–1969	1970–1974		1965–1969	1970–1974
<20	0.249	0.253	1.02	19/76,338	18/71,242
20–24	0.197	0.253	1.28	52/264,005	56/221,364
25–29	0.421	0.301	0.71	90/213,594	64/212,429
30–34	0.515	0.517	1.00	60/116,523	47/90,891
35–39	1.513	1.976	1.31	93/61,485	66/33,405
40–44	4.282	5.715	1.33	75/17,514	48/8,399
≥45	15.873	15.748	0.99	15/945	8/508
All ages	0.538	0.481		404/750,608[b]	307/638,466[b]

[a]For ≥ 35, $\chi^2 = 4.78$, d.f. $\cong 1$, $p = 0.02$. The Mantel-Haenszel summary odds ratio = 1.29 for change in the two time periods.

For all ages, $\chi^2 = 0.89$, d.f. = 1, p = N.S. The Mantel-Haenszel summary odds ratio = 1.08 for change in the two time periods.

[b]Includes not stated.

[c]Rates are slightly lower if those of all races are included, but trends are the same.

Table 21.   Comparison of direct age-standardized rates of Down syndrome in Manitoba and New York State, 1965–1974[a]

Location	1965–1969	1970–1974	1975	1976	1977
Manitoba[b]					
Mothers <35	0.84	0.85			
Mothers ≥35	4.46	7.38			
All ages	1.18	1.47			
New York State (birth certificate reports)					
Mothers <35	0.33	0.32	0.32	0.33	0.30
Mothers ≥35	2.29	2.98	3.46	2.40	2.22
			(3.51)[c]	(2.81)[c]	(2.81)[c]
All ages	0.52	0.56	0.61	0.53	0.48

[a]For standardization the reference population is Upstate New York live births, 1963–1974 (Hook and Chambers, 1977).

[b]Source is Evans et al. (1978) and Evans (personal communication).

[c]The rates in parentheses are rates adjusting for cases known to have been terminated after prenatal diagnosis. These adjustments assume that only 70% would otherwise have survived to live birth, and of these, only 38% have been reported on birth certificates.

cate reports stratified by maternal age (<35, >35) indicated no difference by age (Hook and Chambers, 1977), but the study did not look at year of birth in the completeness analysis. We are attempting to investigate this question by examining completeness of sources for earlier and later years.[4]

The Atlanta data are available only for birth from 1969 on. Comparison of 1969 alone with 1970–1974 is unstable because of small numbers in 1969. There is a suggestion of an increase at all ages judged by summary relative odds, but the trend is not significant in any age bracket, or for the entire data source (Table 22).

---

[4]Since this was written, analysis has indicated that selective changes in reporting do not explain the apparent change (Hook and Cross, in preparation).

Table 22.   Atlanta: All races

Maternal age (years)	1969	1970–1974	Ratio
≤ 25	0.51	0.74	1.4
25–29	0.69	0.95	1.4
30–34	2.03	1.38	0.7
≥ 35	2.82	5.68	2.0

Summary relative odds (M.H.) = 1.33, $p \cong\ = 0.17$, for all ages. For ages ≥ 35, $p \cong\ = 0.18$. Data not available for years before 1969. Analysis is of data from Erickson (personal communication). There are insufficient data on those 35 or over to allow a more refined breakdown in analyses.

BIRTH ORDER

There is a crude association of Down syndrome with birth order because of the association with advanced maternal age. After correction for maternal age, however, the data are conflicting. As Tonomura et al. (1966) noted, "birth order is a very tricky factor."

Perhaps the most refined analysis is that of Stark and Mantel (1966), who found, after extensive evaluation, no evidence for any birth order defect. These data and analyses have been reanalyzed by Fleiss (1973), who considered them in textbook illustrations of standardization of rates. By indirect and direct standardization, rates in firstborn and fifth-born are "about the same" after correction for maternal age, but it is of interest that with both methods there is a trend to slightly greater rate in firstborns. (The comparison is 93.3×10^{-5} versus 84.7×10^{-5} by indirect standardization, ratio = 1.1; and 92.5×10^{-5} versus 75.7×10^{-5} by direct standardization, ratio = 1.2).

Tonomura et al. (1966) found a 68% increase in firstborn children in Japan after correction for the maternal age effect (with lower than expected rates in those of higher birth order), and Smith and Record (1955) also noted an excess in firstborns (see Table 23).

Matsunaga (1967) found not only an increase with lower birth order for Down syndrome but found the same effect for mentally retarded people without Down syndrome in institutions. He concluded that the birth order effect was due to an artifact of "social selection practiced by parents who bring their children to institutions." This source of bias would be most prominent in studies of individuals selected from studies of institutions, as well as, perhaps, surveys like those of Tonomura et al.

Table 23.   Down syndrome and birth order in a U.K. study

Birth order	Number observed	Number expected
1	61	42.7
2	50	58.1
3	34	34.0
4	26	27.9
≥ 5	46	54.3

Data from Smith and Record (1955).

(1966) that involved cases primarily from large hospitals in one area. Parents may be particularly likely to bring affected firstborns to institutions or to hospitals.[5] Tono- mura et al. also noted two other possible sources of bias that might have contributed to their observed birth order effect: differential mortality according to birth rank among affected newborns, and selection of patients in the study from specific areas where practice of birth control was particularly high.

The only study in which low birth order (primogeniture) was negatively asso- ciated with Down syndrome, i.e., lower rates occurred in firstborns, was to my knowledge that of Harlap (1973). This study is noteworthy in the number of unique associations reported: e.g., ethnic difference, socioeconomic status, and biphasic seasonality, in addition to the birth order effect, so that the variant finding may be at- tributable to the contribution of the non-European Jews (non-Ashkenazi) in this study (see Table 24).

SOCIOECONOMIC STUDIES

There is no strong evidence for any association of socioeconomic factors with mater- nal age-specific rates of Down syndrome, nor are there specific data on socioeco- nomic gradients in crude rates (with one exception, noted later), but a trend is likely to emerge because of socioeconomic variation in relative age-specific fertility rates. For example, low social class, at least in some studies, is generally associated with a higher proportion of births to very young mothers, so this might contribute to a spu- rious negative correlation of crude rates with socioeconomic status, even though maternal age-specific rates may be independent of social class. Differentials in rela- tive age-specific fertility rates contribute to higher crude rates of Down syndrome in whites than in blacks, independent of any putative age-specific differences in rates.

In addition, in groups where fertility control is not widely available or, if avail- able, not widely practiced, there is likely to be a much higher fertility rate in older mothers than elsewhere, and consequently a higher proportion of live births to older mothers. This will result in a high crude rate of Down syndrome. This may account for the rate of 1.8 per 1000 live births in Quebec reported by McDonald (1972b), as well as for the apparent high prevalence rates in isolates of the old-order Amish in the U.S. and of an isolate in Northern Sweden. Another extrinsic factor that is likely to have bigger impact in the future may result from socioeconomic differentials in utili- zation of prenatal diagnosis of Down syndrome. Again, there are no specific data on socioeconomic gradients in utilization, but, as with any elective medical procedure in the U.S., there is likely to be such variation, and greater relative utilization of pre- natal diagnosis by the higher socioeconomic groups can be expected. Social factors related to religious beliefs, among other variables, are also likely to result in variation in utilization of prenatal diagnosis.

Such variation is likely to result in lower crude and maternal age-specific rates of Down syndrome live births (especially among those 35 or over) in upper socioeco-

---

[5]This would tend to result in phenotypic surveys also underestimating the maternal age effect, particu- larly at the oldest maternal ages, because children of later birth order would tend to be selectively underas- certained, and higher birth order is associated with higher maternal age. Perhaps this accounts for the level- ing effect seen at the upper ages reported in some of the older surveys (Hook and Lamson, 1980).

Table 24.   Birth order effect in Israeli study

Birth order	Cases	Age-adjusted ratio of observed/expected cases
1	6	0.44
2–3	34	1.16
4–6	25	0.94
≥7	37	1.12

Data from Harlap (1973).

nomic strata (after controlling for other factors) and higher rates in those groups opposed to abortion (after controlling for other factors).

Considering data from the era before selective pregnancy termination was available, studies that found no evidence for any significant socioeconomic association are those of Cohen et al. (1977), Juberg, Goshen, and Sholte (1973), and Sigler et al. (1967). The best data source is probably that from the U.S. collaborative study, in which there was no significant difference in the socioeconomic levels of patients and controls (Sever et al., 1970).

The lack of a strong social class gradient of the disorder in the populations investigated in these studies is some indirect evidence against an environmental agent of strong effect playing a significant etiological role in these populations in live births, although these considerations are not pertinent to the possible effect of an environmental factor without strong socioeconomic variation.

Alberman et al. (1976) found higher social class (I and II) was second only to maternal age as a factor of importance associated with the proportion of cytogenetically abnormal spontaneous abortuses. (There were about 38% in classes I and II compared to 20% in class III and 23% in classes IV and V.) This may reflect, however, only that lower socioeconomic class is associated with a higher absolute rate of spontaneous abortion without cytogenetic abnormality; so among the smaller number of total abortuses to upper social classes, proportionally more have cytogenetic abnormalities.

The only study reporting evidence for a socioeconomic effect upon maternal age-specific rates of Down syndrome is that of Harlap (1973), in which a trend to association with lower socioeconomic class (judged by father's years of schooling) is cited (see Table 25). As noted, however, there were much higher maternal age-specific rates of Down syndrome in non-European than in European Jews (Hook and Harlap, 1979) and the former tend to be of lower socioeconomic class. A socioeconomic effect cannot be distinguished from an ethnic or cultural one in this population based on reports to date.

Table 25.   Age-adjusted ratios of observed/expected cases by father's education in Israeli study

Years of education of father	0–4	5–8	9–12	13+
<35	1.97	1.04	0.90	0.68
≥35	1.15	1.18	1.04	0.77

Data from Harlap (1973).

EVIDENCE PERTAINING TO NONINDEPENDENT OCCURRENCE
OF CHROMOSOMAL ABNORMALITIES IN INDIVIDUALS AND FAMILIES

This section deals primarily with data from studies of live births. In addition to recurrence risks, investigations of consanguinity, the occurrence of double aneuploidy in individuals, and the weak evidence for occurrence of different cytogenetic defects in families, or what may be termed *heteroaneuploidy* (Hecht, 1977), are also considered.

It is well known empirically that women who have a Down syndrome live birth at a younger age have a higher risk for recurrence than women who do not. After the cytogenetic era, it was discovered that the main component of this risk was for parents who were translocation carriers or cryptic mosaics. Nevertheless, even after this class was excluded, among families in which both parents ostensibly have normal karyotypes, there was still a higher recurrence risk if a 47,trisomy 21 child was born to a younger mother (Hamerton et al., 1961). The mechanism for this increased risk is still unknown. There are at least two possible explanations. One is cryptic mosaicism for trisomy 21 in one of the parents, the other is a genetic predisposition to nondisjunction in one of the parents because of autosomal recessive genes, "polygenic" inheritance, or other analogous factors.[6] The latter category may also explain instances of double aneuploidy and of heteroaneuploidy. However, although genes predisposing to meiotic nondisjunction are well known in many lower organisms (see Baker et al., 1976, for extensive review), there is no definitive evidence for such in humans; in fact, most evidence from studies of consanguinity in parents or grandparents of individuals is "negative."

Recurrence Risks for 47,Trisomy 21

Irrespective of mechanism, recurrence risks remains an important question, if only because of its pertinence to accurate genetic counseling.

All of the available pertinent data on live births were compiled by Stene (1970). This was a reanalysis of Hamerton et al.'s (1961) review of some observations of Carter and Evans (1961), as well as data of Oster (1956), subsequently reanalyzed by Mikkelsen (1966). The observations appear in Table 26. Combining results from both series, for a woman under 30 who has had one 47,trisomy 21 child, the estimated risk of a future affected child born to her when under age 30 is $3/211 = 1.4\%$ (95% confidence interval $= 0.29\% - 4.2\%$). (Stene, 1970, in analyzing Oster and Mikkelsen's data, gives $2/91 = 2.2\%$, a higher but not significantly different rate.) These calculations assume implicitly either that the same father is involved or that paternal factors, including age, are not significant.

For a woman over 30 who has had one 47,trisomy 21 child, the reported risk of a future affected child was 0.4% (95% confidence interval $= 0.06\% - 1.7\%$; note that this figure spans all ages at birth of first affected infant) (Table 27).

---

[6]The list is not exclusive. Recurring putative environmental causes could also be invoked.

Table 26.   Data bearing on recurrence of Down syndrome after birth of affected child[a]

Maternal age (pregnancy at risk)	< 30	30–34	35–39	≥ 40
Proportion of affected cases	3/211 (1.4%)	1/145 (0.7%)	0/165 (0%)	1/112 (0.9%)

Calculations are from data in Stene (1970), which are originally from Mikkelsen (1966), Oster (1956), Carter and Evans (1961), and Hamerton et al. (1961) (see Stene, 1970).
[a]Excluding known translocations and parental mosaicism.

This analysis provides the answer to only one of the at least three counseling situations for which data are required. The other situations are: 1) the proband was born to a woman under age 30 who is considering pregnancy over age 30, and 2) the proband was born to a woman over age 30 who is considering subsequent pregnancy. (The break at age 30 here is somewhat arbitrary.)

Unfortunately, all the data in the literature and the data cited previously and in Table 26 for those with pregnancy at risk after age 30 are pooled, so that it is difficult to tell what proportion of women in each class is included in the table. From another perspective, the recurrence risk for those over 30 would, it seems likely, depend both on age of the mother at birth of the affected child and on the age of the mother at time of pregnancy, but the data available do not allow a separate examination of these factors.

Theoretically, there are some grounds for believing that older women who had an affected child when under 30 should have a higher maternal age-specific recurrence risk than the older woman whose affected child was born at age 30 or over.

The fact that in both groups pooled, the recurrence was $2/422 = 0.4\%$ (95% confidence interval $= 0.06\% - 1.7\%$) may have suggested to the original authors that both categories of women do not have significantly higher recurrence risks than those of the general population. However, it may be that the first category of women is significantly underrepresented in the combined series, so that a "negative" inference about this group is based only on a few data.

Optimally, all data of this type should be presented in a matrix by 1-year interval, with columns indicating the age at risk and rows indicating age of birth of proband, in order to derive the maximum useful information.

Table 27.   Recurrence risk for Down syndrome based on data in Table 26

Maternal age at birth of first case	Maternal age at risk	
	< 30	≥ 30
< 30	1.4%[a]	0.4%[b, c]
≥ 30	—	

[a]95% confidence level $= 0.29\% - 4.2\%$.
[b]95% confidence level $= 0.06\% - 1.7\%$.
[c]Note that this figure is derived from studies of those at all ages at birth of the first case.

The number of live born children between birth of the affected child and the pregnancy at risk is likely to be significant, since the more pregnancies with normal outcome that have occurred, the lower the likelihood of recurrence, analogous to the situation for multifactorial inheritance.

In reviewing the literature on genetic counseling, it became evident that variable and somewhat contradictory interpretation was given to these data. The following excerpts apply to the "standard" counseling situation, i.e., one child with 47,trisomy 21, both parents with normal karyotypes (see Table 28).

Mikkelsen and Stene (1970) stated: "Stene...estimated the risk to be between 1% and 2% for women who have had their affected child before the age of 30 years. No increased risk was found for a woman who had her first affected child after the age of 30." As I interpret the paper of Stene, however, his data warrant the inference that the risk is high only for mothers under 30 *who are pregnant again under age 30.*

It is particularly surprising, moreover, that textbooks on genetic counseling differ considerably on this point. For example, Stevenson and Davison (1976) stated: "Observations suggest that these factors [inherited mosaicism and genetic predisposition] determine that...risks to subsequent sibs are about twice as high as to children born to mothers of the same age who have not previously had a mongol child." A table projects a doubling of risks at all ages, with estimated risk for mothers under age 30 as $1/500 = 0.2\%$, about one-eighth the estimate from the data.

Murphy and Chase (1978) commented on the data summarized by Stene: "It would be unwarranted to extrapolate...uncritically to a population of older mothers. It might be proper to assume conservatively that the elements of risk from age and from the occurrence of a previous trisomy 21 are additive." They then gave an example in which they added 1% to the risk figure. By implication this would be done at all maternal ages.

Fuhrman and Vogel (1976) essentially restated conclusions given in Stene's original analysis.

Smith and Berg (1976) stated that the risks for future sibs are the same as those for parents in the general population, "but allowance may be made for a slight additional risk." No statement on the interaction with maternal age at time of the first affected child appears.

Table 28.   Comparison of implications of advice in texts on genetic counseling recurrence risk for Down syndrome at maternal age 40 and for those under 30[a]

Reference	Advice	Risk cited	
		Age < 30	Age 40
Stevenson and Davison (1976)	Double the risk	0.2%	2%
Murphy and Chase (1978)	Add 1%	1.1%	2%
Fuhrman and Vogel (1976)	Age interaction (<30, 1%–2%; ≥30, same as population)	1%–2%	1%

[a]Instances of 47, + 21 Down syndrome only, in which neither parent is a known 47, + 21 mosaic, using as baseline data rounded figures from Table 5.

These discrepancies in interpretation of the data in the literature are perplexing. Murphy and Chase's (1978) suggestion appears the most plausible approach.

Consanguinity and Inbreeding in Parents of Down Syndrome Children and Other Evidence on Genetic Predisposition

In an extensive review of the genetic control of meiosis, Baker et al. (1976) discussed disjunction-defective meiotic mutants in *Drosophila,* in which a clear genetic predisposition to meiotic nondisjunction is found (see also L. Sandler, this volume). In *Drosophila* females, it appears that most mutants affecting meiosis disrupt the disjunction of more than one specific chromosome. There is, however, a tendency for these events to result in substantial meiotic chromosome loss. Of particular interest, for meiosis-II, is that there are at least two mutants that increase nondisjunction in both sexes and affect only the chromosome they are on (Baker et al., 1976, p. 94). Furthermore, there is a group of male-specific meiotic mutants affecting chromosome behavior in *Drosophila,* and most of these, which act during meiosis I, affect only a subset of chromosomes, not all of them. Two alleles on the second chromosome in particular affect chromosome 4 only. (It should be noted that *Drosophila* males in most species lack genetic recombination, unlike humans, so that some sex differences in *Drosophila* with regard to the effects of meiotic mutants are not likely to provide models for species in which both sexes undergo crossing over.)

These data provide some plausible grounds for expecting mutations in humans that may predispose to nondisjunction and in particular to an increased recurrence risk of 47,trisomy 21.

Hecht (1977) has distinguished two different types of effects such genes may have. They may result in homoaneuploidy (tendency for recurrence of the same chromosomal aneuploidy in families) or heteroaneuploidy (tendency for recurrence of the same or other chromosome aneuploidy). In *Drosophila,* both types of mutants have been detected.

The recurrence risk for Down syndrome is suggestive but only weak evidence for genes predisposing to homoaneuploidy for trisomy 21, because such effects could readily arise from cryptic mosaicism in one parent, resulting in secondary nondisjunction.

More convincing evidence, at least for recessive genes, would arise from studies of Down syndrome in relation to inbreeding. There are several studies analyzing the rate of consanguinity among the parents and grandparents of affected persons. It is difficult to visualize how homozygosity of the zygote would be likely to result in trisomic condition of the fetus, so that the relevance of data from such studies on parental consanguinity would seem less pertinent evidence for genetic effects than data on grandparental consanguinity.[7] The latter could result in potentially homozygous conditions in one parent that might predispose to meiotic nondisjunction.

---

[7]Nevertheless, it is conceivable that genes carried by the zygote itself could affect its eventual manifestation as a trisomic live birth. Such genes might result in mitotic nondisjunction, for example, in the first zygote cell division, resulting in a 45, $-21/47, +21$ mosaic, with subsequent cell death of the 45, -21 cell line. Alternatively, the genetic composition of the zygote might affect fetal survival of the trisomy 21 fetus.

Penrose (1961) was apparently the first to suggest that genes in humans predisposing to nondisjunction could be responsible for some familial instances of trisomy 21. Penrose (Penrose and Smith, 1966, p. 165) claimed that if the gene were rare, a detectable increase in consanguinity in maternal grandparents as compared to paternal grandparents would be noted. (This assumes, presumably, recessive genes and of course preferential maternal origin.) Penrose and Smith stated, "In a series of many hundreds of mongols whose family histories were investigated by Penrose...there were five instances of parental consanguinity (mean age of mother 39.0 years) and five of paternal grandparental consanguinity (mean age of mother 35.6 years). Maternal grandparents were consanguineous in 12 cases (mean age of mother 33.5 years) but the excess here above 5 expected is not statistically very remarkable." Forssman and Akesson (1967a) cited further data on Penrose's observations.[8] There were about 700 affected cases. Of the five parental consanguineous cases, only one involved first cousins. Four out of five consanguineous paternal grandparents were first cousins, 5 out of 12 consanguineous maternal grandparents were first cousins, and 2 were cousins of unknown degree. At least the trend is in the direction Penrose predicted. He subsequently expressed the view that a search for such factors was a "wild goose chase" however (Penrose, 1967), in view of the report of the study of Forssman and Akesson (1967a), among others. Among 1079 children with Down syndrome in Sweden, most registered at institutions for the retarded between 1955 and 1959, Forssman and Akesson reported nine cases in which parents were first cousins or closer, including one case of a brother-sister incest—a frequency of 0.8%, probably about the same frequency as in the general Swedish population during the same period. For paternal grandparents the frequency was 14/820 = 1.7%, and for maternal grandparents, 12/821 = 1.5%. (The lower frequency in parents than in grandparents is attributed to a diminishing number of marriages between consanguineous persons in Sweden.) The absence of good control data from the general population renders these "negative" results less than conclusive.

Matsunaga (1967) analyzed Koseki records from Japan and observed that of 104 children with Down syndrome born to mothers under age 30, 6 children, 10 fathers, and 12 mothers had related parents (first and second cousins). Apparently, 8 of the mothers had first-cousin parents. Matsunaga stated that these data exclude a putative recessive gene whose frequency is 3% (or greater) with high confidence. However, they are compatible with lower gene frequencies in the population and, in any event, control data are not provided for comparison.

Berg (1967) examined data on consanguinity in parents of children with Down syndrome and other types of mental retardation in the greater London area in the previous decade. He noted 2 of 302 subjects (0.7%) with Down syndrome who had first-cousin parents. For the other types of mental retardation there were 12/714 = 1.7% cases of consanguineous parents (11 first-cousin marriages, one brother-sister incest). In comparison, Berg cited Bell's 1940 data on hospital patients with consanguineous parents in England, which gave a frequency of 0.6%–0.7%.

---

[8]They discussed his data in a report of their own. Apparently, Penrose, who was at the conference and heard their report, made these further observations available to them, but never reported formally himself.

Polani (1967) reported similar data. In 208 affected children, two parents and three pairs of grandparents were first cousins.

These data, particularly those of Forssman and Akesson, are sufficient to make it unlikely that maternal inbreeding (consanguineous maternal grandparents) plays a more significant role in recurrence than paternal inbreeding. However, they are not adequate to exclude a recessive gene with homozygous effects in either parent, nor do they exclude recessive genes with effect in the zygote itself. The lack of adequate control data and the relatively small number of observations in most series make it difficult to make strong statements about the absence of any inbreeding effects.

Other data pertinent to the possible effect of autosomal recessive genes could come from studies of inbred populations.

Two studies of Amish groups in the U.S. have been published. Juberg and Davis (1970) found that the mean inbreeding coefficients (f) of 16 Down syndrome children, their parents, and 12 other more remote ancestors in an Indiana isolate did not significantly differ from that of matched controls. In fact, the mean value of f for the Down syndrome cases was less than that of the controls for 12 of 15 groups. While these data do not suggest any inbreeding effect, they involve small numbers of cases in a population isolate in which pertinent genes may not be segregating.

Kwitterovich, Cross, and McKusick (1966) reported on the prevalence of Down syndrome in the Old Order Amish in Holmes County, Ohio. The rate was 16 cases in an estimated population of 10,000 cytogenetically confirmed cases, 15 of which were 47, + 21. The lack of a significantly higher prevalence rate than apparently was expected was interpreted by the authors as providing "no support for a genetic factor in etiology." The data, however, are difficult to invoke against the hypothesis of genetic (recessive) etiology. Since this was a prevalence study and the subjects ranged in age from 1 to 29, the crude frequency was much higher than would be expected from other surveys during this period because of the high mortality rate with age. The median age of this group of 16 was about 11 years (the mean, 12.3), and one would expect a 50% to 75% mortality by this age. The 95% confidence interval for the observed prevalence rate of 16/10,000 was about 0.9×10^{-3} to 2.6×10^{-3}. (Counting only the 47, + 21 cases, the 95% interval is $0.8 \times 10^{-3} - 2.5 \times 10^{-3}$). The lower limit is greater than the expected prevalence of a group of Down syndrome with this median age. It would be helpful to have current and historical data on the maternal age structure of the population, since it is possible that the crude incidence and prevalence rates are elevated only because of a very high proportion of older mothers in this population. Nevertheless, the data, as presented, must be regarded as prima facie evidence for a higher crude prevalence in this inbred group than in other studies.

Because of these considerations, I reexamined the data of Juberg and Davis (1970). Their 16 cases of Down syndrome were found in a population of approximately 5500, resulting in a prevalence rate of 2.9×10^{-3}, with 95% confidence interval of 1.66×10^{-3} to 4.72×10^{-3}. The median age in this group was even older, 14.6 years (the mean, 12.1). There is no reason to assume diminished mortality of Down syndrome in the Amish compared to other populations studied in this period (e.g., those of Fabia and Drolette, 1970). Therefore, one may assume that the crude prevalence rate in this population reflects a crude incidence rate of about twice this value, i.e., 5.8×10^{-3}. Again, it is possible that a very high proportion of older mothers in this population explains the high crude rates here. Alternatively, the case-control method of Juberg and Davis (1970) is not sensitive enough to detect an effect of inbreeding upon this trait in this population, or the higher crude rate is due to social and/or environmental differences between the Amish and other populations. At least the data of Juberg and Davis (1970) and, to a lesser extent, those of Kwitterovich et al. (1966) are consistent in an increase in prevalence and crude incidence rates in two different Amish populations compared to outbred populations of European background.

In a study from Northeastern Sweden of an inbred population isolate, Böök (1953) found a crude prevalence rate of 10/8981, or 1.1 per 1000, but noted that significant underascertainment had occurred. Assuming all 10 living subjects were those under age 10 then alive in the community and, adjusting for underascertainment, he estimated the incidence to be 3.8/1000. A minimum figure was derived by considering all 13 subjects known to have been born in 1929–1948, which provides a minimum incidence rate of 2.5/1000. He stated that the true rate is probably between these two rates, but it could even be higher. The (minimum) maternal age-specific incidence rates of Down syndrome were given as 0.6/1000 in those under 40 and 21.2/1000 in those over 40. He also stated, "The incidence of women aged 40 and above giving birth to children was nine percent for the rural parts of Norrbolten County against 7.5 percent for all rural districts in Sweden." If "incidence" in this context means fertility rate, it is extraordinarily high, if the denominator includes women beyond the usual childbearing ages. However, he may mean by "incidence" the proportion of mothers in this age bracket having live births, with which the figures of 7.5% and 9% appear more consistent. As in the Amish, the high crude (real) incidence rate of Down syndrome in the Swedish group may be attributable to a high proportion of older mothers in the population, but this explanation remains conjectural.

So far only autosomal recessive factors that may predispose to nondisjunction have been considered. However, it is at least possible, as Penrose (1967) noted, that dominant genes may also predispose to nondisjunction and, by implication, 47, + 21 Down syndrome as well. There seem to be no good data that allow evaluation of this possibility. Such data could come from systematic studies of "collateral" relatives (e.g., cousins), in which the intermediate relatives in the pedigree (e.g., siblings, which are parents of the cousins) hypothetically could be carriers of dominant genes with diminished penetrance or expressivity. (Studies of other combinations of relatives, e.g., uncle-aunt, nephew-niece, would also be pertinent.)

However, dominant inheritance with reduced penetrance and expressivity may be operationally difficult, if not impossible, to distinguish from polygenic or multifactorial inheritance. Indeed, it would be of interest to analyze the recurrence risk data in siblings from the perspective of a multifactorial model, making appropriate adjustments for maternal age and the number of normal siblings. It would appear plausible that the processes that result in a 47, + 21 live birth are in fact multifactorial in many instances, in the sense in which that term is usually understood in human genetics.

Heteroaneuploidy

The evidence for genes that predispose to nondisjunction for more than one chromosome in humans can be of at least three sorts:

1. Data on inbreeding and consanguinity of the type discussed previously
2. Data on multiple affected sibs (or other relatives if a dominant gene or multifactorial model applies) with different cytogenetic conditions
3. Data on individuals who have double aneuploidy

There seem to be no data or analyses in the literature on the first category. With regard to the second category, a large number of families have been reported in which siblings are affected with different cytogenetic conditions (see Baker et al., 1976; Hecht, 1977, for citation of cases). Some pedigrees involving affected cousins consistent with a dominant gene (with reduced penetrance) have also been noted (Penrose, 1967). The difficulty is that many of these instances involve anecdotal case reports, and in the few series the possibility of selective ascertainment of affected relatives appears likely. Even selective publication cannot be excluded.

While there may well be Mendelian genes that predispose to multiple affected sibs in humans, the available evidence to date seems to also be consistent with chance effects, ascertainment bias, and selective publication.

With regard to the third category of evidence, a higher frequency of double aneuploidy in persons than expected is not, in itself, complete proof of genetic predisposition, because environmental events inducing nondisjunction of different chromosomes could also result in such an observation. The evidence concerning the frequency of double aneuploidy in a person with trisomy 21 is surprisingly inconclusive.

The most suggestive evidence comes from the data on the simultaneous occurrence of 47,trisomy 21 with extra X chromosomes—in particular, the XXY genotype.

Hamerton et al. (1965) reported pooled data from three series. In these there were 3 XXYs in 616 Down syndrome cases, which (indirectly calculated) is equivalent to a doubling of the expected rate of XXYs. They also summarized four sex chromatin surveys and noted that among 18,718 people screened, there were 2 with XXY, + 21. Both of these were in the Taylor and Moores (1967) study, which included 4934 males. Only one of the two cases was cytogenetically confirmed. (No double aneuploidy was noted in 4754 females, apparently). On the basis of these data, Hamerton (1971) concluded there is little doubt that double trisomics occur with greater frequency than would be expected by chance.

Mikkelsen (1970), however, found no sex chromosome abnormality among 322 males with Down syndrome. (Among 310 females there was one case of 47,XX, + 21/47 isoXq,21 + .) The subjects in this series were apparently predominantly in their childhood years and born primarily to younger mothers. They had been actively sought out in communities for cytogenetic investigation. In the same report, Mikkelsen cited an earlier sex chromatin screening study of hers in which there were no sex chromosome abnormalities among 607 males with Down syndrome (nor among 555 females with Down syndrome).

The differences in results between Hamerton's institutional series and Mikkelsen's sex chromatin surveys and major screening study "may reflect a younger age group examined by Hamerton, or the hospital selection of his cases. Patients with a double trisomy may be more severely affected. . ." (Mikkelsen, 1970) and thus more likely to be hospitalized or institutionalized. Of course, it could be argued they might be more likely to die sooner and thus be missed in studies of older persons.

It is difficult to determine whether the 632 cases reported by Mikkelsen in 1970 are included in or overlap with the 235 cases of Down syndrome that she and co-workers reported in 1976, which included infants born from January 1, 1960, to December 31, 1971, in Copenhagen. Of these 235 cases, 177 "unselected" subjects with Down syndrome were cytogenetically diagnosed and include 1 48,XXY, + 21, 1 48,XXY, + 21/47, + 21, and 1 48,XYY, + 21 case. (Fifty-eight were not cytogenetically studied because their parents refused permission. The remainder died before they could be studied.) The number of males and females studied is not stated but there clearly appears to be an increase in heteroaneuploidy in males with Down syndrome (minimum rate = 3/177) in this series compared to males in earlier studies (0/929), a difference that is significant at the 0.05 level. At face value the results of these two publications from the same laboratory seem discrepant, and some ad hoc explanation—such as temporal cluster of double trisomies in Copenhagen—would have to be invoked to explain the differences. However, this would tend to imply that environmental rather than genetic factors are more likely to explain the difference.

Because both the XXY genotype (and XXX) and 47, + 21 increase with maternal age, the frequency of double trisomy expected on the basis of "chance" alone is not simply the product of their crude frequencies (about 10^{-3} each) but must be adjusted for the maternal age composition of the populations involved and of Down syndrome cases detected. (The data necessary for this analysis are not always provided in surveys so that it is sometimes difficult to evaluate the results.) Thus, the expectations of double trisomy involved in Down syndrome given in Smith and Berg (1976, p. 209) are all too low, and must be adjusted upward.

The study of Hecht et al. (1969) is one of the few to make the adjustment. These authors studied the sex chromatin of 772 patients with Down syndrome and found one XXY, + 21. From knowledge of maternal age in this population they calculated an expected number of 3.14. With regard to 1257 other subjects reported in the literature from six other series, including one of Hamerton, they reported a frequency of 2 in 1257 cases. Assuming the same maternal age distribution in this group as in the other (which they suggest is a conservative assumption), they derived the expected number of cases of 9.25 in the combined series compared to an observed number of 3. Thus, the observed frequency was below that expected for a population of comparable maternal age. The interpretation given is that while there is a high frequency at birth (because of Taylor and Moores', 1967, study—see below, however, for discussion of newborn data), there is strong selection subsequently against XXY, + 21 cases, in view of their own data.

Another observation of interest is that cases of double aneuploidy for extra X and extra number 21 chromosomes have preferentially been reported in males. Mikkelsen et al.'s (1976) data regarding this have already been cited. Additional evidence is derived from Smith and Berg's (1976, pp. 207–208) review, which lists all cases known to them of double aneuploidy with Down syndrome. These include (counting twins as one case) 17 cases of XXY, three XXY/XY mosaics, three XXXs, and three mosaic XXX/XYs. In addition, there are five XYYs and one XXX/XX/XO mosaic. The excess of XXYs in this group may be attributable to the (putative) greater phenotypic severity of the Down syndrome male with an extra X than the Down syndrome female with an extra X (similar to the known greater phenotypic severity of 47,XXY compared to 47,XXX) and consequently a higher probability of ascertainment. If, however, the excess of +21,XXY cases is due to meiotic or cytological factors, it may mean that: 1) double nondisjunction is particularly likely to occur in male first division meiosis, 2) human ova that are +X,21 are more receptive to fertilization by Y bearing sperm, or 3) some other type of preferential fertilization occurs, e.g., +21,Y sperm to +X ova. Alternatively, factors related to differential fetal survival could also be involved. In any event, it would be interesting to investigate the sources of the extra X and extra 21 chromosomes in these double aneuploid people to determine if they came from the same parent and same meiotic stage.

The reports in the literature are so heterogeneous that it may be helpful to restate some points. Several types of biases can enter into studies of the frequency of XXY,+21 cases in postnatal surveys. Among others, these involve the putative greater phenotypic effect and putative greater mortality of XXY,+21 persons compared to 47,+21 persons. Earlier mortality would result in underascertainment of cases. However, a more severe phenotypic effect that cannot be separated entirely from an effect upon mortality (e.g., greater level of retardation or high frequency of congenital heart defect) might also result in greater likelihood of ascertainment of such cases in institutions and hospitals. The overall direction of the resultant of the combination of these two biases cannot be predicted, and it is perhaps noteworthy that there are many studies that report discordant results. The best data on live-birth prevalence would come from live-birth studies, with due attention to the possibility of differentials in fetal mortality.

Taylor and Moores' (1967) newborn survey (two XXY,+21 cases in 4934 males) remains the only one to report any evidence for an excess. For example, in a study of 37,233 male births, Bell and Corey (1974) found no XXY,+21 cases (Bell, personal communication), although there were 40 XXYs. Similarly, in 37,779 newborn males in newborn studies summarized by Hook and Hamerton (1977) there were no XXY,+21 cases, although there were 35 XXYs. (There was also no XXY,+21 or XXX,+21 in these series). The numbers in the latter studies may still be too small to allow a strong negative statement, however. Thus, on this question of heteroaneuploidy, on which the most data are available in live births, not even a tentative inference is warranted.

This illustrates how a generally accepted view on the epidemiology of Down syndrome may be undermined by close examination of the pertinent evidence.

It is somewhat ironic, however, that the available data from studies of abortuses are consistent with a heteroaneuploid effect.

Alberman et al. (1975) (Table 29) found a 10- to 20-fold increase in the rate of Down syndrome over the rate expected in live-born children among previous pregnancies of couples who were first detected because they had a spontaneous abortus with (any) trisomy. (There was no such increased risk among those with abortus with

Table 29.   Previous Down syndrome among sibs of abortuses in a U.K. study

Abortus outcome	Siblings with Down syndrome	All siblings	%
Abnormal karyotype	5	476	1.1%[a]
Karyotype not known	6	2474	0.2%
Normal karyotype	0	1042	0%
Live-born controls	0	1072	0%

Data from Alberman et al. (1975).

[a]5/244 = 2.1% among siblings of a trisomic abortus.

normal chromosomes or nontrisomic cytogenetic abnormality.) There is a suggestion that recurrence of abortion is more likely among mothers who have cytogenetically normal fetuses. However, among mothers with a cytogenetically abnormal abortus, if they have another abortus, it is much more likely to be cytogenetically abnormal. Data on this point have been summarized by Jacobs (1979) from five studies of 103 women with two spontaneous abortions and known karyotype. Of 27 cases where the first abortion was trisomic, the second was trisomic in 22. Of 55 cases where the first abortion was not trisomic, the second was trisomic in only 6. Considering only trisomic and normal cases, the relative odds of a second abortus being trisomic if the first one is, is 84.0 (see Tables 30 and 31). The risk of a second trisomic abortus, given a first trisomic abortus, is increased at all maternal ages but is particularly high for older mothers. These data strongly suggest that women known to have had a trisomic conceptus are at increased risk to have another, but the precise risk of a Down syndrome live birth cannot be gauged. As Jacobs noted, however, the history of a trisomic abortus should be regarded as grounds for amniocentesis.

The mechanism for this effect is uncertain but may be due to genetic factors discussed previously. It would be of interest to collect data on ancestral inbreeding in such instances, where possible.

Of all the available data, these are the most convincing for a heteroaneuploid effect in humans.

FEMALE SEX HORMONES

Observations by Carr (1976) concerning the association of triploidy and, possibly, other chromosome aberrations in abortuses with previous parental exposure to female sex hormones led to interest in the possibility that such hormones also predispose to abnormalities in live births, particularly Down syndrome.

Among studies of the presence of defects in children born to former users of oral contraceptives, Peterson (1969) found one case of Down syndrome in 401 users compared to 3/641 in controls. Robinson's (1971) study does not mention Down syndrome among the outcomes observed in former users. The Royal College of General Practitioners (RCGP, 1976) found 5 cases among 4522 former users (1.11×10^{-3}) compared to 9 in 9617 controls (0.94×10^{-3}), a slightly but not significantly higher rate. Janerich, Flink, and Keogh (1976) found a lower rate of former birth control pill users among mothers of children with Down syndrome compared to controls (18/103 = 17.5% versus 26/103 = 25.2%), a trend in the direction of a protective ef-

Table 30. Trisomics in second abortion by cytogenetic data on first abortus

Maternal age at time of first abortus	First abortus	Second abortion			
		Normal	Trisomic	Other	Total
≤30	Normal	31	4	5	40
	Trisomic	3	4	0	7
	Other	6	4	4	14
		40	12	9	61
30–34	Normal	7	0	2	9
	Trisomic	1	4	1	6
	Other	1	2	0	3
		9	6	3	18
≥35	Normal	4	2	0	6
	Trisomic	1	14	1	16
	Other	0	1	1	2
		5	17	2	24
Total		54	35	14	103

From Jacobs (1979); reprinted by permission. See also Table 30.

Table 31.   Selected data from analysis of Jacobs (1979)

First abortion	Second abortion		
	Trisomic	Normal	Total
Trisomic	22	5	27
Normal	6	42	48

Relative odds of second abortus being trisomic, given that the first abortus is trisomic, are 84.0.

fect of former pill use. They noted that "the deficiency of pill users...was actually quite large.... Using the marginal χ^2 test, the value fell just short of formal significance $(0.10 > p > 0.05)$." The authors did not indicate the relative odds for former pill use among those with a Down syndrome birth, but these may be calculated as 0.63, with a standard error of 0.22 (the 95% confidence interval, however, is about 0.3–1.3.) The authors noted that the unusual deficiency of former pill users among mothers of Down syndrome infants was concentrated among the older mothers.

The results of this study are very reassuring concerning the lack of effect of pill use upon the subsequent occurrence of Down syndrome.

Harlap and Davies (1978), however, in a cross-sectional study of births, found a rate of Down syndrome births in birth control pill users of $10/2994 = 3.34 \times 10^{-3}$ compared to $24/13,832 = 1.74 \times 10^{-3}$ ($\chi^2 = 3.14$, $p < 0.08$) in non-pill users. (The total rate was $34/16,826 = 2.02 \times 10^{-3}$.) The trend was particularly noteworthy in thinner women, an effect present after age adjustment. (There was a four- to five-fold excess in thin pill users.) It is hard to judge the significance of the trend in the data of Harlap and Davies because they studied numerous pregnancy outcomes, and it is not unexpected that suggestive associations with pill use should be observed for some of them. Moreover, the overall trend for Down syndrome was not nominally significant at the 0.05 level, although the authors indicated that the trend to an effect in thinner mothers was significant (Table 32).

Alberman et al. (1976) reported about a 20% excess in the proportion of abnormal karyotypes in abortuses to those using oral contraceptives over 18 months, but not if they were used for a shorter period. "The small increase...applied to nearly every type of [cytogenetic] anomaly." No reports on the results for trisomy 21 specifically are reported in this series.

It appears that at least the data on live births—with the exception of the report of Harlap and Davies (1978)—are consistent with no effect of prior use of oral contraceptives, although the data on spontaneous abortuses are counter to this.

PATERNAL FACTORS[9]

It is clear that about 20% to 25% of 47,trisomy 21 is of paternal origin (e.g., see Hansson and Mikkelsen 1978; Magenis et al., 1977; Wagenbichler et al., 1976). Holmes (1978a) has implied that because of this, paternal age is very likely to be a risk factor for Down syndrome. This, however, is a nonsequitur. For example, the extra Y chromosome of the XYY genotype is of paternal origin, but there is no evidence for increasing rate with increasing parental age for this genotype (Carothers et al., 1978).

---

[9]See also chapter by Magenis, this volume.

Table 32.   Percent (subsequent) offspring with Down syndrome in pill users and non-users

Study	Pill users	Non-users
Cross-sectional		
Peterson (1969)	0.25%	0.47%
	(401)[a]	(641)
RCGP (1976)	0.11%	0.09%
	(4522)	(9617)
Harlap and Davies (1978)	0.33%	0.17%
	(2994)	(13,832)
Case-control		
Janerich et al. (1976)	40.9%	52.5%
	(44)	(162)

[a]Parentheses = N.

All statistical analyses have shown that maternal age is much stronger than paternal age as a risk factor for Down syndrome (e.g., see Penrose and Smith, 1966, p. 158). This does not mean, however, that paternal age makes no contribution as a weak risk factor in addition to maternal age. Two studies (Matsunaga et al., 1978; Stene et al., 1977) have reported that for fathers ages 55 or over, the risks of a Down syndrome birth are about twice that expected after adjustment for mother's age, but they reported no evidence for a paternal age effect under 55. Erickson (1978), however, studying a very large sample of cases, found no evidence for a paternal age effect at any age, although his sample may not have been representative of particular age categories of marriages (Stene and Stene, 1978). Case-control studies in which maternal ages are matched and paternal ages compared have revealed no evidence whatsoever for a paternal age effect (Cohen et al., 1977; Sigler et al., 1967). The latter studies, however, may not have had power to exclude an effect at the very oldest ages.

On the basis of the evidence to date, it seems likely that paternal age is not a risk factor of any significant magnitude for men under 55, and certainly not for those under 50, and that for ages 55 and over, there may be a doubling in risk. Although such an effect must be confirmed in other investigations before it can be regarded as ubiquitous, at present there appears to be no alternative but to cite this putative risk in counseling men ages 55 or over.[10]

---

[10]*Addendum:*   Since this was written, Erickson (1979) published an analysis of two more data sets. In Atlanta for the period 1968–1976, he found no overall significant paternal age effect but suggestive evidence for an increase in men 50 and over married to women under 35, but not to older women. For United States birth certificate data for 1974, he found no significant effect, but if anything a trend to a decrease in older men. Our unit in the Birth Defects Institute has recently completed an analysis of three other data sets. In birth certificate reports in Upstate New York for 1963–1974 there was no evidence for an increase at older ages (Regal et al., in press). In British Columbia data for 1952–1963 there was no evidence for a paternal age effect. In British Columbia data for 1964–1976, however, two distinct statistical analyses (regression and case-control) revealed a statistically significant paternal age effect, albeit of modest size (about 0.5 years in the case-control analysis). The effect is qualitatively different from those reported by others in that there was evidence of a slight general upward trend with paternal age from age 20 on (Hook et al., in preparation). The data appear likely to be close to complete with regard to affected cases. The precise implications of these findings for counseling are still being analyzed. Variations between the results in this data set and the others discussed may possibly be attributable to geographic and temporal variation in a putative paternal effect, to artifacts of (incomplete) sampling of some affected populations, and/or to statistical fluctuation.

Data pertinent to parental age effects from reports of ages in those cases where parental origin has been assigned cytogenetically are presented in Table 33. These studies are likely to be heterogeneous in the category of cases included for study. For example, the paternal ages of those studied by Wagenbichler et al. (1976) are considerably higher than those reported by Magenis et al. (1977) and Hansson and Mikkelsen (1978). Perhaps Wagenbichler et al., in contrast to the other two, reported parental ages at the time of study, not at birth, or else studied older children who were born when mean parental age was much higher than it is now. In any event, it is noteworthy that the midparental ages (probably the best variable for comparison of the two categories) is, in general, higher for those of maternal than of paternal origin. Unfortunately, the methods of case selection are not sufficiently described to allow any inferences on what the appropriate parental or midparental ages should be in a control population. It appears likely that it will be some time before population inferences about the magnitude of a paternal age effect will be possible from such cytogenetic studies.

SOME OTHER PUTATIVE CAUSAL FACTORS: THYROID DISEASE AND AUTOANTIBODIES, HEPATITIS, RADIATION

Since the topics of this section have been reviewed in detail elsewhere, these putative causal factors are reviewed only briefly.

The work of Fialkow (1969, 1970; Fialkow et al., 1971) on thyroid disorders is of particular interest because his data suggest a familial predisposition to thyroid autoimmunity in mothers of Down syndrome children. Although there are many positive studies, only two negative studies of the association of thyroid autoantibodies and Down syndrome have appeared (McDonald, 1972a, which includes an extensive review of earlier work; Wren et al., 1967). McDonald, however, did find a higher frequency of thyroid disease in parents of Down children compared to controls (11/100 versus 3/100). The biological reasons for the associations remain unexplained. Conceivably, some other factors, such as a specific HLA genotype or other related immunological variable, may mediate the association of Down syndrome and maternal thyroid autoimmunity, if it is not attributable directly to thyroid autoantibodies or some other thyroid-related product or function. (Studies of HLA A and B haplotypes in Down syndrome reveal no deviation from control distributions (Segal et al., 1975).) Moreover, those with other chromosome abnormalities, in particular XO mosaicism or X isoX, have what appears to be an even stronger association with thyroid autoimmunity than those with Down syndrome (see Fialkow, 1969).

There has been voluminous discussion of Stoller and Collman's proposal (1965) that the pattern of Down syndrome incidence in Victoria, Australia, between 1953 and 1964 followed that for infectious hepatitis, with a 9-month lag. Many were unable to confirm these reports in other jurisdictions (see references in Cohen et al., 1977; Lilienfeld, 1969), and the statistical analysis was challenged both by Kogon, Kronmal, and Peterson (1968) and Stark and Mantel (1967). The graphs presented by the original authors appeared to be so suggestive of a strong association, and by inference a causal one, that the entire episode illustrates the need for caution before ac-

Table 33. Parental ages in three studies where parental origin of extra chromosome in 47, +21 persons was determined

Origin	Number of cases	Maternal age		Paternal age		Midparental age		Study
		Mean	S.D.	Mean	S.D.	Mean	S.D.	
Paternal								
Meiosis I	5	29.20	10.47	30.20	7.01	29.70	8.47	Magenis et al. (1977)
	3	29.00	8.72	30.00	8.72	29.50	8.72	Hansson and Mikkelsen (1978)
Subtotal	8	29.13	9.19	30.13	2.06	29.63	7.92	
Meiosis II	2	26.50	3.54	28.50	2.12	27.50	2.12	Magenis et al. (1977)
	4	27.75	4.57	28.75	2.87	28.25	3.66	Hansson and Mikkelsen (1978)
Subtotal	6	27.33	7.23	28.67	2.42	28.00	3.13	
Not stated or known	8	28.75	7.91	33.88	10.20	31.31	8.83	Wagenbichler et al. (1976)
Total	14[a]	28.36	7.23	29.50	5.45	28.93	6.18	Magenis et al. (1977), Hansson and Mikkelsen (1978)
Maternal								
Meiosis I	23	30.00	7.42	32.70	8.80	31.35	7.92	Magenis et al. (1977)
	9	30.78	6.28	33.11	8.31	31.94	7.07	Hansson and Mikkelsen (1978)
Subtotal	32	30.22	7.03	32.81	8.53	31.52	7.58	
Meiosis II	1	41.00	0.00	42.00	0.00	41.50	0.00	Magenis et al. (1977)
	6	25.83	6.01	30.17	4.79	28.00	5.37	Hansson and Mikkelsen (1978)
Subtotal	7	28.00	7.94	31.86	6.26	29.93	7.07	
Not stated or known	4	28.00	6.73	30.25	10.59	29.13	8.61	Hansson and Mikkelsen (1978)
	10	37.10	7.03	38.80	6.00	37.95	6.28	Wagenbichler et al. (1976)
Total	43[a]	29.65	7.05	32.42	8.24	31.03	7.45	Magenis et al. (1977), Hansson and Mikkelsen (1978)

[a]Excludes cases of Wagenbichler et al. because the parental age of the population sampled is so clearly discrepant from the other two reports.

cepting as ubiquitous what appear to be "obvious" and strongly suggestive purported associations. (It does appear likely, however, that infectious hepatitis type B surface antigen is increased in those with Down syndrome itself (Blumberg, 1978).)

Only some ad hoc hypothesis(es) other than simply chance deviations can reconcile the differences between the studies that show positive association between Down syndrome and parental exposure to ionizing irradiation (e.g., Uchida, 1977) and the studies that show no association (e.g., Cohen et al., 1977). The nature of the radiation, some interaction with time and/or dose, or some methodological factor is likely to contribute to these differences. The reader is referred to the papers cited here and in Hook and Porter (1977) (see also Uchida, this volume). Interesting hypotheses that may explain some of the negative studies are those of Wald, Turner, and Borges (1970), who postulated a dose interaction effect, and Alberman et al. (1972), who suggested that a time delay is necessary for effect to manifest.

EPIDEMIOLOGY OF DOWN SYNDROME
ASSOCIATED WITH STRUCTURAL CHANGES[11]

Of the approximately 5% of Down syndrome cases associated with a structural rearrangement, about 50%–60% have D/21 "interchanges," about 40%–50% have G/21 interchanges, and a minuscule proportion, probably no more than 5%, has some other structural rearrangements, such as tandem duplication. All have in common three doses of the 21q arm (or a subregion of the 21q arm) represented somewhere in the genome of the affected person. Of the G/21 interchanges, most involve 21/21 interchanges and thus cannot be distinguished operationally from 21 isochromosomes, but throughout the discussion G/21 interchanges are designated as "translocations," which is the usual convention.

About 90%–95% of G/21 interchange Down syndrome cases are de novo; the remainder have "inherited" their translocation from a carrier parent. The father may be the source slightly more freqently than the mother.

Somewhere between 50% and 65% of D/21 interchange Down syndrome cases are de novo, and almost all (at least 95%) of the remainder have inherited their translocations from a carrier mother.

In general there is little, if any, evidence for a phenotypic difference between the translocation and trisomic cases of Down syndrome. (See Hook, 1978a, for discussion of the evidence bearing on this.) The only notable differences are the higher parental age associated with trisomic cases compared to a parental age distribution about the same as the general population for interchange trisomics and the greater likelihood that an interchange case of Down syndrome has an affected relative. (Of course, it is just affected subjects whose translocations are inherited that have this higher likelihood. The recurrence risk for a de novo interchange trisomy appears to be much lower than for a 47,trisomy 21 case). Estimates of the likelihood that a Down syndrome case ascertained randomly is the consequence of an inherited translocation have been made by Albright and Hook (in press). As may be expected, these values diminish with increasing maternal age.

---

[11]See also the chapter by Hamerton in this volume.

The mutation rate for translocations resulting in interchange trisomic Down syndrome is approximately $2.0 - 2.5 \times 10^{-5}$ per gamete resulting in a live birth (Hook and Albright, 1978; Kikuchi et al., 1969; Polani et al., 1965). (It should be recalled that the prevalence in live births is one-half the mutation rate.)

Recently, evidence for a temporal trend in mutation rates for interchange Down syndrome was noted in New York State. The rate increased from 1968–1972 (about 1.8×10^{-5}) to 1973–1977 (about 3.0×10^{-5}) (Hook and Albright, in preparation). (The marked increase in mutation rate, however, was confined to infants born to mothers under age 30.) In data from newborn chromosome series (Hook and Hamerton, 1977) there was 1 case in 56,952 infants, a mutation rate of 0.9×10^{-5}, with wide 95% confidence limits (0.04×10^{-5} to 9.8×10^{-5}).

Higher mutation rates for de novo G/21 (1.42×10^{-5}) than for de novo D/21 (0.62×10^{-5}) interchange trisomics were observed by Polani et al. (1965), and a slight trend in this direction was also noticed by Kikuchi et al. (1969) (1.14×10^{-5} versus 1.01×10^{-5}). For the data of Hook and Albright (1978) the rates were (1.44×10^{-5} versus 1.08×10^{-5}).

Polani et al. (1965) also noted a higher frequency of all Down syndrome interchange trisomics in live births to younger mothers. Although age-specific mutation rates are not given, they may be estimated from their data as approximately 2.3×10^{-5} for women under 32 and 1.6×10^{-5} for women 30 or over. (All sporadic interchanges in those 30 or over were in the G/21 category in their series.) In Hook and Albright's (1978) data, the estimated mutation rate was about 2.5×10^{-5} in those under 30 and 2.4×10^{-5} in those 30 or over.

It is difficult to evaluate the statistical significance of these apparent age differences; only data from other sources will allow judgments on whether these apparent trends are consistent.

Regarding parental age, Matsunaga and Tonomura (1972) presented data that suggest a very slight younger maternal age effect (1.6 years) for sporadic 21/D interchange and slightly older maternal age for sporadic G/21 interchanges, 1.5 years, both of which differences, albeit slight, are of nominal statistical significance ($p < 0.05$) and questionable biological significance. There is no evidence for any parental age effect for interchange trisomics due to inherited translocations.

REFERENCES

Abramson, F. D. 1971. Spontaneous fetal death in man: A methodological and analytical evaluation. Doctoral dissertation, University of Michigan, Ann Arbor.

Alberman, E., Creasy, M., Elliot, M., and Spicer, C. 1976. Maternal factors associated with fetal chromosomal anomalies in spontaneous abortions. Br. J. Obstet. Gynaecol. 83: 621–627.

Alberman, E., Elliot, M., Creasy, M., and Dhadial, R. 1975. Previous reproductive history in mothers presenting with spontaneous abortions. Br. J. Obstet. Gynaecol. 82:366–373.

Alberman, E., Polani, P. E., Fraser Roberts, J. A., Spicer, C. C., Elliot, M., and Armstrong, E. 1972. Parental exposure to X-irradiation and Down's syndrome. Ann. Hum. Genet. 36: 195–208.

Albright, S. G., and Hook, E. B. Estimates of the likelihood that a Down's syndrome child of unknown genotype is a consequence of an inherited translocation. J. Med. Genet. In press.

Ament, R. P. 1976. Reanalysis of seasonal trend in incidence of Down's syndrome in West Jerusalem. Am. J. Epidemiol. 103:342–343.

Apgar, V. (ed.). 1970. Down's syndrome (mongolism). Ann. N.Y. Acad. Sci. 171:303–688.

Aula, P., Leisti, J., and von Koskull, H. 1973. Partial trisomy 21. Clin. Genet. 4:241–251.

Baker, B. S., Carpenter, A. T. C., Esposito, M. S., Esposito, R. E., and Sandler, L. 1976. The genetic control of meiosis. Annu. Rev. Genet. 10:53–134.

Bell, A. G., and Corey, P. N. 1974. A sex chromatin and Y body survey of Toronto newborns. Can. J. Genet. Cytol. 16:239–250.

Beolchini, P. E., Bariatti, A. B., and Morganti, G. 1962. Indagini genetico statistiche sulle fratrie di 432 soggetti mongoloidi. Acta Genet. Med. Gamell. 11:430–449.

Berg, J. M. 1967. Discussion in mongolism. In G. E. W. Wolstenholme and R. Porter (eds.), CIBA Foundation Study Group No. 25, p. 32. J. & A. Churchill, London.

Blumberg, B. S. 1978. Characteristics of the Hepatitis B virus. In N. E. Norton and C. S. Chung (eds.), Genetic Epidemiology, (pp. 529–538). Academic Press, New York.

Bochkov, N. P., Kuleshov, N. P., Chebotarov, A. N., Alekhin, V. I., and Midian, S. A. 1974. Population cytogenetic investigation of newborns in Moscow. Humangenetik 22:139–152.

Böök, J. A. 1953. A genetic and neuropsychiatric investigation of a north-Swedish population. II. Mental deficiency and convulsive disorders. Acta Genet. 4:345–414.

Bowen, P., Chermak, B. C., Campbell, D. J., and Rouget, A. 1974. Mild characteristics of Down's syndrome with normal karyotype in cultured lymphocytes and skin fibroblasts. Birth Defects Orig. Art. Ser. 10(10):42–48. Alan R. Liss, New York.

Carothers, A. D., Collyer, S., DeMey, R., and Frackiewicz, A. 1978. Parental age and birth order in the aetiology of some sex chromosome aneuploidies. Ann. Hum. Genet. 41:277–287.

Carr, D. H. 1976. Chromosome anomalies as a cause of spontaneous abortion. Am. J. Obstet. Gynecol. 97:283–293.

Carr, D. H., and Gedeon, M. 1977. Population cytogenetics of human abortuses. In E. B. Hook and I. H. Porter (eds.), Population Cytogenetics: Studies in Humans, pp. 1–10. Academic Press, New York.

Carter, C. O., and Evans, K. A. 1961. Risk of parents who have had one child with Down syndrome (mongolism) having another child similarly affected. Lancet 2:785–788.

Christianson, R. G. 1976. Down syndrome and maternal age. Lancet 2:1198.

Cohen, B. H., Lilienfeld, A. M., Kramer, S., and Hyman, L. C. 1977. Parental factors in Down's syndrome—Results of the second Baltimore case-control study. In E. B. Hook and I. H. Porter (eds.), Population Cytogenetics: Studies in Humans, pp. 301–352. Academic Press, New York.

Collman, R. D., and Stoller, A. 1962. A survey of mongoloid births in Victoria, Australia, 1942–1957. Am. J. Pub. Health 52:813–829.

Collman, R. D., and Stoller, A. 1969. Shift of childbirth to younger mothers and its effect on the incidence of mongolism in Victoria, Australia 1939–1964. J. Ment. Defic. Res. 13:13–19.

Creasy, M. R., and Crolla, J. A. 1974. Prenatal mortality of trisomy 21 (Down's syndrome). Lancet 1:473–474.

Day, R. W., and Miles, C. P. 1965. Familial Down's syndrome with undetected translocation. J. Pediatr. 67:399–409.

Erickson, J. D. 1978. Down's syndrome, paternal age, maternal age and birth order. Ann. Hum. Genet. 41:289–298.

Erickson, J. D. 1979. Paternal age and Down syndrome. Am. J. Hum. Genet. 31:489–497.

Evans, J. A., Hunter, A. G. W., and Hamerton, J. L. 1978. Down's syndrome and recent demographic trends in Manitoba. J. Med. Genet. 15:43–47.

Fabia, J. J. 1970. Down's syndrome (mongolism): A study of 2421 cases born alive to Massachusetts residents 1950–1966. Doctoral thesis, Harvard University School of Public Health, Cambridge, Mass.

Fabia, J., and Drolette, M. 1970. Life tables up to age 10 for Mongols with and without congenital heart defect. J. Ment. Defic. 14:235–242.

Ferguson-Smith, M. A. 1976. Prospective data on risk of Down's syndrome in relation to maternal age. Lancet 2:252.

Ferguson-Smith, M. A. 1978. Maternal age and Down syndrome. Lancet 2:213.

Fialkow, P. J. 1969. Genetic aspects of autoimmunity. Prog. Med. Genet. 11:117–167.

Fialkow, P. J. 1970. Thyroid autoimmunity and Down's syndrome. Ann. N.Y. Acad. Sci. 171: 500–511.

Fialkow, P. J., Thuline, H. C., Hecth, F., and Bryant, J. 1971. Familial predisposition to thyroid disease in Down's syndrome: Controlled immunoclinical studies. Am. J. Hum. Genet. 23:67–85.

Fleiss, J. L. 1973. Statistical Methods for Rates and Proportions. John Wiley & Sons, New York. pp. 158–164.

Forssman, H., and Akesson, H. O. 1965. Mortality in patients with Down's syndrome. J. Ment. Defic. Res. 9:146–149.

Forssman, H., and Akesson, H. 1967a. Consanguineous marriages and mongolism. In G. E. W. Wolstenholme and R. Porter (eds.), CIBA Foundation Study Group No. 25, pp. 23–29. J. & A. Churchill, London.

Forssman, H., and Akesson, H. O. 1976. Note on mortality in patients with Down's syndrome. J. Ment. Defic. Res. 11:106–109.

Fuhrman, W., and Vogel, F. 1976. Genetic counseling. Springer-Verlag, Berlin. p. 61.

Gardner, R. J. M., et al. 1973. A survey of 972 cytogenetically examined cases of Down's syndrome. N. Z. Med. J. 78:403–409.

Goad, W. B., Robinson, A., and Puck, T. T. 1976. Incidence of aneuploidy in a human population. Am. J. Hum. Genet. 28:62–68.

Goff, C., Mellman, W. J., and Zackai, E. H. 1973. Evidence for seasonal variation on the birth of maternal-age independent trisomy 21. Am. J. Hum. Genet. 25:29A.

Greenberg, R. C. 1963. Two factors influencing the births of mongols to younger mothers. Med. Off. 109:62–64.

Gustavson, K. H. 1964. Down's syndrome—A clinical and cytogenetical investigation. Institute for Medical Genetics, Uppsala, Sweden.

Halevi, H. S. 1967. Congenital malformation in Israel. Br. J. Prev. Soc. Med. 21:66–77.

Hall, B. 1964. Mongolism in newborns. Acta. Paediatr. 154(suppl.).

Hamerton, J. L. 1971. Human Cytogenetics, Vol. 11: Clinical Cytogenetics. Academic Press, New York. pp. 1–544.

Hamerton, J. L., Briggs, S. M., Giannelli, F., and Carter, C. O. 1961. Chromosome studies in detection of parents with high risk of second child with Down's syndrome. Lancet 2: 788–791.

Hamerton, J. L., Giannelli, F., and Polani, P. E. 1965. Cytogenetics of Down's syndrome (mongolism). I. Data on a consecutive series of patients referred for genetic counseling and diagnosis. Cytogenetics 4:171–185.

Hamerton, J. L., Jagiello, G. M., and Kirman, B. H. 1962. Sex chromosome abnormalities in a population of mentally defective children. Br. Med. J. 1:220–223.

Hansson, A., and Mikkelsen, M. 1978. The origin of the extra chromosome 21 in Down syndrome. Cytogenet. Cell Genet. 20:194–203.

Harlap, S. 1973. Down's syndrome in West Jerusalem. Am. J. Epidemiol. 97:225–232.

Harlap, S. 1974. A time-series analysis of the incidence of Down's syndrome in West Jerusalem. Am. J. Epidemiol. 99:210–217.

Harlap, S., and Davies, A. M. 1978. The Pill and Births: The Jerusalem Study. Final Report, Contract No. NO1-HD-4-2853. Center for Population Research, National Institute of Child Health and Human Development, National Institutes of Health, Bethesda, Md. pp. 69–73.

Hashem, N., and Sakr, R. 1961. Mongolism among Egyptian children. Proc. 2nd Int. Cong. Ment. Retard. Part L.:387–403.

Hay, S., and Barbano, H. 1972. Independent effects of maternal age and birth order on the incidence of selected congenital malformations. Teratology 6:271–279.

Hecht, F. 1977. The non-randomness of human chromosome abnormalities. In E. B. Hook and I. H. Porter (eds.), Population Cytogenetics: Studies in Humans, pp. 237–250. Academic Press, New York.

Hecht, F., Nievaard, J. E., Duncanson, N., et al. 1969. Double aneuploidy: The frequency of XXY in males with Down's syndrome. Am. J. Hum. Genet. 21:352–359.

Heston, L. L. 1977. Alzheimer's disease, trisomy 21, and myeloproliferative disorders: Associations suggesting a genetic diathesis. Science 196:322–323.

Higurashi, M., Matsui, I., Nakagome, Y., and Naganuma, M. 1969. Down's syndrome: Chromosome analysis in 321 cases in Japan. J. Med. Genet. 6:401–404.

Holmes, L. B. 1978a. Genetic counseling for the older pregnant woman: New data and questions. New Engl. J. Med. 298:1419–1421.

Holmes, L. B. 1978b. Genetic counseling for the older pregnant woman. New Engl. J. Med. 299:836.

Hook, E. B. 1977. Exclusion of chromosomal mosaicism: Tables of 90%, 95% and 99% confidence limits and comments on use. Am. J. Hum. Genet. 29:94–97.

Hook, E. B. 1978a. Differences between rates of trisomy 21 (Down's syndrome) and other chromosomal abnormalities diagnosed in live births and in cells cultured after 2nd trimester amniocentesis—Suggested explanations and implications for genetic counseling and program planning. In D. Bergsma and R. L. Summitt (eds.), Proceedings of the National Foundation—March of Dimes Symposium, Memphis, 1977. Birth Defects Orig. Art. Ser. 14(6C): 249–267. Alan R. Liss, New York.

Hook, E. B. 1978b. Rates of Down's syndrome in livebirths and at midtrimester amniocentesis. Lancet 1:1053.

Hook, E. B. 1978c. Models and assumptions in calculating the probabilities of detecting chromosomal mosaicism. Hum. Genet. 40:235–239.

Hook, E. B. 1978d. Spontaneous deaths of fetuses with chromosomal abnormalities diagnosed prenatally. New Engl. J. Med. 299:1036–1038.

Hook, E. B. 1978e. Genetic counseling for the older pregnant woman. New Engl. J. Med. 299:835–836.

Hook, E. B., and Albright, S. G. 1978. Mutation rates for translocation Down's syndrome—Apparent temporal change. Am. J. Hum. Genet. 30:111A.

Hook, E. B., and Chambers, G. M. 1977. Estimated rates of Down's syndrome in livebirths by one year maternal age intervals for mothers aged 20 to 49 in a New York State study— Implications of the "risk" figures for genetic counseling and cost benefit analysis of prenatal diagnosis programs. In D. Bergsma, R. B. Lowry, B. K. Trimble, and M. Feingold (eds.), Numerical Taxonomy on Birth Defects and Polygenic Disorders. Birth Defects Orig. Art. Ser. 13(3A): 123–141. Alan R. Liss, New York.

Hook, E. B., and Cross, P. K. Temporal increase in the rate of Down's syndrome live births to older mothers in New York State. In preparation.

Hook, E. B., Cross, P. K., Lamson, S. H., Regal, R. R., Baird, P. A., and Uh, S. H. Paternal age and Down's syndrome in British Columbia: Evidence for an effect independent of maternal age in 1964–1976 livebirths. In preparation.

Hook, E. B., and Fabia, J. J. 1978. Frequency of Down syndrome by single-year maternal age interval: Results of a Massachusetts study. Teratology 17:223–228.

Hook, E. B., and Hamerton, J. L. 1977. The frequency of chromosome abnormalities detected in consecutive newborn studies—Differences between studies—Results by sex and severity of phenotypic involvement. In E. B. Hook and I. H. Porter (eds.), Population Cytogenetics: Studies in Humans, pp. 63–79. Academic Press, New York.

Hook, E. B., and Harlap, S. 1979. Differences in maternal age-specific rates of Down syndrome between Jews of European origin and North African or Asian origin. Teratology 20: 243–248.

Hook, E. B., and Lamson, S. H. 1980. Dates of Down's syndrome at the upper extreme of maternal-age—Absence of a leveling effect and evidence for artifacts resulting from analysis of rates by five year maternal age intervals. Am. J . Epidemiol. 111:78–80.

Hook, E. B., and Lindsjo, A. 1978. Down's syndrome in livebirths by single year maternal age interval in a Swedish study: Comparison with results from a New York State study. Am. J. Hum. Genet. 30:19–27.

Hook, E. B., and Porter, I. H. 1977. Human population cytogenetics—Comments on racial differences in frequency of chromosome abnormalities, putative clustering of Down's syndrome, and radiation studies. In E. B. Hook and I. H. Porter (eds.), Population Cytogenetics: Studies in Humans, pp. 353–365. Academic Press, New York.

Hook, E. B., Woodbury, D. F., and Albright, S. G. 1979. Rates of trisomy 18 in livebirths, stillbirths, and at amniocentesis. In C. J. Epstein, C. J. R. Curry, S. Packman, S. Sherman, and B. D. Hall (eds.), Proceedings of the National Foundation—March of Dimes Birth Defects Conference, San Francisco, 1978. Birth Defects Orig. Art. Ser. XV(5C). Alan R. Liss, New York.

Jacobs, P. A. 1979. Recurrence risks for chromosomal abnormalities. In C. J. Epstein, C. J. R. Curry, S. Packman, S. Sherman, and B. D. Hall (eds.), Proceedings of the National Foundation—March of Dimes Birth Defects Conference, San Francisco, 1978. Birth Defects Orig. Art. Ser. XV(5C):71–80. Alan R. Liss, New York.

Jacobs, P. A., Melville, A., Ratcliffe, S., Keay, A. J., and Syme, J. 1974. A cytogenetic study of 11,680 newborn infants. Ann. Hum. Genet. 37:359–376.

Janerich, D. T., Flink, E. M., and Keogh, M. D. 1976. Down's syndrome and oral contraceptive usage. Br. J. Obstet. Gynaecol. 83:617–620.

Janerich, D. T., and Jacobson, H. 1977. Seasonality in Down's syndrome. Lancet 1:515–516.

Jervis, G. A. 1970. Premature senility in Down's syndrome. Ann. N.Y. Acad. Sci. 171:559–561.

Jongbloet, P. H. 1971. Month of birth and gametopathy: An investigation into patients with Down's, Klinefelter's and Turner's syndrome. Clin. Genet. 2:315–330.

Juberg, R. C., and Davis, L. M. 1970. Etiology of non-disjunction: Lack of evidence for genetic control. Cytogenetics 9:284–293.

Juberg, R. C., Goshen, C. R., and Sholte, F. G. 1973. Socioeconomic and reproductive characteristics of the parents of patients with the G1 trisomy syndrome. Soc. Biol. 20:404–415.

Kaplan, S. D., and Ament, R. P. 1975. Seasonal trend in Down's syndrome. PAS reporter 13(8):1–5.

Kardon, N., Krauss, M., Silverberg, G., and Davis, J. 1978. Aneuploidy and the older gravida: Which risk to quote. Lancet 1:1305–1306.

Kikuchi, O., Oishi, H., Tonomura, A., Yamada, K., Tanaka, Y., Kurita, T., and Matsunaga, E. 1969. Translocation of Down's syndrome in Japan: It's frequency, mutation rate of translocation and parental age. Jap. J. Hum. Genet. 14:93–106.

Klinger, H. P., Glasser, M., and Kara, H. W. 1976. Contraceptives and the conceptus. I. Chromosome abnormalities of the fetus and neonate related to maternal contraceptive history. Obstet. Gynecol. 48:40–48.

Kogon, A., Kronmal, R., and Peterson, D. R. 1968. The relationship between infectious hepatitis and Down's syndrome. Am. J. Pub. Health 58:305–311.

Kuleshov, N. P., Alekhin, N. I., Egolina, N. A., and Karetnikova, N. A. 1975. Frequency of chromosome abnormalities among infants who died during the perinatal period. Genetika 11:107–113.

Kuroki, Y., Yamamoto, Y., Matusi, I., and Kurita, T. 1977. Down syndrome and maternal age in Japan, 1950–1973. Clin. Genet. 12:43–46.

Kwitterovich, P. O., Cross, H. E., and McKusick, V. A. 1966. Mongolism in an inbred population. Bull. Johns Hopkins Hosp. 119:268–275.

LaMarche, P. H., Heisler, A. B., and Kronemer, N. S. 1967. Disappearing mosaicism: Suggested mechanism is growth advantage of normal over abnormal cell population. R. I. Med. J. 50:184–189.

Lamson, S. H., and Hook, E. B. A simple function for maternal age specific rates of Down's syndrome in the 20–49 age interval and its biological implications. Am. J. Hum. Genet. In press.

Lander, E., Forssman, H., and Akesson, H. O. 1964. Seasons of birth and mental deficiency. Acta Genet. 14:265–280.

Leck, I. 1966. Incidence and epidemicity of Down's syndrome. Lancet 2:457–460.

Lilienfeld, A. 1969. Epidemiology of Mongolism. Johns Hopkins Press, Baltimore. p. 145.

Lindsjo, A. 1974. Down's syndrome in Sweden. Acta Paediatr. Scand. 63:571–576.

Lowry, R. B., Jones, D. C., Renwick, D. H. G., and Trimble, B. K. 1976. Down syndrome in British Columbia, 1952–1973: Incidence and mean maternal age. Teratology 14:29–34.

Lunn, J. G. 1959. A survey of mongol children in Glasgow. Scot. Med. J. 4:368–376.

McDonald, A. D. 1972a. Thyroid disease and other maternal factors in mongolism. Can. Med. Assoc. J. 106:1085–1089.

McDonald, A. D. 1972b. Yearly and seasonal incidence of mongolism in Quebec. Teratology 6:1–4.

Machin, G. A., and Crolla, J. A. 1974. Chromosome constitution of 500 infants dying during the perinatal period. Humangenetik 23:183–198.

Magenis, R. E., Overton, K. M., Chamberlin, J., Brady, T., and Lovrien, E. 1977. Parental origin of the extra chromosome in Down's syndrome. Hum. Genet. 37:7–16.

Mantel, N., and Stark, E. R. 1966. Paternal age in Down's syndrome. Am. J. Ment. Defic. 71: 1025.

Marmol, J. G., Scriggins, A. L., and Vollman, R. F. 1969. Mothers of mongoloid infants in the collaborative project. Am. J. Obstet. Gynecol. 104:533–543.

Matsunaga, E. 1967. Parental age, livebirth order and pregnancy-free interval in Down's syndrome in Japan. In G. E. W. Wolstenholme and R. Porter (eds.), CIBA Foundation Study Group No. 25, pp. 6–22. J. & A. Churchill, London.

Matsunaga, E., and Fujita, H. 1977. A survey on maternal age and karyotype in Down's syndrome in Japan, 1947–1975. Hum. Genet. 37:221–230.

Matsunaga, E., and Tonomura, A. 1972. Parental age and birthweight in translocation Down's syndrome. Ann. Genet. 36:209–219.

Matsunaga, E., Tonomura, A., Oishi, H., and Kikuchi, Y. 1978. Reexamination of paternal age effect in Down's syndrome. Hum. Genet. 40:259–268.

Mikkelsen, M. 1966. Familial Down's syndrome: A cytogenetical and genealogical study of twenty-two families. Ann. Hum. Genet. 30:125–146.

Mikkelsen, M. 1967. Down's syndrome at young maternal age: Cytogenetical and genealogical study of eighty-one families. Ann. Hum. Genet. 31:51–69.

Mikkelsen, M. 1970. A Danish survey of patients with Down's syndrome born to young mothers. Ann. N.Y. Acad. Sci. 171:370–378.

Mikkelsen, M., Fischer, G., Stene, J., Stene, E., and Petersen, E. 1976. Incidence study of Down's syndrome in Copenhagen, 1960–1971: With chromosome investigation. Ann. Hum. Genet. 40:177–182.

Mikkelsen, M., and Stene, J. 1970. Genetic counseling in Down's syndrome. Hum. Hered. 20: 457–464.

Moran, P. A. P. 1974. Are there two maternal age groups in Down's syndrome? Br. J. Psychiatry 124:453–455.

Morris, R. Z. 1971. Down's syndrome in New Zealand. N.Z. Med. J. 73:195–198.

Murphy, E. A., and Chase, G. A. 1978. Principles of Genetic Counseling. Year Book Medical Publishers, Chicago, p. 316.

Newcombe, H. B., and Tavendale, O. G. 1964. Maternal age and birth order correlations. Problems of distinguishing mutational from environmental components. Mutat. Res. 1: 446–467.

NICHD National Registry for Amniocentesis Study Group. 1976. Midtrimester amniocentesis for prenatal diagnosis—Safety and accuracy. JAMA 236:1471–1476.

Oakley, G. P. 1978. Natural selection, selection bias, and the prevalence of Down's syndrome. New Engl. J. Med. 299:1068–1069.

Oster, J. 1953. Mongolism. Danish Science Press, Copenhagen.

Oster, J. 1956. The causes of mongolism. Dan. Med. Bull. 3:158–164.

Papp, Z., Osztovics, M., Schuler, D., Mehes, K., Czeizel, E., Horvath, L., Szemere, G., and Laszlo, J. 1977. Down's syndrome: Chromosome analysis of 362 cases in Hungary. Hum. Hered. 27:305–309.

Penrose, L. S. 1933. The relative effects of paternal and maternal age in mongolism. J. Genet. 27:219–224.

Penrose, L. S. 1934. A method of separating the relative aetiological effects of birth order and maternal age with special reference to mongolian imbecility. Ann. Eugen. 6:108–122.

Penrose, L. S. 1961. Mongolism. Br. Med. Bull. 17:184–189.

Penrose, L. S. 1967. Discussion. G. E. W. Wolstenholme and R. Porter (eds.), CIBA Foundation Study Group No. 25, p. 31. J. & A. Churchill, London.

Penrose, L. S. 1968. Studies of mosaicism in Down's anomaly. In G. A. Jervis (ed.), Mental Retardation. Charles C Thomas Publisher, Springfield, Ill.

Penrose, L. S., and Smith, G. F. 1966. Down's anomaly. J. & A. Churchill, London.

Peterson, W. F. 1969. Pregnancy following oral contraceptive therapy. Obstet. Gynecol. 34: 363–367.

Polani, P. E. 1967. Discussion on mongolism. In G. E. W. Wolstenholme and R. Porter (eds.), CIBA Foundation Study Group No. 25, pp. 32–33. J. & A. Churchill, London.

Polani, P. E., Alberman, E., Berry, A. C., Blunt, S., and Singer, J. D. 1976. Chromosome abnormalities and maternal age. Lancet 2:516–517.

Polani, P. E., Hamerton, J. L., Giannelli, F., and Carter, C. O. 1965. Cytogenetics of Down's syndrome (mongolism). III. Frequency of interchange trisomies and mutation rate of chromosome interchanges. Cytogenetics 4:193–206.

Record, R. G., and Smith, A. 1955. Incidence and sex distribution of mongoloid defectives. Br. J. Prev. Soc. Med. 9:10–15.

Regal, R. R., Cross, P. K., Lamson, S. H., and Hook, E. B. A search for evidence for a paternal age effect independent of a maternal age effect in birth certificate reports in New York State. Am. J. Epidemiol. In press.

Richards, B. W. 1969. Mosaic mongolism. J. Ment. Defic. Res. 13:66–83.

Robinson, S. C. 1971. Pregnancy outcome following oral contraceptives. Am. J. Obstet. Gynecol. 109:354–358.

Rothman, K. J. 1976. Detecting cyclic variation. Am. J. Epidemiol. 104:585–586.

Rothman, K. J., and Fabia, J. J. 1976. Place and time aspects of the occurrence of Down's syndrome. Am. J. Epidemiol. 103:560–564.

Royal College of General Practitioners (RCGP) 1976. The outcome of pregnancy in former oral contraceptive users. Br. J. Obstet. Gynaecol. 83:609–616.

Segal, D. J., Schlant, J. W., Pabst, H. F., McCoy, E. E., and Dossetor, J. B. 1975. HL-A frequencies in Down's syndrome. Humangenetik 27:45–48.

Sergovich, F. R., Valentine, G. H., Carr, D. H., and Soltan, H. C. 1964. Mongolism (Down's syndrome) with atypical clinical and cytogenetic features. J. Pediatr. 65:197–199.

Sever, J. L., Gilkeson, M. R., Chen, T. C., Ley, A. C., and Edmunds, D. 1970. Epidemiology of mongolism in the collaborative project. Ann. N.Y. Acad. Sci. 171:328–340.

Shiono, H., Kadowaki, J., and Nakao, T. 1975. Maternal age and Down's syndrome. Clin. Pediatr. 14:241–244.

Sigler, A. T., Cohen, B. H., Lilienfeld, A. M., Westlake, J. E., and Hetznecker, W. H. 1967. Reproductive and marital experience of parents of children with Down's syndrome (Mongolism). J. Pediatr. 70:608–614.

Singer, R. B., and Levinson, L. (eds.). 1976. Medical risks: Patterns of mortality and survival. D.C. Health 1976: 2-26-2-27.

Slater, B. C. S., Watson, G. I., and McDonald, J. C. 1964. Seasonal variation in congenital abnormalities: Preliminary report of a survey conducted by the Research Committee of Council of the College of General Practitioners. Br. J. Prev. Soc. Med. 18:1–7.

Smith, A., and Record, R. G. 1955. Maternal age and birth rank in aetiology of mongolism. Br. J. Prev. Soc. Med. 9:51–55.

Smith, G. F., and Berg, J. M. 1976. Down's Anomaly. 2nd Ed. J. & A. Churchill, London.

Spielman, R. J., Mellman, W. J., and Zackai, E. H. 1975. Seasonal variation in trisomy 21 incidence. Am. J. Hum. Genet. 27:84A.

Stark, C. R., and Mantel, N. 1966. Effects of maternal age and birth order on the risk of mongolism and leukemia. J. Nat. Cancer Inst. 37:687–698.

Stark, C. R., and Mantel, N. 1967. Lack of seasonal or temporal-spatial clustering of Down's syndrome births in Michigan. Am. J. Epidemiol. 86:199–213.

Stark, C. R., and White, N. B. 1977. Cluster analysis and racial differences in risk of Down's syndrome. In E. B. Hook and I. H. Porter (eds.), Population Cytogenetics: Studies in Humans, pp. 275–283. Academic Press, New York.

Stein, Z. A., Susser, M., Klein, J., and Warburton, D. 1977. Amniocentesis and selective abortion for trisomy 21 in the light of the natural history of pregnancy and fetal survival. In E. B. Hook and I. H. Porter (eds.), Population Cytogenetics: Studies in Humans, pp. 257–274. Academic Press, New York.

Stene, J. 1970. Detection of higher recurrence risk for age-dependent chromosome abnormalities with an application to trisomy G (Down's syndrome). Hum. Hered. 20:112–122.

Stene, J., Fischer, G., Stene, E., Mikkelsen, M., and Petersen, E. 1977. Paternal age effect in Down's syndrome. Ann. Hum. Genet. 40:299–306.

Stene, J., and Stene, E. 1978. On data and methods in investigations in parental age effects. Ann. Hum. Genet. 41:465–468.

Stevenson, A. C., and Davison, B. C. C. 1976. Genetic counseling. William Heinemann Medical Books, London. pp. 124–125.

Stevenson, A. C., Johnston, H. A., Stewart, M. I. P., and Golding, D. R. 1966. Congenital malformations: A report of a study of series of consecutive births in 24 centers. Bull. WHO 34(suppl.):9–127.

Stoller, A., and Collman, R. D. 1965. Incidence of infective hepatitis followed by Down's syndrome nine months later. Lancet 2:1221–1223.

Sutherland, G. R., Carter, R. F., Bauld, R., Smith, I. I., and Bain, A. D. 1978. Chromosome studies at the pediatric necropsy. Ann. Hum. Genet. 42:173–181.

Sutherland, G. R., Cliasy, S. R., Bloor, G., and Carter, R. F. 1979. The South Australian Down syndrome survey. Med. J. Aust. 2:58–61.

Sutherland, G. R., Fitzgerald, M. G., and Danks, D. M. 1972. Difficulty in showing mosaicism in the mother of three mongols. Arch. Dis. Child. 47:970–971.

Tarjan, G., Eyman, R. K., and Miller, C. R. 1969. Natural history of mental retardation in a state hospital, revisited. Am. J. Dis. Child. 117:609–620.

Taylor, A. I. 1968. Cell selection in vivo in normal/G trisomic mosaics. Nature 219:1028–1030.

Taylor, A. I. 1970. Further observations of cell selection in vivo in normal/G trisomic mosaics. Nature 227:163.

Taylor, A. I., and Moores, E. C. 1967. A sex chromatin survey of newborn children in two London hospitals. J. Med. Genet. 4:258–259.

Taysi, K., Kohn, G., and Mellman, W. J. 1970. Mosaic mongolism. II. Cytogenetic studies. J. Pediatr. 76:880–885.

Tonomura, A., Oishi, H., Matsunaga, E., and Kurita, T. 1966. Down's syndrome: A cytogenetic and statistical survey of 127 Japanese patients. Jap. J. Hum. Genet. 11:1–16.

Trimble, B. K., and Baird, P. A. 1978. Maternal age and Down syndrome: Age-specific incidence rates by single-year intervals: Am. J. Med. Genet. 2:1–5.

Uchida, I. A. 1977. Maternal radiation and trisomy 21. In E. B. Hook and I. H. Porter (eds.), Population Cytogenetics: Studies in Humans, pp. 285–299. Academic Press, New York.

Verresen, H., van den Berghe, H., and Creemers, J. 1974. Mosaic trisomy in a phenotypically normal mother of mongol. Lancet 1:526.

Wagenbichler, P., Killian, W., Rett, A., and Schnedl, W. 1976. Origin of the extra chromosome no. 21 in Down's syndrome. Hum. Genet. 32:13–16.

Wahrman, J., and Fried, K. 1970. The Jerusalem prospective newborn survey of mongolism. Ann. N.Y. Acad. Sci. 171:341–360.

Wald, N., Turner, J. H., and Borges, W. 1970. Down's syndrome and exposure to X-irradiation. Ann. N.Y. Acad. Sci. 171:454–466.

Warkany, J., Weinstein, E. D., Soukup, S. W., Rubinstein, J. H., and Curless, M. C. 1964. Chromosome analyses in a children's hospital, selection of patients and results of studies. Pediatrics 33:454–465.

Wren, P. J., Evans, D. A. P., Vetters, J. M., and Chow, A. 1967. Autoimmune antibodies in mongol families. Lancet 2:186–188.

Zellweger, H., Abbo, G., Nielsen, M. K., and Wallwork, K. 1966. Mosaic mongolism with normal chromosomal complement in white blood cells. Humangenetik 4:323–327.

Zellweger, H., and Simpson, J. 1973. Is routine prenatal karyotyping indicated in pregnancies of very young women. J. Pediatr. 82:675–677.

The Abortus As a Predictor of Future Trisomy 21 Pregnancies

Eva D. Alberman

Before discussing the value of the abortus as a predictor of future trisomy 21 pregnancies, one needs to set into perspective the risks of abortion (early fetal loss) in general, and in trisomies and trisomy 21 in particular.

First, what is the overall incidence of early fetal loss of all recognized pregnancies, that is, the loss of a conception before 28 weeks of gestation? Figure 1 is derived from data from a longitudinal study of pregnancies, some ascertained a month after the last menstrual period (French and Bierman, 1962). This shows that the risk of loss is extremely high in the second month of pregnancy but falls sharply after this time, so that the estimate of overall risk of loss will vary with the time of ascertainment. French and Bierman estimated that 24% of pregnancies that had reached 4 weeks of gestation ended as a fetal loss. Estimates of losses of fertilized ova before this gestational age are still based on data published by Hertig and Rock (Hertig, 1967), who suggested that very early losses were extremely common.

It is also clear that fetal loss at different stages of gestation varies qualitatively as well as quantitatively, the earliest losses including a large proportion of chromosomally anomalous fetuses, the later abortions far less (Figure 2). Specific anomalies also seem to have a characteristic gestational age at which they tend to be expelled. If we accept the theory that autosomal monosomic conceptions occur as often as do trisomics, nearly all such conceptions must be lost very early in pregnancy, because autosomal monosomics have only rarely been found in abortion series. On the other hand, other nonlethal anomalies, for instance, the XXY karyotype, are also rarely found, because they tend to survive pregnancy. The mean age at expulsion of different anomalies has been described by several groups, the largest series having been collected in France (Boué, Boué, and Lazar, 1975).

The results from different abortions series, if one allows for their different gestational age distributions, are remarkably similar. Overall, the percentage of chromosomally abnormal varies from 61% in the series weighted by very early losses

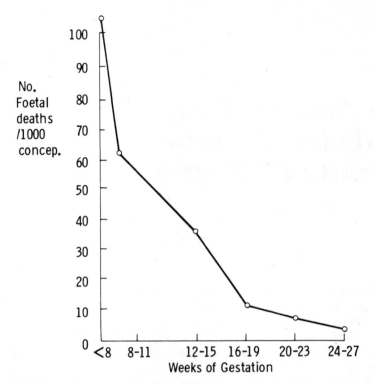

Figure 1.   Estimated fetal death rate at different periods of gestation. (Derived from French and Bierman, 1962.)

(Boué et al., 1975) to 22% and 24% in series that included fetal losses after 20 weeks (Carr, 1967; Dhadial, Machin, and Tait, 1970). There is general agreement that the autosomal trisomies account for about half of all the anomalies found. The relative frequency with which the different trisomies are found also is consistent from series to series, trisomy 16 being strikingly more common than any other (Creasy, 1977). Trisomies 21 and 22 appear with almost equal frequency in abortion studies (Figure 3).

One question of concern is whether the incidence of trisomies in all autosomes is similar but differential prevalence in abortion series occurs because some are lethal in very early development, or whether some trisomies arise more commonly than others. Certainly we know that, among the anomalies we can detect, prenatal viability varies. Thus, trisomy 22 is lethal, although it has been calculated that of all conceptions trisomic for trisomy 21, only 65%–70% are lethal before 28 weeks (Creasy and Crolla, 1974).

Another important question is whether the conceptions with trisomy 21 that prove lethal in utero differ in other aspects from those that survive, or whether they just form different ends of a spectrum of the same condition. Macroscopically, the

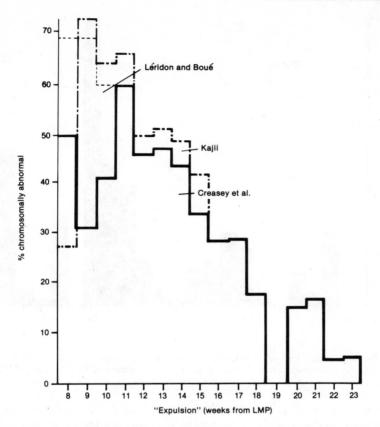

Figure 2. Percentage of chromosomal abnormalities in abortuses lost after different periods of gestation in three studies (Creasy, Crolla, and Alberman, 1976; Kajii, personal communication; Léridon and Boué, 1971). (Reprinted with permission from Creasy, 1977.)

clinical features of trisomic 21 fetuses are similar to those seen in survivors, and in all epidemiological aspects that have been examined, the trisomy 21 abortions seem to behave in a way similar to the survivors. They show the same raised maternal age as the survivors and the same tendency to occur more commonly after preconceptual radiation (Alberman et al., 1972a, b). We may conclude that there is probably no major etiological difference between the abortions and the survivors with this anomaly.

This is important to establish from a practical point of view as well as for academic interest, because one of the most interesting points that has emerged from the study of abortuses has been the suggestion that recurrence of chromosomal anomalies in the same parents is very much more common than originally suspected but that many are lost before birth.

Table 1 shows abortion data from Alberman et al. (1975) and Boué and Boué (1973) of the outcome of two karyotyped abortions from the same mother. On the

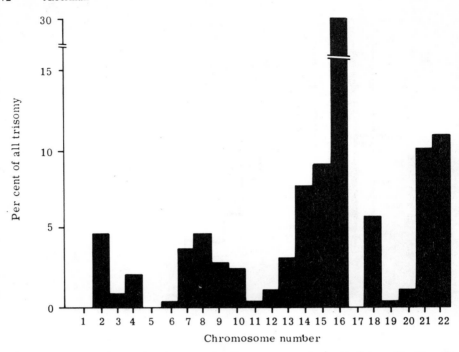

Figure 3.   Percentage distribution of different trisomies in three large abortion studies (Creasy et al., 1976; Kajii, personal communication; Therkelsen et al., 1973). (Reprinted with permission from Creasy, 1977.)

whole there is concordance between the karyotypes, as far as the distinction between normal or abnormal is concerned. Similarly, trisomies tend to recur, but they are not always identical.

The data in Table 2 include the abortion pairs concordant for trisomy shown in Table 1, but added to these are five pairs from the Alberman et al. (1975) study and one from the Boués' (1973) study in which a trisomic fetus was preceded by a sibling with Down syndrome; additional cases where a third pregnancy with a trisomy (or double trisomy) was identified; and one more case from a recent follow-up of the Guy's Hospital (London) study (Alberman et al., 1975), where a trisomy 16 (not banded) abortion was followed by the birth of an infant with Edwards syndrome, who died in the neonatal period. No general conclusion can be drawn from these highly selected data, except the demonstration of what seems to be a nonspecific, nondisjunctional tendency in certain mothers. This is similar to the frequent case reports of recurrences of trisomies in siblings, sometimes but not always concordant for chromosomal type.

More challenging is the suggestion that certain apparently unrelated anomalies, for instance, triploidy and trisomy, may occur in the same sibship more often than expected by chance, but larger numbers are needed to test this hypothesis.

Based on the recurrence risks in the combined data (Table 1), Alberman et al. (1975) made a crude estimate, illustrated in Table 3, of the risk of other chromosomal anomalies in sibships where the propositus was a normal baby, a chromosom-

Table 1.   Mothers with two abortions karyotyped

First abortion	Second abortion					
	Normal	Monosomy	Trisomy	Polyploidy	Translocation	All
Normal	24	1	5	4	0	34
Monosomy	3	0	1	1	0	5
Trisomy	3	1	14	1	0	19
Polyploidy	1	0	3	1	0	5
Translocation	0	0	0	0	3	3
All	31	2	23	7	3	66

Combined results of Alberman et al. (1975) and Boué and Boué (1973).

Table 2.   Recurrences of more than one trisomy (including surviving Down sibs)

Concordant	Partially concordant	Discordant
1 C+/C+	1 G+/E+/E+	1 E+/C+/D+G+
2 D+/D+		1 G+/E+
1 E+/E+(18)		3 G+/C+
1 G+/G+		3 G+/D+
		3 D+/C+
		3 D+/E+
		1 G+/F+

Data from Boué and Boué (1973) and Guy's Hospital (Alberman et al., 1975).

ally normal abortus, and a chromosomally abnormal abortus. This simply illustrates the risk of recurrence of anomalies, which is probably high enough to explain the excess of spontaneous abortions in siblings found both before and after a "marker" abortion of abnormal chromosome constitution.

Because of this tendency to recurrence of trisomies, prenatal diagnosis has been recommended (Alberman et al., 1975) for mothers pregnant again after the loss of a trisomic fetus. We have subsequently followed up some of the mothers in our abortion studies, a minority of whom received amniocentesis; some preliminary results are presented below.

These data are derived from two sources. First, we carried out a systematic follow-up of those mothers who had entered one or both of our own abortion studies (Alberman et al., 1972a, b; Alberman et al., 1976), who had been delivered in a proportion of the collaborating hospitals. We were only able to follow 40% overall; 25% of mothers moved without trace, in 21% no reply was received from the mother or her doctor, and other difficulties accounted for the remainder. The follow-up of those who had had a chromosomally abnormal fetus was better; 62% were interviewed, in part because they were an older group and less likely to move, and in part because they had remained in touch for genetic advice.

We contacted 62 mothers of trisomic abortuses and found that only 47 had become pregnant again after the index abortion. These 47 mothers had subsequently had 65 pregnancies, of which 7 had been terminated for social reasons. Of the remainder, 12 (21%) had aborted spontaneously (2 before a planned amniocentesis could take place), leaving 46 pregnancies that proceeded to term.

Table 3. Risk of other chromosomal anomalies in sibships

| | Pregnancies before propositus | | | | | Chromosomal anomaly recognized or estimated | |
| | Viable | | Aborted | | | | |
Propositus	Apparent chromosomally normal	Recognized chromosomally abnormal	Estimated chromosomally normal	Estimated chromosomally abnormal		Proportion	Percentage
Normal baby ($N=847$)	1072	0	196	77		77/1345	5.7
Abortion, chromosomally normal ($N=992$)	1042	0	505	147		147/1694	8.7
Abortion, chromosomally abnormal ($N=392$)	471	5	62	155		160/693	23.1

Seven of the term births had prenatal diagnostic amniocentesis, and chromosomal results were available for all. All of these were normal and were followed by a normal live birth. Of the remaining births, one, which had not had diagnostic amniocentesis, was the baby with Edwards syndrome, previously mentioned. The others were apparently normal, except for one neonatal death that was delivered at 24 weeks gestation but did not appear to have had any signs of a chromosomal anomaly.

In summary, after excluding terminations and spontaneous abortions, 46 live births were delivered to 38 mothers who had previously had trisomic abortions, of which one was reported to have a chromosomal anomaly (Edwards syndrome).

Besides this planned follow-up we accumulated data on all mothers of trisomic abortions in our series who were referred for amniocentesis in subsequent pregnancies. These included the seven mothers described in the account of the follow-up. In all, amniocenteses were carried out in 34 pregnancies to 29 mothers; results were available for 29, all normal, and an additional two live births followed an unsuccessful amniocentesis. We have no information on outcome of the three remaining cases, done elsewhere. Five additional mothers were referred for amniocentesis; four aborted before this could be done, and one after amniocentesis, but in none of these were chromosomal investigations on the fetus successful.

If we add together all our data on pregnancies after a trisomic abortion, from the planned follow-up and other referrals, we find that of 73 live births that followed a trisomic abortion in 60 mothers, only one was found to be chromosomally abnormal and none was found to have trisomy 21. Not one of the 29 successful amniocenteses carried out proved to be abnormal.

These results are based on small numbers only, but suggest that the yield of viable chromosomal anomalies in pregnancies following a known trisomic abortion is likely to be of the same order as the 1% following the birth of a viable trisomic infant.

Clearly, more data are needed, and these will have to be analyzed allowing for the selection effect of women who decide not to embark on future pregnancies. Recent analyses carried out on a series of pregnancies of women doctors (Roman et al., 1978) suggested that such selection effects can have an important bearing on follow-up studies of reproductive history. It will probably be some years before we have a good estimate of the use of karyotyped abortions as predictors of trisomy 21 survivors.

REFERENCES

Alberman, E., Creasy, M., Elliott, M., and Spicer, C. 1976. Maternal factors associated with fetal chromosomal anomalies in spontaneous abortions. Br. J. Obstet. Gynaecol. 83(8): 621–627.

Alberman, E., Elliott, M., Creasy, M., and Dhadial, R. 1975. Previous reproductive history in mothers presenting with spontaneous abortions. Br. J. Obstet. Gynaecol. 82(5):366–373.

Alberman, E., Polani, P. E., Fraser Roberts, J. A., Spicer, C. C., Elliott, M., and Armstrong, E. 1972a. Parental exposure to X-irradiation and Down's syndrome. Ann. Hum. Genet. 36:195–208.

Alberman, E., Polani, P. E., Fraser Roberts, J. A., Spicer, C. C., Elliott, M., Armstrong, E., and Dhadial, R. K. 1972b. Parental X-irradiation and chromosome constitution in their spontaneously aborted fetuses. Ann. Hum. Genet. 36:185-194.

Boué, J., and Boué, A. 1973. Chromosomal analysis of two consecutive abortuses in each of 43 women. Hum. Genet. 19:275-280.

Boué, J., Boué, A., and Lazar, P. 1975. The epidemiology of human spontaneous abortions with chromosomal anomalies. In R. J. Blandau (ed.), Aging Gametes, pp. 330-348. S. Karger AG, Basel.

Carr, D. H. 1967. Chromosome anomalies as a cause of spontaneous abortion. Am. J. Obstet. Gynecol. 97:283-293.

Creasy, M. R. 1977. The cytogenetics of early human fetuses. Doctoral thesis, University of London, London.

Creasy, M. R., and Crolla, J. A. 1974. Prenatal mortality of Trisomy 21 (Down's syndrome). Lancet 1:473-474.

Creasy, M. R., Crolla, J. A., and Alberman, E. D. 1976. A cytogenetic study of human spontaneous abortions using banding techniques. Hum. Genet. 31:177-196.

Dhadial, R. K., Machin, A. M., and Tait, S. M. 1970. Chromosomal anomalies and spontaneously aborted human fetuses. Lancet 2:20-21.

French, F. E., and Bierman, J. M. 1962. Probabilities of fetal mortality. Pub. Health Rep. 77 (10):835-847.

Hertig, A. T. 1967. The overall problem in man. In K. Benirschke (ed.), Comparative Aspects of Reproductive Failure, pp. 11-41. Springer-Verlag, Berlin.

Léridon, H., and Boué, J. 1971. La mortalité intrauterine d'origine chromosomique. Population 26:113-138.

Roman, E., Doyle, P., Beral, V., Alberman, E., and Pharoah, P. 1978. Fetal loss, gravidity and pregnancy order. Early Hum. Dev. 2(2):131-138.

Therkelsen, A. J., Grunnet, N., Hjort, T., Hyre Jensen, O., Jonasson, J., Lauritsen, J. G., Lindsten, J., and Brunn Petersen, G. 1973. Studies on spontaneous abortions. In A. Boué and C. Thibault (eds.), Chromosomal Errors in Relation to Reproductive Failure. INSERM, Paris.

Parental Origin
of Nondisjunction

R. Ellen Magenis and Jan Chamberlin

Since the advent of quinacrine chromosome banding techniques (Caspersson et al., 1970; Caspersson, Lomakka, and Zech, 1971), acrocentric human autosomes 13–15 and 21–22 have been found to have constant banding patterns of the long arm and surprisingly variable short arms and satellites. The variations in fluorescent staining of the short arm, stalk, and satellite regions of chromosome 21 have been followed in 56 families with Down syndrome with the assumption that they behave as true genetic polymorphisms. To the extent that they represent stable, heritable markers, they can provide information about the parental origin and the meiotic division in which nondisjunction results in a trisomic Down offspring (Figures 1 and 2). Requirements for such a study include: 1) inherent stability of the short arm variation, which implies infrequent or no crossing over within this short-arm marker region of homologues, 2) Mendelian inheritance, and 3) the occurrence of distinguishable heteromorphisms of chromosome 21 at frequencies that allow detection of a reasonable number of parents who are heteromorphic and thus informative.

There are a number of reports (Magenis, Chamberlin, and Overton, 1974; Magenis et al., 1977; Magenis, Donlon, and Wyandt, 1978; Robinson et al., 1976; Verma and Lubs, 1976) using quinacrine fluorescence, C-banding, Giemsa-11 banding, and acridine orange banding that support the assumption that acrocentric short-arm heteromorphisms are stable and heritable. Exceptions include 14 of 99 variants in 10 sibships reported by Craig-Holmes, Moore, and Shaw (1975), one variant in 208 offspring in 32 families reported by Robinson et al. (1978), and one variant in the 56 Down families reported at the University of Oregon Health Sciences Center.

The assumption that acrocentric short-arm heteromorphisms are heritable is not necessarily rejected by these few exceptions until variations due to chromosome compaction and staining techniques are taken into account and until correct assignment of biological parentage is tested using other genetic markers. The assumption of rare or absent crossing over within the short-arm marker region of acrocentric chromosomes is less certain. Hultén (1974) found no chiasma in the short arms of the small acrocentrics in a meiotic study of a normal male and only occasional chias-

Supported by grants from NICHD (HD-07997), Maternal and Child Health Services 920.

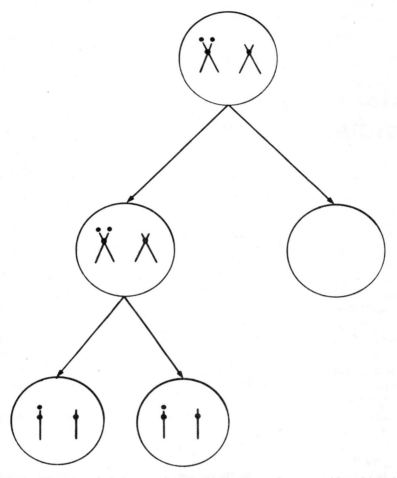

Figure 1.   Diagram meiosis I error, given that the marker regions are stable and inherited.

mata in these regions in studies of infertile males. Chandley, Seuánez, and Fletcher (1976) studied five male translocation carriers; three of these had translocations involving an acrocentric chromosome. They found no chiasma of the short arms of either the short or long acrocentric chromosomes, although chiasmata were seen on the long arms between the centromere and the breakpoints of the translocations. Gimelli et al. (1976) reported "jumping" satellites in three generations of a family with a balanced 10/22 translocation. They found prominent satellites on the normal chromosome 22 in the father; in his daughter and son they were transferred to the translocation chromosome 22. In the third generation, the bright satellites were back on a normal 22. Gimelli et al.'s interpretation was that exchanges had occurred between the short arms of chromosomes 22 at meiotic pairing. However, crossing over in the region between the centromere and the breakpoint on the long arm of the

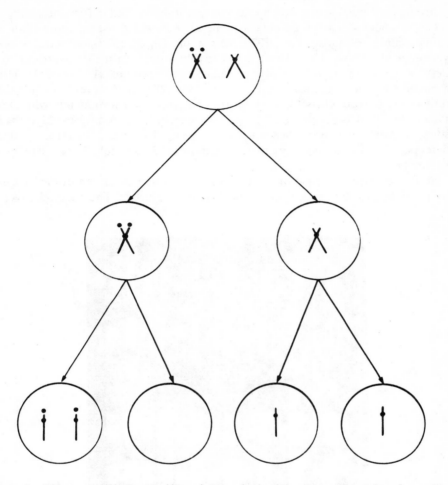

Figure 2.   Diagram meiosis II error, if crossing over in the short-arm satellite regions does not occur.

translocated 22 would give the same result, and from Chandley's data appears more likely.

An intriguing possibility for exchanges of marker short-arm material among nonhomologous chromosomes is suggested from the one exception to Mendelian inheritance in this study. A child trisomic for 21 had a brightly fluorescent satellite on a chromosome 22 unlike that of either parent; other heteromorphisms as well as blood group and serum protein markers were consistent with paternity. The source of the bright marker on chromosome 22 was possibly a chromosome 15 in one parent who had a satellite of similar brilliance and morphology. We were not able to verify this possibility with DAPI staining (Schweizer, Ambros, and Andren, 1978) (which preferentially stains the chromosome 15 short arms), since the child's brightly fluorescing chromosome 22 was DAPI negative.

Methods of maximizing detectable heteromorphism, and in turn increasing the number of conclusions for parental origin, have included use of more than one staining technique (Mattei et al., 1979; Verma and Dosik, 1978) and serial printing (Overton et al., 1976). The latter method involves serial prints of overexposed to underexposed negatives of quinacrine-stained chromosomes 21 (Figure 3). Using this method we have reached conclusions in over 80% of the families studied. In Figure 4, homologous chromosomes 21 from a normal parent of a child with Down syndrome are illustrated. No satellites are visible on either chromosome 21 at the exposure that would usually be chosen for karyotyping. However, when the negative is underexposed, a distinct satellite on one chromosome 21 is visible, but no satellite on the other appears.

Studies of parental origin of de novo translocation in Down syndrome have also been possible by utilizing chromosome heteromorphisms. The method involves

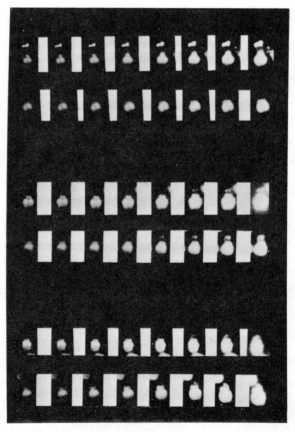

Figure 3.   Serial printing of six different chromosomes 21. Note that no satellite is visible on some 21s at the exposure best for chromosome identification, and that one chromosome 21 has no satellite at any exposure.

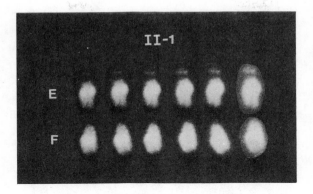

Figure 4.   Serially printed homologous chromosomes 21 from a parent of a child with Down syndrome.

determination of the origin of the "free" 21 in the case of a 21/21 translocation, or the "free" 14 in the 14/21 translocation. Once the parental source of the "free" chromosome is established, the origin of the translocation can be determined by exclusion. Occasionally, the marker regions are intact in the translocation chromosome and the parent of origin can be directly determined, as in Figure 5. In this instance (Table 2, Case 5) the presence of both maternal marker regions suggested a meiosis I error; usually the stage of meiotic error could not be determined for the translocation subjects.

METHODS

Chromosomes were prepared from peripheral blood cultures of 61 Down syndrome patients, their parents, and their siblings, using standard techniques. Slides were stained with the fluorochrome quinacrine mustard (Caspersson et al., 1970) and photographed with a Zeiss photomicroscope II on panatomic-X film. At least 16 metaphase spreads were photographed per subject. The chromosomes 21 from each of these cells were printed at six to eight different exposure times to maximize detection of centromeric, short-arm, and satellite variations (Overton et al., 1976). Comparisons of the markers of the Down subject and parents were made independently by three observers skilled in chromosome marker studies. Conclusions regarding the parent of origin and the timing of the meiotic error were made only when all three observers agreed.

   Blood group, red cell, and serum protein polymorphisms were examined in 52 of the Down offspring and their parents. No assigned paternities were excluded.

RESULTS

Parental origin could be assigned in 49 of 61 Down persons. These included 42 subjects with trisomy 21 from 37 families (Table 1) and 7 subjects with de novo translocations (Table 2). The trisomy 21 data are pooled in Table 3 in two groups for

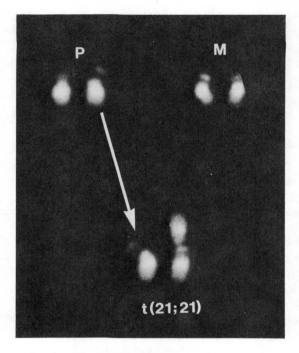

Figure 5.   A 21/21 translocation from a child with Down syndrome.

Down progeny of mothers younger than age 35 and those 35 or older. Subjects 40–42 (Table 1) are excluded, since the mosaic 21 trisomic cell line in subject 40 may have resulted from a mitotic error, and her children (subjects 41 and 42) do not represent "an error" in meiosis if oogenesis involved the trisomic cell line.

DISCUSSION

The results from Tables 1–3 demonstrate a preponderance of first meiotic division errors accounting for trisomy 21 offspring at all parental ages. This is also true for the small but not insignificant (21%) proportion of cases due to paternal nondisjunction.

Langenbeck et al. (1976) suggested that there was a bias toward meiosis II errors in the earlier reported parental origin data. They stated that only two of the five possible types of matings (*ab* × *cd* and *aa* × *bc*) permit detection of meiosis I errors and that the frequency of markers make the *ab* × *cd* mating uncommon. Eight percent of the families we studied were informative for both parental origin and stage of meiosis. The 12 noninformative families had the following parental mating types:

1.   *ab* × *cd*—one couple
     The quality of the culture from the child with Down syndrome was too poor to analyze.

Table 1.   Parental ages at the time of birth of each Down syndrome child, with the stage and parental origin of the meiotic error

Subject	Maternal age	Paternal age	Meiotic division	Parental origin
1	20	23	I	M
2	21	23	I	M
3	21	30	I	P
4[a]	22	22	I[b]	M[b]
5	22	24	I	P
6	22	24	I	P
7	22	25	I	M
8	22	26	I	M
9	22	30	I	M
10	24	27	I	M
11	24	27	II	P
12	26	27	I	M
13	27	27	I	M
14	28	26	I	M
15	28	37	I	M
16	29	29	I	M
17[b]	29	30	II[b]	P[b]
18	29	30	I	M
19	31	26	I	M
20	32	33	I	M
21	33	37	I	M
22	33	39	I	M
23	34	36	I	M
24	38	32	I	P
25	39	39	I	M
26[b]	40	43	I[b]	M[b]
27[c]	41	42	II	M
28	42	49	I	M
29	42	54	I	M
30	43	41	I	P
31[a]	44	44	I[a]	M[a]
32[c]	42	43	II	M
33	33	36	I	M
34	19	21	I	M
35	43	46	I	M
36[d]	20	23	I	M
37	27	26	I	M
38	26	33	I	P
39	25	24	I	M
40[e]	26	33	II or mitotic	P
41[f]	28	55	I	M
42[f]	29	56	I	M

[a]Niece and aunt.

[b]Niece and aunt.

[c]Siblings.

[d]Trisomy 21 sibling still under study.

[e]Mosaic.

[f]Siblings offspring of mosaics.

Table 2. Parental origin of Down syndrome due to de novo translocation

Case	Chromosomes	Maternal age	Paternal age	Parental origin
1	21/21	21	24	M
2	21/21	22	27	M
3	21/21	23	28	P
4	21/21	24	25	P
5	21/21	26	25	M—Meiosis I
6	14/21	24	25	M
7	14/21	33	33	M

Table 3. Meiotic error and parental origin results grouped by maternal age

Parental origin	Meiosis I	Meiosis II	Total
Younger age			
M (ages 20–34)	23	0	23
P (ages 21–39)	4	2	6
Older age			
M (ages 35–44)	6	2	8
P (ages 32–54)	2	0	2
Total	35	4	39

2. $ab \times bc$—five couples
    Offspring were abb and abc.
3. $ab \times bb$—two couples
    Down syndrome offspring were bbb and abb.
4. $ab \times ab$—one couple
5. $aa \times bc$—one couple
6. $aa \times aa$—one couple
    Mediocre quality study.
7. Not determined—one couple
    The quality of study did not allow analysis.

Ten of these 12 had mating types that did not allow conclusions; thus only 10 of the 61 cases had parental types uninformative for meiosis I determinations.

Table 4 summarizes 155 cases with parental origin results from the literature. These do not include translocation Down syndrome cases or those cases in which either parental origin or stage of meiosis were not reported. Thirty-seven (24%) were paternal in origin. Of the 118 maternal errors, 75% occurred in meiosis I; of those paternal in origin, 54% occurred in meiosis II. When only the larger, presumably less biased, published series (Hansson and Mikkelson, 1978; Mattei et al., 1979; Schmidt, Dar, and Nitowsky, 1976; Wagenbichler, 1976) are summarized with results from this study, there are 160 cases. Thirty-six (23%) were of paternal origin; 14 of the 36 (39%) were meiosis II errors. Of the 124 maternal errors, 19 (15%) were meiosis II errors.

Table 4.   Summary of reports[a] by others of parental origin and meiotic error in trisomy 21 Down syndrome

Report	Maternal meiosis		Paternal meiosis		No. conclusions/ studies attempted
	I	II	I	II	
Bott, Sekhon, and Lubs (1975)		3		4	7/59
deGrouchy (1970)		1			1/?
Emberger and Taib (1975)		1			1/?
Giraud, Mattei, and Mattei (1975)	1	2			3/32
Hara and Sasaki (1975)	1	2		1	4/33
Juberg and Jones (1970)		1			1/?
Kajii and Niikawa (1973)	1				1/?
Licznerski and Lindsten (1972)	1				1/6
Mattei et al. (1979)	29	5	4	4	42/61
Mikkelsen, Hallberg, and Poulsen (1976) Hansson and Mikkelsen (1978)	9	6	3	4	22/72
Moore et al. (1976)	1				1/?
Mutton (1973)		1			1/?
Niikawa, Merotto, and Kajii (1977) (abortuses)	3	1			4/7
Punnett and Kistenmacher (1973)	1			1	2/10
Robinson (1973)	4				4/12
Schmidt, Dar, and Nitowsky (1976)	22		1		23/40
Schmidt, Sokol, and Nitowsky (1978)				1	1/?
Smith and Sachdeva (1973)					0/20
Uchida (1973)				1	1/?
Verma and Dosik (1978)			1		1/?
Wagenbichler (1976)	16	6	8	4	34/70
Total	89	29	17	20	155/ >422

[a]Reports that did not state the total numbers of studies attempted are designated by a question mark.

It is of interest that one of the reported cases has XYY in addition to trisomy 21 (Schmidt et al., 1978). The YY error is of necessity a paternal meiosis II error (or mitotic); the extra chromosome 21 in this patient was also a paternal meiosis II error. Carothers et al. (1978) found a small but significant inverse relationship between paternal age and incidence of XYY. If this holds true for all paternal meiosis II errors, then the only likely paternal age effect would be upon paternal meiosis I errors. Many more studies are required for statistical significance.

Nine de novo translocation cases have been reported with parental origin results. Only one of these is a 14/21 translocation; the others are 21/21 translocations (see Table 5). The 14/21 case was due to a meiosis I maternal error; three of the eight 21/21 translocations were of paternal origin. These data combined with ours give a total of 16 cases. All three 14/21 translocation cases were of maternal origin, while 5 of the 13 21/21 translocation cases were paternally derived (38% paternal). This is in contrast to the 20%–25% paternal origin of free trisomy 21. However, the numbers of translocation cases are small, and the trend may change as more cases are studied.

Table 5.   Parental origin of de novo translocation: Reports by others

Report	Case	Chromosomes	Maternal age	Paternal age	Parental origin
Robinson (1973)	1	14/21			Maternal meiosis I
Hara and Sasaki (1975)	2	21/21			Paternal
Schmidt, Dar, and Nitowsky (1975)	3	21/21			Maternal
Verma et al. (1977)	4	21/21 ?reverse tandem	32	32	Paternal
Jacobs, Mayer, and Rudak (1978)	5	21/21	25	31	Maternal
Mattei et al. (1979)	6	21/21			Maternal
	7	21/21			Maternal
	8	21/21			Maternal
	9	21/21			Paternal

It is clear that there is an increased risk for a Down syndrome offspring once one has been born (Milunsky, 1973; Uchida, 1970). Unanswered questions include: 1) Is the recurrence risk different when the nondisjunction is paternal rather than maternal, or due to a meiosis I or II error? 2) Is there a common cause for either meiosis I or II errors? 3) Does the same type of error recur in familial cases—is there a familial predisposition?

We have studied five families with more than one trisomy 21 offspring with these questions in mind. Two families have an affected aunt and niece. In one family (Figure 6), both errors were of maternal origin and occurred in meiosis I; in the other, one was due to a maternal meiosis I error in an older mother and the other was a paternal meiosis II error (Figure 7). Two families have affected siblings; in one, the errors were both maternal meiosis II errors, and the mother was over 40 years at the birth of both affected offspring. In the other family, one was due to a meiosis I maternal error in a young mother; evaluation of the other is not yet complete. In the fifth family, with three affected trisomy 21 offspring (two studied for origin), the cause was found to be maternal meiosis I. However, the mother has two cell populations, one normal and the other trisomy 21. The latter cell line comprises approximately 10% of the total, and contains two identical paternally derived chromosomes (Figure 8). The trisomic line could be meiotically derived, but as a minor population it is more likely due to a mitotic nondisjunctive event involving a chromosome inherited from her father. Thus, all the familial cases are different and do not yet permit generalizations.

With parental origin known, a more definitive search for factors contributing to the nondisjunctive event is possible. Hypotheses include delayed fertilization (German, 1968; Juberg, 1976; Moscati and Becak, 1978), physiological changes in the female reproductive tract (Ford, 1973), seasonality and preovulatory overripeness (Jongbloet, 1971), accelerated aging in young mothers (Emanuel et al., 1972), maternal thyroid antibodies (Fialkow et al., 1971), environmental agents (Stoller and Collman, 1965; Uchida, Holunga, and Lawler, 1968), parental mosaicism (Hsu et al., 1971) α_1 antitrypsin heterozygosity (Fineman et al., 1976), interchromosomal effects (Nielsen et al., 1974), and paternal age (Stene et al., 1977). Since fertilization

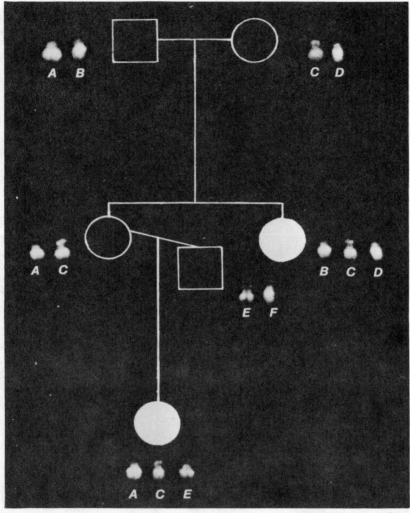

Figure 6.   Meiosis I maternal error in aunt and niece. (From Magenis et al., 1977, *Human Genetics 37:* 7-16.)

occurs after meiosis I in the ovum and since most maternal errors appear to have oc-curred in meiosis I, those hypotheses involving delayed fertilization and Fallopian tube malfunction can be eliminated as major factors. Those hypotheses suggesting maternal causative factors that might affect the ovum before ovulation (such as x-irradiation, thyroid antibodies, and interchromosomal effect) can now be tested further in those of known maternal origin. The frequent finding, however, of two Y bodies (meiosis II error), and of two chromosome 9 or two chromosome 1 hetero-chromatin bodies in sperm (Pearson, Geraedts, and Pawlowitski, 1973), and the in-cidence of paternal errors in this study indicate that fathers should be included in further exploration of some of these hypotheses. We have preliminary data regard-

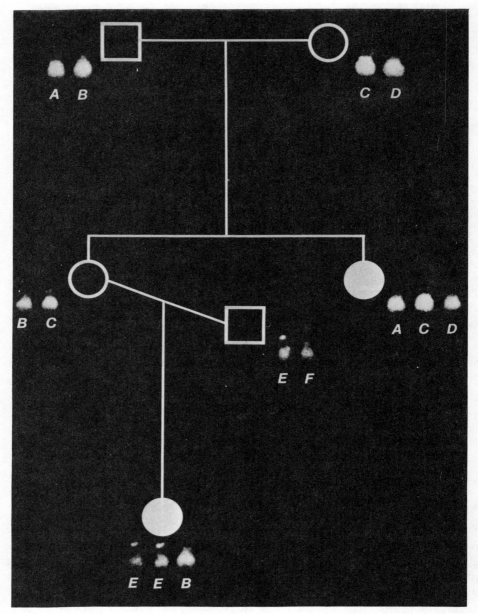

Figure 7.   Maternal meiosis I error in a maternal aunt; meiosis II paternal error in a niece. (From Magenis et al., 1977, *Human Genetics* 37:7–16.)

ing thyroid antibodies in 22 mothers and 12 fathers tested. Four of the mothers had thyroid antibodies. Three of these were the source of the nondisjunction; two of the three were under age 35, the third was older. In the fourth case, the parental origin

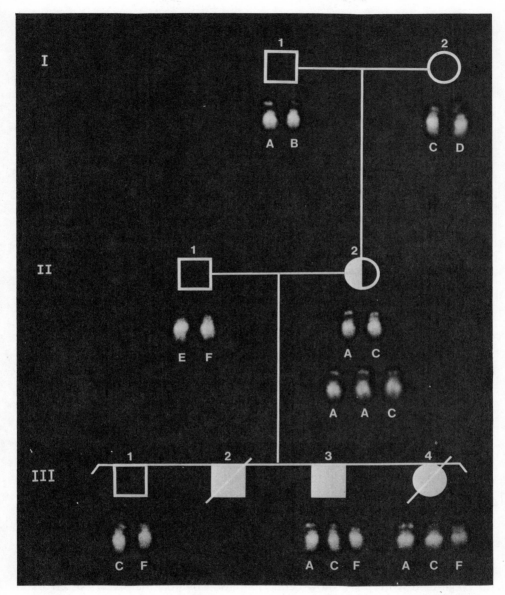

Figure 8. Mosaic mother with three trisomy 21 offspring. Two were available for study and were due to maternal errors. The extra chromosome in the trisomic population in the mother was meiosis II paternal or mitotic in origin.

study is incomplete. Only 1 of the 12 fathers had thyroid antibodies; he was age 57. His Down offspring was the result of a maternal meiosis I nondisjunctive event, apparently unrelated to either his age or thyroid status.

Nielsen et al. (1974) postulated an increased risk of nondisjunctive events in families with large heterochromatin variants, particularly of chromosome 9. We

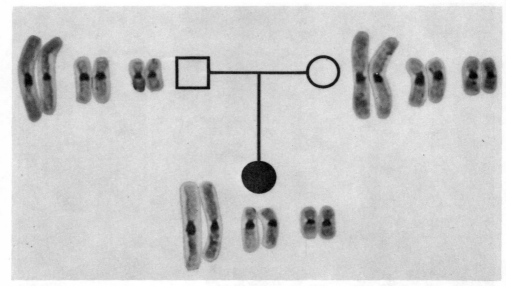

Figure 9.   Segregation of 1qh, 9qh, and 16qh C-band regions in a family with a trisomy 21 Down child of maternal meiosis I origin.

have begun a study of the inheritance of C-band variants in Down syndrome, particularly of chromosomes 1, 9, and, 16, with the idea that an interchromosomal effect in disjunction would result in nonrandom segregation of the larger marker regions in the Down syndrome offspring (Figure 9). Data thus far are not conclusive.

SUMMARY

Stable, heritable heteromorphisms of human chromosomes 21 can be used to trace the parental origin and the meiotic division accounting for trisomic 21 offspring. From 20% to 25% of these errors are of paternal origin, as judged from informative matings in which one or both parents have distinguishably different chromosomes 21. About 75% of the errors occur in meiosis I. These heteromorphisms can also be used to determine the parental origin of de novo translocations leading to Down syndrome. The numbers of cases are small, but there is a suggestion that there is a higher rate of paternal origin (38%) among 21/21 translocation Down syndrome than of simple trisomy 21 Down syndrome. Knowledge of the parent of origin and the stage of division may allow better resolution of potential causes of errors in meiotic segregation of these two homologues.

Our data presented in this summary paper include new cases and cases previously published (Magenis et al., 1977).

ACKNOWLEDGMENTS

We thank the Clinical Cytogenetics Laboratory (Douglas Hepburn and Marvin Yoshitomi), who did the initial studies of the affected patients; Diane Plumridge, who aided in ascertaining, counseling, and following the families; and Everett Lovrien, Shirley Rowe, and Nancy Lamvik, who performed the gene marker studies. We also thank Dr. Horace Thuline, Michael Begleiter, and Dr. Patricia Howard Peebles, who allowed us to study their families with Down siblings. We especially thank Kathleen Overton who helped originate this work, and all the families who contributed to the study.

REFERENCES

Bott, C. E., Sekhon, G. S., and Lubs, H. A. 1975. Unexpected high frequency of paternal origin of trisomy 21. Paper presented at the American Society of Human Genetics 27th annual meeting, October 8–11, Baltimore.

Carothers, A. D., Collyer, S., DeMay, R., and Frackiewicz, A. 1978. Parental age and birth order in the aetiology of some sex chromosomes aneuploidies. Ann. Hum. Genet. 41:277–287.

Caspersson, T., Hultén, M., Lindsten, J., and Zech, L. 1970. Distinction between extra G-like chromosomes by quinacrine mustard fluorescence analysis. Exp. Cell Res. 63:240–243.

Caspersson, T., Lomakka, G., and Zech, L. 1971. The 24 fluorescence patterns of the human metaphase chromosomes—Distinguishing characters and variability. Hereditas 67:89–102.

Chandley, A. C., Seuánez, H., and Fletcher, J. M. 1976. Meiotic behavior of five human reciprocal translocations. Cytogenet. Cell Genet. 17:98–111.

Craig-Holmes, A. P., Moore, F. B., and Shaw, M. W. 1975. Polymorphism of human C-band heterochromatin. II. Family studies with suggestive evidence for somatic crossing over. Am. J. Hum. Genet. 27:178–189.

deGrouchy, J. 1970. 21p— maternal en double exemplaire chez un trisomique 21. [A maternal 21p— in two copies in a trisomy 21.] Ann. Genet. 13:52–55.

Emanuel, I., Sever, L. E., Milham, S., Jr., and Thuline, H. 1972. Accelerated aging in young mothers of children with Down's syndrome. Lancet 2:361–353.

Emberger, J. M., and Taib, J. 1975. 21p+ maternal en double exemplaire chez un trisomique 21. [A maternal 21p+ in two copies in a trisomy 21.] J. Genet. Hum. 23(suppl.):98–101.

Fialkow, P. J., Thuline, H. C., Hecht, F., and Bryant, J. 1971. Familial predisposition to thyroid disease in Down's syndrome: Controlled immunochemical studies. Am. J. Hum. Genet. 23:67–86.

Fineman, R. M., Kidd, K. K., Johnson, A. M., and Breg, W. R. 1976. Increased frequency of heterozygotes for α_1 antitrypsin variants in individuals with either sex chromosome mosaicism or trisomy 21. Nature 260:320–321.

Ford, J. H. 1973. Induction of chromosomal errors. Lancet 1:54.

German, J. 1968. Mongolism, delayed fertilization and human sexual behavior. Nature 217:516–518.

Gimelli, G., Porro, E., Santi, F., Scappaticci, S., and Zuffardi, O. 1976. "Jumping" satellites in three generations: A warning for paternity tests and prenatal diagnosis. Hum. Genet. 34:315–318.

Giraud, F., Mattei, J.-F., and Mattei, M. G. 1975. Etude chromosomique chez les parents d'enfants trisomiques 21. Chromosome marqueurs, remaniements, cassures et aneuploidies. [Chromosome study of parents of children with trisomy 21. Chromosome markers, rearrangements breaks, and aneuploidies.] Lyon Med. 223(3):241–251.

Hansson, A., and Mikkelsen, M. 1978. The origin of the extra chromosome 21 in Down's syndrome. Cytogenet. Cell Genet. 20:194–203.

Hara, Y., and Sasaki, M. 1975. A note on the origin of extra chromosomes in trisomies 13 and 21. Proc. Jap. Acad. 51:295–299.

Hsu, L. Y. F., Gertner, M., Leiter, E., and Hirschhorn, K. 1971. Paternal trisomy 21 mosaicism and Down's syndrome. Am. J. Hum. Genet. 23:592–601.

Hultén, M. 1974. Chiasma distribution at diakinesis in the normal human male. Hereditas 76:55–78.

Jacobs, P. A., Mayer, M., and Rudak, E. 1978. Structural abnormalities in Down syndrome: A study of two families. Cytogenet. Cell Genet. 20:185–193.

Jongbloet, P. H. 1971. Month of birth and gametopathy, and investigation into patients with Down's, Klinefelter's and Turner's syndrome. Clin. Genet. 2:315–330.

Juberg, R. C. 1976. Origin of chromosomal abnormalities: Evidence for delayed fertilization in meiotic nondisjunction. In International Congress of Human Genetics, Vol. 5., p. 132. Excerpta Medica, Amsterdam.

Juberg, R. C., and Jones, B. 1970. The Christchurch chromosome (Gp–) mongolism, erythroleukemia and an inherited Gp– chromosome (Christchurch). New Engl. J. Med. 282:292–297.

Kajii, T., and Niikawa, N. 1973. Personal communication to M. Sasaki and Y. Hara. Lancet 2:1257–1258.

Langenbeck, U., Hansmann, I., Hinney, B., and Hönig, V. 1976. On the origin of the supernumerary chromosome in autosomal trisomies—With special reference to Down's syndrome. Hum. Genet. 33:89–102.

Licznerski, G., and Lindsten, J. 1972. Trisomy 21 in man due to maternal nondisjunction during the first meiotic division. Hereditas 70:153–154.

Magenis, R. E., Chamberlin, J., and Overton, K. 1974. Sequential Q and C-band variants: Inheritance in four generations of a family. Paper presented at the Somatic Cell Genetics 13th annual conference, December, Virgin Islands.

Magenis, R. E., Donlon, T. A., and Wyandt, H. E. 1978. Giemsa-11 staining of chromosome 1: A newly described heteromorphism. Science 202:64–65.

Magenis, R. E., Overton, K. M., Chamberlin, J., Brady, T., and Lovrien, E. 1977. Parental origin of the extra chromosome in Down's syndrome. Hum. Genet. 37:7–16.

Magenis, R. E., Palmer, C. G., Wang, L., Brown, M., Chamberlin, J., Parks, M., Merritt, A. D., Rivas, M. L., and Yu, P. L. 1977. Heritability of chromosome banding variants. In E. B. Hook and I. H. Porter (eds.), Population Cytogenetics: Studies in Humans. Academic Press, New York.

Mattei, J.-F., Mattei, M. G., Ayme, S., and Giraud, F. 1979. Origin of the extra chromosome in trisomy 21. Hum. Genet. 46:107–110.

Mikkelsen, M., Hallberg, A., and Poulsen, H. 1976. Maternal and paternal origin of extra chromosome in trisomy 21. Hum. Genet. 32:17–21.

Milunsky, A. 1973. The Prenatal Diagnosis of Hereditary Disorders. Charles C Thomas Publisher, Springfield, Ill. p. 25.

Moore, C. M., Arbisser, A. I., Simon, F. A., and Morris, F. H., Jr. 1976. Maternal first meiotic nondisjunction in a case of monozygous twins with Down's syndrome. In International Congress of Human Genetics, Vol. 5., p. 142. Excerpta Medica, Amsterdam.

Moscati, I. M., and Becak, W. 1978. Down syndrome and frequency of intercourse. Lancet 2:629–630.

Mutton, D. E. 1973. Origin of the trisomic 21 chromosome. Lancet 1:375.

Nielsen, J., Friedrich, U., Hreidarsson, A., and Zeuthen, E. 1974. Frequency of 9qh+ and risk of chromosome aberrations in the progeny of individuals with 9qh+. Humangenetik 21:211–216.

Niikawa, N., Merotto, E., and Kajii, T. 1977. Origin of acrocentric trisomies in spontaneous abortuses. Hum. Genet. 40:73–78.

Overton, K. M., Magenis, R. E., Brady, T., Chamberlin, J., and Parks, M. 1976. Cytogenetic darkroom magic: Now you see them, now you don't. Am. J. Hum. Genet. 28:417–419.

Pearson, P. L., Geraedts, J. P. M., and Pawlowitski, I. H. 1973. Chromosomal studies on human male gametes. In A. Boué and C. Thibault (eds.), Les Accidents Chromosomiques de la Reproduction, pp. 219–229. [Chromosomal Accidents of Reproduction.] Inserm, Paris.

Punnett, H. H., and Kistenmacher, M. L. 1973. The origin of the extra chromosome in trisomy 21. Genetics 74(suppl.):222.

Robinson, J. A. 1973. Origin of extra chromosome in trisomy 21. Lancet 1:131–133.

Robinson, J. A., Buckton, K. E., Evans, H. J., and Robson, E. B. 1978. A possible mutation of a fluorescence polymorphism. Ann. Hum. Genet. 41:323–328.

Robinson, J. A., Buckton, K. E., Spowart, G., Newton, M., Jacobs, P. A., Evans, H. J., and Hill, R. 1976. The segregation of human chromosome polymorphisms. Ann. Hum. Genet. 40:113–121.

Schmidt, R., Dar, H., and Nitowsky, H. M. 1975. Origin of extra 21 chromosome in patients with Down syndrome. Pediatr. Res. 9(4):318.

Schmidt, R., Dar, H., and Nitowsky, H. M. 1976. Apparent parental mosaicism for 21 trisomy as a predisposing factor for children with Down's syndrome. In International Congress of Human Genetics, Vol. 5, p. 151. Excerpta Medica, Amsterdam.

Schmidt, R., Sokol, S., and Nitowsky, H. M. 1978. Origin of extra chromosomes in 48,XYY, + 21 aneuploidy. Am. J. Hum. Genet. 30:93A.

Schweizer, D., Ambros, P., and Andren, M. 1978. Modification of DAPI banding on human chromosomes by prestaining with a DNA-binding oligopeptide antibiotic, distamycin A. Exp. Cell Res. 3:327–332.

Smith, G. F., and Sachdeva, S. 1973. Origin of extra chromosome in trisomy 21. Lancet 1: 487.

Stene, J., Fischer, G., Stene, E., Mikkelsen, M., and Petersen, E. 1977. Paternal age effect in Down's syndrome. Ann. Hum. Genet. 40:299–306.

Stoller, A., and Collman, R. D. 1965. Virus aetiology for Down's syndrome (mongolism). Nature 208:903–904.

Uchida, I. A. 1970. Epidemiology of mongolism: The Manitoba study. Ann. N.Y. Acad. Sci. 171:361–369.

Uchida, I. A. 1973. Paternal origin of the extra chromosome in Down's syndrome. Lancet 2: 1258.

Uchida, I. A., Holunga, R., and Lawler, C. 1968. Maternal radiation and chromosomal aberrations. Lancet 2:1045–1049.

Verma, R. S., and Dosik, H. 1978. Trisomy 21 in a child due to paternal nondisjunction as determined by RFA technique. Jap. J. Hum. Genet. 23:17–21.

Verma, R. S., and Lubs, H. A. 1976. Inheritance of acridine orange R variants in human acrocentric chromosomes. Hum. Hered. 26:315–318.

Verma, R. S., Peakman, D. C., Robinson, R., and Lubs, H. A. 1977. Two cases of Down syndrome with unusual de novo translocation. Clin. Genet. 11:227–234.

Wagenbichler, P. 1976. Origins of the supernumerary chromosome in Down's syndrome. In International Congress of Human Genetics, Vol. 5, p. 167. Excerpta Medica, Amsterdam.

Relation of Maternal Age Effect in Down Syndrome to Nondisjunction

John A. Sved and L. Sandler

The common understanding of the observation that the frequency of trisomy 21 is much higher in offspring born to older, as compared to younger, mothers is that the probability of meiotic nondisjunction of homologous chromosomes increases with the age of the female. An obviously related question—Does the probability of non-disjunction increase similarly with the age of the male?—has, following Penrose (1933), usually been answered in the negative. This difference between the sexes, moreover, finds a ready physiological basis in the dictyotene stage, which is charac-teristic of female, but not of male, meiosis.

In the light of these generalities, however, the results of cytological determina-tions of the parental origin of the extra chromosome in trisomy 21 individuals are somewhat puzzling. In the series developed by Magenis et al. (1977) and by Magenis and Chamberlin (this volume), 39 trisomy 21 persons are reported for whom an une-quivocal determination of the parental origin of the extra chromosome was made. Of this total, 31 (79%) proved to be the result of maternal nondisjunction—a figure in agreement with Magenis et al.'s tabulation of the total of all other such determi-nations (73 maternal nondisjunctions among 97 cases = 75%). It seems, therefore, that some 75% of Down syndrome cases result from nondisjunction in the mother. Note that a proportion of paternal nondisjunction is not, by itself, incompatible with the simultaneous existence of a maternal age effect and absence of a paternal age effect.

However, in this same series, 29 of the 39 trisomy 21 infants were born to young (<34 years) mothers and 10 to older (35–44 years) mothers. Among the trisomic off-spring born to the young mothers, 23 (79%) resulted from maternal nondisjunction; among the trisomics born to older mothers, 8 (80%) involved maternal nondisjunc-tion. Thus, although there are few data, it appears that the percentage of trisomic offspring resulting from paternal nondisjunction is similar in trisomic offspring born to younger and to older mothers. It seems difficult to reconcile this observation with the idea that the probability of meiotic nondisjunction increases with maternal, but not with paternal, age.

In particular, assume that, among young mothers, a fraction p of affected persons is the result of paternal nondisjunction. Then, if there is no age effect in males but there is a 10-fold increase in nondisjunction frequency between young and old females, it follows that the probability of paternal nondisjunction among affected offspring of old females is $p/10$. Taking the observed numbers 23/6 in young females and 8/2 in old, the value of p giving the best fit to all the data is found by maximum likelihood to be 0.253, which is close to the overall figure mentioned previously. A χ^2 test can then be made. The 1 d.f. χ^2 corrected for continuity is 6.45, corresponding to a probability of only about 1% that all the data can be accounted for by an age effect on the frequency of nondisjunction in the mother only.

It would appear, therefore, that one of three things must be true: 1) the few extant data may be misleading, and older mothers only rarely give birth to trisomics resulting from paternal nondisjunction; 2) contrary to the conventional wisdom, there may be an increase in the rate of nondisjunction in males with increasing paternal age comparable to the situation in females; 3) the maternal age effect may not be the result of an increase in the rate of nondisjunction with increasing maternal age but, rather, may reflect some postmeiotic age-related change in females.

Whether there may be a paternal age effect for Down syndrome has received considerable contemporary attention. Unfortunately, this has not led to any unequivocal conclusions. Stene et al. (1977) and Matsunaga et al. (1978) reported a significant increase in the incidence of Down syndrome among offspring of very old (>55 years) fathers. In contrast, Erickson (1978, 1979) found no paternal age effect in two large, although relatively poorly ascertained samples and one smaller, well-ascertained sample.

The reason for the difficulty in demonstrating a paternal age effect is, of course, the close correlation between maternal and paternal ages. In order to test for a paternal effect, it is necessary to first remove the large maternal effect, and most of the information is lost during this process. However, the cytogenetic information on the parental origin of the nondisjunction now available gives us a way of estimating the amount of information that a sample provides on maternal and paternal age effects. The important statistic here is that about 75% of trisomics result from female nondisjunction and 25% from male nondisjunction. We can, therefore, ask how likely it is that a paternal age effect similar to the maternal age effect will be undetected because of the numerically greater number of cases contributed by the female.

If the increase in nondisjunction with parental age is linear, some information can be deduced analytically. It can be readily shown that if the *proportionate* increases in nondisjunction are comparable in females and males, then the *overall* linear regression of trisomy incidence against parental age is three times (0.75/0.25) as high in the females as in the male. The chance of detecting a significant male age effect is, therefore, considerably lower than that for detecting a female age effect. In addition, the variances of both partial regression coefficients are increased over the regular regression coefficients by a factor $1/(1-r^2)$, where r is the correlation of female and male ages.

To get numerical estimates of the chance of detecting a paternal age effect, it is most convenient to turn to computer simulation. The reason for this is partly that the assumption of linearity introduces considerable biases (Stene and Stene, 1977), and use of computer simulation removes the need for making this assumption.

We chose to analyze simulated data according to the procedure outlined by Erickson (1978), which divides the data into single-year age classes according to female age and tests for an overall effect of young versus old males. We assumed that the proportional increase of nondisjunction against age of females follows the form of the well-ascertained sample of Erickson (1979, Figure 1). We then tested the effect of allowing a corresponding increase in males, but the overall rate of production of trisomics in the two cases was an approximate 3/1 ratio. The much larger sample of control ages in Erickson's (1979) NIS sample (his Appendix Tables 2, 3) was used to give more accurate estimates of the proportion of the population in the various parental age classes.

The overall population size was chosen to produce approximately 200 affected births. These data were then analyzed to test for young versus old male parents in the manner indicated by Erickson, using both 40 and 55 years as the ages of separation into young and old males. This procedure was then repeated 1000 times to generate a population of probability values.

In almost every case (977/1000), the sample of 200 trisomics was sufficient to enable a male effect to be detected at a 5% confidence level when the division between old and young males was 40 years. In other words, an age effect in males comparable to that in females ought to be detected in a sample of 200. The fact that it was not in the data analyzed by Erickson indicates that there is not an age effect in males comparable to that in females.

It is interesting that the result for the comparison between males above and below 55 years of age was equivocal. In only approximately two-thirds of cases, would a significant effect have been detected. The reason for the lower probability of detection is the paucity of cases in the higher age groups. This is precisely the area where there has been disagreement between Stene and Stene (1977, 1978) and Erickson (1978, 1979). That Erickson found no effect at this age level does not, therefore, rule out the possibility of an age effect in old males. The considerably higher numbers tested in Erickson's other samples would, however, convincingly rule out this possibility (although Stene and Stene, 1978, argued that there may be an ascertainment bias in those data).

We used the generated data to test for a difference in the statistical procedures adopted by Stene and Stene and by Erickson. We found that the procedure of grouping female age classes does not obviously increase the power of the statistical test. Nor, on the other hand, does it introduce a very significant bias in a sample size of 200. We showed this by generating data in which there was no male age effect and finding that the procedure failed to introduce one. Erickson (1978) has, however, shown that a significant bias may be produced in samples of larger size.

It is worth considering the question of what extra information is given by studying the paternal age distribution of cases classified, on cytological grounds, as coming from nondisjunction in the male. If no age effect is found, the conclusion is clear. If, however, there is a significant regression on male age, then, unfortunately, the cytological classification helps little in resolving whether the increase is due to increased nondisjunction in the male or to increased risk due to some property of the female. Just as with data unclassified by parental origin, the high correlation of female and male ages makes this question difficult to answer.

Overall, therefore, the available data do not rule out an age effect in very old fathers, although they do exclude age effects comparable to those in the female. Magenis's observation of two instances of paternal nondisjunction among older mothers might, therefore, be explained by such an age effect in very old males. Because of the paucity of data, there seems little point at present in trying to estimate what rates of increase in old males would be compatible with both the cytologically classified and the overall data.

In summary, then, if it proves to be true that the frequency of meiotic nondisjunction in males does not substantially increase with the age of the male, and if in the future the data continue to imply that a substantial proportion of Down syndrome offspring born to older women is the result of nondisjunction in the father, then it will be necessary to conclude that the maternal age effect for trisomy 21 (and, by inference, for the other trisomies as well) is the result of a postmeiotic, age-related change in the female. None of the statistical data, of course, suggests just what such an age-related change in the female might be. However, the observation that the majority of trisomy 21 fetuses do not come to term (Alberman, this volume) suggests the possibility that the female age effect might be the consequence of older women more often carrying such fetuses to term. Precisely this suggestion has been made by Erickson (1978). Although it may seem strange that older women should be more successful in carrying Down syndrome offspring, this differential may really reflect a breakdown with age of a mechanism that has evolved to *prevent* the birth of aneuploids. Such a mechanism would also account for the observation of a maternal age effect for trisomies in addition to trisomy 21.

REFERENCES

Erickson, J. D. 1978. Down syndrome, paternal age, maternal age and birth order. Ann. Hum. Genet. 41:289–298.
Erickson, J. D. 1979. Paternal age and Down syndrome. Am. J. Hum. Genet. 31:489–497.
Magenis, R. E., Overton, K. M., Chamberlin, J., Brady, T., and Lovrien, E. 1977. Parental origin of the extra chromosome in Down's syndrome. Hum. Genet. 37:7–16.
Matsunaga, E., Tonomura, A., Oishi, H., and Kikuchi, Y. 1978. Reexamination of paternal age effect in Down's syndrome. Hum. Genet. 40:259–268.
Penrose, L. E. 1933. The relative effects of paternal and maternal age in mongolism. J. Genet. 27:219–224.
Stene, J., Fischer, G., Stene, E., Mikkelsen, M., and Peterson, E. 1977. Paternal age effect in Down's syndrome. Ann. Hum. Genet. 40:299–306.
Stene, J., and Stene, E. 1977. Statistical methods for detecting a moderate paternal age effect on incidence of disorder when a maternal one is present. Ann. Hum. Genet. 40:343–353.
Stene, J., and Stene, E. 1978. On data and methods in investigations on parental-age effects. Ann. Hum. Genet. 41:465–468.

Frequency of Mosaicism, Translocation, and Other Variants of Trisomy 21

John L. Hamerton

As early as 1932, Waardenburg suggested that Down syndrome might be caused by a chromosome abnormality. Penrose (1939) concluded that "mongolism and some other malformations may have their origins in chromosome abnormalities." Mittwoch (1952) was the first to carry out meiotic studies on a patient with Down syndrome and found 24 bodies in the primary spermatocytes. She concluded that these represented the normal human chromosome number, which was thought to be 48 at that time. Lejeune (1959) and Lejeune, Gautier, and Turpin (1959) were the first to demonstrate that patients with Down syndrome had an additional small chromosome thought to be number 21. This was rapidly confirmed by Ford et al. (1959) and Jacobs et al. (1959), and it has now been amply confirmed that the basic chromosome defect in Down syndrome is trisomy for chromosome 21.

The advent of chromosome banding techniques in 1969 and their application to human cytogenetics allowed this chromosome to be specifically identified as the smaller of the two G chromosomes, which had an intensely fluorescent proximal segment and a distal pale segment, and also allowed the demonstration that it was most probably a triplication of the distal pale segment (q22), which is the cause of Down syndrome phenotype (see Summitt, this volume, for review).

The demonstration of a chromosome abnormality by Lejeune and his colleagues in 1959 unleashed numerous cytogenetic studies. Polani et al. (1960) were the first to demonstrate a Robertsonian translocation in a child with Down syndrome born to a young mother; in the same year the familial transmission of such translocations was demonstrated (Carter et al., 1960; Penrose, Ellis, and Delhanty, 1960).

Before, but more significantly since, the advent of chromosome banding, other usually reciprocal translocations involving chromosome 21 and another autosome have been identified as associated with the Down syndrome phenotype, and it is these rearrangements in which the break points have been specifically identified that have led to the implication of band q22 as the specific Down syndrome segment (see Summitt, this volume, for review).

Mixoploids, or chromosome mosaics, had been demonstrated in the late 1950s and early 1960s in patients with sex chromosome abnormalities (Ford, 1961), and Clarke, Edwards, and Smallpiece (1961) reported the first mixoploid 46,XX/47, XX, + G girl—"an intelligent child with some mongoloid characteristics" whose overall picture at 11 months "was thought to be against the diagnosis of mongolism."

Since then many other mixoploids have been reported with a full Down syndrome phenotype, others with a milder expression, and still others with an essentially normal phenotype (see Smith and Berg, 1976, for review). Some parents of Down syndrome infants, themselves normal, have been shown to have a trisomic cell line along with their normal chromosomes (see Jagiello, this volume).

Finally, in this brief review of Down syndrome cytogenetics something should be said about the numerous cytogenetic associations that have been reported. These range from associations with other trisomics and sex chromosome abnormalities in the same subject or in different subjects in the same sibship or family (see Smith and Berg, 1976, for review). These suggest perhaps some constitutive nondisjunctional error in these cases.

More interesting, and perhaps more important, if the biological significance of minor variants were less obscure, are the numerous associations that have been reported or suggested between the minor chromosome variants, satellites, short arms, fluorescence variation, or centric heterochromatin and the occurrence of trisomy 21 (see Hamerton, 1971; Smith and Berg, 1976, for review). The major problems in the study of such variants are related to the high frequency in the general population, definition of the variant, ascertainment bias, properly controlled studies, and the need to study large numbers of persons if significant results on true biological associations are to be obtained. This particularly applies to the study of association between events occurring with such a high frequency as trisomy 21 on the one hand and certain variants on the other, particularly when the latter shows no apparent clinical effect in most cases. Nonetheless, if real associations could be demonstrated, they might be of immense value in genetic counseling. A small amount of new data on this topic, obtained by Dr. H. S. Wang at the Division of Genetics, University of Manitoba, are presented.

In this brief review we have seen that a cytogenetic study of Down syndrome has revealed a whole spectrum of chromosome abnormalities and that many problems still await a solution, some of which receive further attention in this volume. Next the frequency of some of the different chromosome abnormalities found in Down syndrome are reviewed.

CLASSIFICATION

A simple classification of chromosome abnormalities found in Down syndrome follows. A division into numerical and structural abnormalities is proposed, and these are then subdivided according to the origin of the abnormality (Rieger, Michaelis, and Green, 1976):

A. Numerical—Resulting from an error in mitosis or meiosis
1. Primary trisomy
2. Mixoploidy
B. Structural—Resulting from chromosome rearrangement combined with malsegregation
1. Secondary trisomy (extra chromosome has two identical arms)—Origin
may be the result of:
a. isochromosome formation
b. translocation between homologous chromosomes
2. Tertiary trisomy (extra chromosome results from a reciprocal or Robertsonian translocation between two standard chromosomes)—Origin may be
the result of:
a. Robertsonian translocation
b. reciprocal translocation
c. tandem translocation

Numerical Abnormalities

Primary Trisomy (47,XX or XY, + 21)   In 57,000 consecutive newborn babies
studied in six separate surveys, an overall frequency of about 1/800 babies with
Down syndrome was obtained (Hook and Hamerton, 1977) (Table 1). The frequencies in different populations ranged from a high of about 1/700 to a low of about
1/1400. This range compares well with the figures given by Smith and Berg (1976),
who reviewed data from 34 studies and showed that 28 studies fell in the range 1/500
to 1/1000, whereas 5 studies gave a frequency of less than 1/1000 and only one a frequency of greater than 1/500 (Table 2). These figures do not take into account the
highly significant effect of maternal age, which Hook discusses in detail (this
volume).

Mixoploidy or Chromosome Mosaicism   The true frequency of mixoploidy is
difficult, if not impossible, to establish because theoretically it is impossible to rule
out the presence of a second cell line in any study. Arbitrary limits must be placed,
therefore, on the numbers of cells required to establish the presence of a second cell
line. Penrose (1967) proposed arbitrary limits of not less than 9% and not more than
91% of cells counted having a trisomic constitution. Ford (1969) proposed a statistical approach to the determination of mosaicism. Except in specific studies, such
approaches are rarely taken in the routine cytogenetic study of patients with Down
syndrome, most of which are made for diagnostic purposes. In such instances a

Table 1.   Primary trisomy 21 in newborn chromosome surveys

Survey	No. of babies	Trisomy 21	Frequency
Edinburgh	11,680	17	1/687
Arhus	11,148	16	1/696
London	2,081	2	1/1040
Winnipeg	13,939	14	1/995
Boston	13,751	19	1/723
New Haven	4,353	3	1/1451
Total	56,952	71	1/802

Table 2.   Down syndrome incidence at
birth (34 studies)[a]

Incidence	No. of reports
<1/1000	5
1/1000–1/700	18
1/699–1/500	10
>1/500	1

Data from Lilienfeld (1969) and Smith
and Berg (1976).

[a]20 studies, hospital data; 4 studies, general population; 1 study, sibs of non-Down
retardates.

limited number of cells is usually examined from only one tissue, so that any estimates of mixoploidy obtained from such studies will be minimal.

The original mixoploid reported by Clarke et al. (1961) was a patient with minimal stigmata of Down syndrome and in whom the clinical diagnosis was in doubt.
This has of course resulted in the introduction of further ascertainment bias, namely, that the majority of deliberate searches for mosaicism have been in patients in
whom the diagnosis was doubtful.

Despite these problems, some estimates of the frequency of mosaicism have
been made. Hamerton, Giannelli, and Polani (1965) and Richards (1969) reported
an incidence of detected mosaicism of between 1% and 2% at all maternal ages, and
although this figure is undoubtedly low it might be said to present a baseline minimal figure. Among patients referred because of diagnostic doubt, the incidence of
mosaicism may be as high as 10%. The proportion of mosaic cells is highly variable
from person to person and from tissue to tissue. It has been reported in a number of
studies, however, that the frequency of trisomic cells is greater in fibroblasts than in
lymphocytes (Richards, 1974). No correlation between the expression of the clinical
phenotype and proportion of trisomic cells has been consistently found, although
where there is some doubt about the clinical diagnosis, the finding of mixoploidy
may be more likely if appropriate studies are made. Grosse, Hopfengartner, and
Schwanitz's (1971) and Priest, Verhulst, and Siskin's (1973) studies suggested that a
correlation may exist between the proportion of trisomic cells and features diagnostic for Down syndrome, particularly the dermal index score. Ford (1964) suggested
that the finding of a higher frequency of trisomic cells in fibroblasts rather than lymphocytes may be due to the normal cells having a selective advantage and replacing
the trisomic cells in the more rapidly dividing tissues. Taylor's (1968) longitudinal
study and other subsequent studies have not confirmed this hypothesis (see Hamerton, 1971; Smith and Berg, 1976, for review).

Several mothers of one or more Down syndrome infants have been reported to
have mosaic chromosomes (see Hamerton, 1971; Jagiello, this volume; Smith and
Berg, 1976, for reviews) and eight phenotypically normal fathers of affected children who themselves have mixoploid trisomy 21 are reported by Smith and Berg
(1976). In general, Richards (1974) has shown that, as might be expected, mixoploid
parents of children affected with Down syndrome have a lower proportion of tri-

Table 3.   Down syndrome (D.S.) frequency of patients with Robertsonian translocations[a]

Series	Total D.S. patients	% Robertsonian translocations
Hamerton (1971)	2594	3.5
Mikkelsen (1970)		
Matsunaga and Tonomura (1972)	4330	5.0
Giraud and Mattei (1975)	4760	4.8

[a]The figures should not be summed to obtain a mean value because overlap of cases occurs between different studies.

somic cells than mixoploid patients with the Down syndrome phenotype. In this study, 16 out of 17 parents had less than 30% trisomic cells. These findings clearly indicate that especially, although not exclusively, in families where more than one patient with Down syndrome has been found and the parental chromosomes are normal, an extensive search for mixoploidy may be warranted.

In conclusion, mixoploidy is well established among the cytogenetic causes of what may be a milder form of Down syndrome phenotype, and in some cases mixoploidy may be demonstrated in the absence of the Down syndrome phenotype. This no doubt depends not only on the numbers of trisomic cells present but also on the distribution. Similarly, the risk in such parents of producing a child with Down syndrome will depend on the extent to which the germ line is involved in mixoploidy.

Robertsonian Translocations   Between 3% and 5% of patients with Down syndrome at all maternal ages have Robertsonian translocations (Table 3); of these, about 50% are D;21q and 50% are G;21q. Of patients with D;21q translocations, about 50% are inherited and 50% are sporadic, whereas about 90% of G;21q are inherited and only 10% are sporadic (Table 4). The overall frequency of translocation differs among Down syndrome patients born to mothers under 30 (8%) when compared to those over 30 (1.5%) (Table 5) (Hamerton, 1971), and this simply reflects the higher frequency of Down syndrome among families in which a translocation is present and in which there is, therefore, no maternal age effect.

The advent of banding techniques has allowed us to identify the chromosomes involved in Robertsonian translocations. We can see from Table 6 that t(14q21q) is the most frequent of the t(Dq21q) types (59%) and that the t(21q21q) or i(21) occurs with a frequency of 83% among the G;21q types.

Table 4.   Types of Robertsonian translocation

Series	t(Dq21q)	t(Gq21q)	t(Dq21q) Inherited	Sporadic	t(Gq21q) Inherited	Sporadic
Hamerton (1971)	44	56	51	49	94.4	5.6
Mikkelsen (1970)						
Matsunaga and Tonomura (1972)	55.3	44.7	55	45	9.3	8.7

Data from Hamerton (1971) and Smith and Berg (1976).

Table 5. Robertsonian translocations among Down syndrome patients[a] born to mothers expressed according to maternal age

Maternal age (years)	% Robertsonian translocation
< 30	8.0
> 30	1.5

Data from Hamerton (1971, Table 5.11).

[a]$N = 1527$.

Reciprocal Translocations   A wide variety of reciprocal translocations involving chromosome 21 have been reported (see deGrouchy and Turleau, 1977; Hamerton, 1971; Smith and Berg, 1976), some of which have resulted in the birth of a child with Down syndrome, others in the birth of children with duplication or deletion of other chromosome segments. The study of such translocations has led to the assignment of 21q22 as the segment primarily responsible for the Down syndrome phenotype, whereas duplication of band q21 has a relatively normal phenotype with moderate mental retardation (Aula, Leisti, and von Koskull, 1973; Niebuhr, 1974; O'Donnell et al., 1975; Raoul et al., 1976; Wahrman et al., 1976; Williams et al., 1975). Several nonfamilial tandem translocations involving fusion of 21q centromere to telomere giving rise to the Down syndrome phenotype have been reported by several authors (see Smith and Berg, 1976, for review).

There are few data on the frequency of reciprocal translocations associated with Down syndrome. It is clear, however, that compared to the Robertsonian translocation, they are extremely rare, no such translocations being reported among 56,952 newborn infants reviewed by Hook and Hamerton (1977).

ASSOCIATIONS WITH OTHER CHROMOSOME ABNORMALITIES

Trisomy 21 or other cytogenetic variants of trisomy 21 have been shown to be associated with a wide variety of other chromosome abnormalities (see Hamerton, 1971; Smith and Berg, 1976, for reviews), and it has been suggested that such

Table 6. Chromosomes involved in Robertsonian translocations[a]

Type	%
t(14q21q)	58.5
t(13q21q)	22.0
t(15q21q)	19.5
t(21q21q)	83.3
t(21q22q)	16.6

[a]$N = 4760$.

associations may occur with a frequency greater than might be expected by chance. The best-established situation is for Klinefelter syndrome and Down syndrome, first described by Ford et al. (1959), in which the overall combined frequency based on a chance association should be 0.31×10^{-5} (Hamerton et al., 1965). Hamerton et al. observed three double trisomics in a series of 616 primary males with trisomy G, an incidence estimated at 0.53×10^{-5} (Hamerton, 1971). On the other hand, in six sex chromatin surveys of the newborn comprising 23,229 liveborn males, 47 were chromatin positive and two were double trisomics (48,XXY, G+), an incidence of 8.62×10^{-5}, or 18 times greater than the indirect estimate for the general population and 30 times higher than expected based on chance association (Taylor and Moores, 1967). Among 38,000 newborn males studied in six consecutive newborn chromosome studies, no double aneuploids were found (Hook and Hamerton, 1977). Thus, the question of whether a higher incidence of double aneuploidy is present at birth than might be expected by chance is still open.

Of greater interest than the association with other major chromosome abnormalities is the possible significance of minor variants. There have been tentative suggestions that such minor variants occur with a greater frequency than might be expected by chance among patients with Down syndrome and their families (Hamerton, 1971; Hamerton et al., 1965; Smith and Berg, 1976). A recent study in our laboratory (Wang and Hamerton, 1979) examined the C-band polymorphism of chromosomes 1, 9, and 16, and showed a significant association ($p < 0.001$) between "partial" and "total inversion" of the C-band of chromosome 9 in a group of 93 patients with Down syndrome compared to the control group, which consisted of normal consecutive babies and three groups of non-Down syndrome mentally retarded patients. One group of mentally retarded patients (patients with idiopathic mental retardation without congenital malformations) also showed a significant excess of "inversions" over controls ($p < 0.05$). The biological significance of this finding is by no means clear, and properly designed further studies are clearly needed. No other significant association was seen nor was there any change in size distribution of the C-bands studied between the three groups.

Little that is new has been presented here. It is clear, however, that a vast body of knowledge has been built up since Lejeune first demonstrated a chromosome abnormality in 1959. No well-documented exceptions to the presence of trisomy for a whole chromosome or a significant segment of chromosome 21 have been documented. These studies clearly provide a basis for future work to try and determine the mechanisms whereby the chromosome abnormality gives rise to the specific phenotype.

REFERENCES

Aula, P., Leisti, J., and von Koskull, H. 1973. Partial trisomy 21. Clin. Genet. 4:241.

Carter, C. O., Hamerton, J. L., Polani, P. E., Gunalp, A., and Weller, S. D. V. 1960. Chromosome translocation as a cause of familial mongolism. Lancet 2:678–680.

Clarke, C. M., Edwards, J. H., and Smallpiece, V. 1961. 21-trisomy/normal mosaicism in an intelligent child with some mongoloid characteristics. Lancet 2:1028–1030.

deGrouchy, J., and Turleau, C. 1977. Clinical Atlas of Human Chromosomes. John Wiley & Sons, New York.

Ford, C. E. 1961. Human chromosome mosaics. In W. M. Davidson and D. R. Smith (eds.), Human Chromosomal Abnormalities, pp. 23–27. Staples Press, London.

Ford, C. E. 1964. Selection pressure in mammalian cell populations. Symp. Int. Soc. Cell Biol. 3:27–45.

Ford, C. E. 1969. Mosaics and chimaeras. Br. Med. Bull. 25:104–109.

Ford, C. E., Jones, K. W., Miller, O. J., Mittwoch, U., Penrose, L. S., Ridler, M., and Shapiro, A. 1959. The chromosome in a patient showing both mongolism and the Klinefelter syndrome. Lancet 1:709–710.

Giraud, F., and Mattei, J.-F. 1975. Aspects épidémiologiques de la trisomie 21. [Epidemiological aspects of trisomy 21.] J. Hum. Genet. 23:1–30.

Grosse, K. P., Hopfengartner, F., and Schwanitz, G. 1971. Doppelte aneuploidie: 46,XX/45, XO/47,XX,G$^+$. Kasuistische mitteilung. Humangenetik 13:333.

Hamerton, J. L. 1971. Human Cytogenetics, Vol. 2. Academic Press, New York.

Hamerton, J. L., Giannelli, F., and Polani, P. E. 1965. Cytogenetics of Down's syndrome (mongolism). I. Data on a consecutive series of patients referred for genetic counselling and diagnosis. Cytogenetics 4:171–185.

Hook, E. B., and Hamerton, J. L. 1977. The frequency of chromosome abnormalities detected in consecutive newborn studies—Differences between studies—Results by sex and by severity of phenotypic involvement. In E. B. Hook and I. H. Porter (eds.), Population Cytogenetics: Studies in Humans, pp. 63–79. Academic Press, New York.

Jacobs, P. A., Baikie, A. G., Court Brown, W. M., and Strong, J. A. 1959. The somatic chromosomes in mongolism. Lancet 1:710.

Lejeune, J. 1959. Le mongolisme. Premier exemple d'aberration autosomique humaine. [Mongolism. First example of human autosomal aberration.] Ann. Genet. Semaine Hop. 1:41–49.

Lejeune, J., Gautier, M., and Turpin, R. 1959. Etude des chromosomes somatiques de neuf enfants mongoliens. [Study of somatic chromosomes in nine mongoloid infants.] Compt. Rend. 248:1721–1722.

Lilienfeld, A. M. 1969. Epidemiology of Mongolism. Johns Hopkins Press, Baltimore.

Matsunaga, E., and Tonomura, A. 1972. Parental age and birth weight in translocation Down's syndrome. Ann. Hum. Genet. 36:209–219.

Mikkelsen, M. 1970. A Danish survey of patients with Down's syndrome born to young mothers. Ann. N.Y. Acad. Sci. 171:370.

Mittwoch, U. 1952. The chromosome complement in a Mongolian imbecile. Ann. Eugenics 17:37.

Niebuhr, E. 1974. Down's syndrome. The possibility of a pathogenetic segment on chromosome no. 21. Humangenetik 21:99.

O'Donnell, J. J., Hall, B. D., Conte, F. A., Romanowski, J. C., and Epstein, C. J. 1975. Down's syndrome: Localization of locus to distal portion of long arm of chromosome 21. Ped. Res. Abst. 9:315.

Penrose, L. S. 1939. Maternal age, order of birth and developmental abnormalities. J. Ment. Sci. 85:1141–1150.

Penrose, L. S. 1967. Studies of mosaicism in Down's anomaly. In G. A. Jarvis (ed.), Mental Retardation. Charles C Thomas Publisher, Springfield, Ill.

Penrose, L. S., Ellis, J. R., and Delhanty, J. D. A. 1960. Chromosomal translocations in mongolism and in normal relatives. Lancet 2:409–410.

Polani, P. E., Briggs, J. H., Ford, C. E., Clarke, C. M., and Berg, J. M. 1960. A mongol girl with 46 chromosomes. Lancet 1:721–724.

Priest, J. H., Verhulst, C., and Siskin, S. 1973. Parental dermatoglyphics in Down's syndrome. A ten year study. J. Med. Genet. 10:328.

Raoul, O., Dutrillaux, B., Carpenter, S., Mallet, R., Lejeune, J. 1976. Trisomies partielles du chromosome 21 par translocation maternelle t(15;21)(q26.2;q21). Ann. Genet. 19:187–190.

Richards, B. W. 1969. Mosaic mongolism. J. Ment. Defic. Res. 13:66.

Richards, B. W. 1974. Investigation of 142 mosaic mongols and mosaic parents of mongols; cytogenetic analysis and maternal age at birth. J. Ment. Defic. Res. 18:199–208.

Rieger, R., Michaelis, A., and Green, M. M. 1976. Glossary of genetics and cytogenetics. 4th Ed. Springer-Verlag, Berlin.

Smith, G. F., and Berg, J. M. 1976. Down anomaly. 2nd Ed. Churchill-Livingstone, London.

Taylor, A. I. 1968. Cell selection *in vivo* in normal/G trisomic mosaics. Nature 219:1028.

Taylor, A. I., and Moores, E. C. 1967. A sex chromatin survey of newborn children in two London hospitals. J. Med. Genet. 4:258.

Waardenburg, P. J. 1932. Das menschliche Auge und seine Erbanlangen. Bibliog. Genet. 7.

Wahrman, J., Gostein, R., Richler, C., Goldman, B., Akstern, E., and Chaki, R. 1976. The mongoloid phenotype in man is due to trisomy of the pale G band of chromosome 21. In P. L. Pearson and K. R. Lewis (eds.), Chromosomes Today, Vol. 5. John Wiley & Sons, New York.

Wang, H. S., and Hamerton, J. L. 1979. C band polymorphisms of chromosomes 1, 9, and 16 in four subgroups of mentally retarded patients and a normal control. Hum. Genet. 51:269–275.

Williams, J. D., Summitt, R. L., Martens, P. R., and Kimbrell, R. A. 1975. Familial Down syndrome due to t(10;21) translocation: Evidence that the Down phenotype is related to trisomy of a specific segment of chromosome 21. Am. J. Hum. Genet. 27:478.

MEIOSIS

Chiasmata, Down Syndrome, and Nondisjunction
An Overview

Paul E. Polani

Chiasmata seem relevant to a number of aspects of Down syndrome but especially to the origin of trisomy 21. The following propositions can be made: 1) that normal chromosome disjunction demands pairing, which 2) is generally followed by crossing over with genetic exchange, and so by chiasma formation, 3) that maintenance of pairing between homologous chromosome segments, during the prophase of the first meiotic division to first meiotic metaphase, is essential to—although it may not be sufficient for—regular chromosome disjunction, 4) that this final maintenance of pairing generally depends on the presence of chiasmata, and 5) that in the absence of these interactions between homologues, malsegregation, nondisjunction and, at times, other chromosome, disturbances at meiotic anaphase may result.

However, it does not follow that genetic exchange and its correlates—genetically, recombination and, cytologically, chiasma formation—are absolute guarantees of regular chromosome disjunction, or are the only requirements for regular disjunction of homologous chromosomes, or of chromatids. Other processes, such as the regular function of the centromeres or the meiotic spindle, either at first or second meiotic divisions or at both, are required for regular segregation, which may also be hampered in abnormal circumstances by factors in the chromosomes that prevent their regular separation. The evidence on which these summary statements are based has been accumulated over almost three-quarters of a century from work in plant and animal genetics and cytogenetics, and it rests on these foundations rather than on direct observation of human meiosis. It follows that much that we know of human chromosome behavior and misbehavior is generally pieced together from information gleaned from other organisms and that only some pieces in the mosaic are genuinely human.

CHIASMATA IN MAN AND MICE

Many workers have studied chiasmata of human meiotic cells from males with allegedly normal spermatogenesis (Eberle, 1966; Edwards, 1970; Ferguson-Smith, 1976; Ford and Hamerton, 1956; Hultén, 1974; Hultén and Lindsten, 1970; Kjessler, 1966; Lange, Page, and Elston, 1975; Luciani, 1970; McDermott, 1973; McIlree, Tulloch, and Newsam, 1966; Skakkebaek, Bryant, and Philip, 1973).

The data suggest a mean chiasma count per cell at "diakinesis" of the human male of about 50, with averages ranging from 44 to 56, although there is significant variation between different investigators (Lange et al., 1975). Chiasma counts for individual bivalents of the human male, identified by banding, are given by Hultén (1974), and similar data have been tabulated by Page and Ferguson-Smith (Lange et al., 1975; Ferguson-Smith, 1976). Hultén's chiasmata on individual bivalents ranged from a high mean of 3.90 for chromosome 1 to a low of 1.05 for chromosome 21 (all in the long arm), with the longer acrocentrics averaging about two chiasmata per bivalent long arm. The distribution of chiasmata of meiotic chromosomes is of considerable interest and has been worked out in detail by Hultén (1974) in one human male whose 500 metaphases I and diakineses were studied and in whom 41 complete, well-banded cells were fully analyzed (Table 1). In general, chiasmata were more often distal, and especially terminal, than proximal in chromosome arms, an observation made also by McDermott (1973), who found a terminalization coefficient of about 0.60 (ranging from 0.52 to 0.72). Hultén could not determine whether there was or was not progressive terminalization from diplonema to metaphase I, but she thought, although with uncertainty, that her findings pointed in that direction. Hultén's findings suggested (not unexpectedly) the existence of an obligate chiasma also in the human male, because the shorter chromosomes had a higher mean

Table 1.   Average chiasmata per bivalent in man

Bivalent number	Females (26–49 years)[a]	Males 1 subject (86 years)[b]	Males 21 subjects (mean age 28.29 years)[c]
1–3	4.00–2.89	3.90 (1)–2.92 (3)	4.01 (1)–3.12 (3)
4–5	2.46–2.11	2.85 (5)–2.79 (4)	3.01 (4)–2.84 (5)
X	2.76		
6–12	2.22–1.67	2.74 (7)–2.21 (11)	2.65 (6)–2.28 (12)
13–15	1.55–1.45	2.05 (15)–1.85 (13)	2.02 (13)–1.87 (15)
16–18	1.55–1.34	2.16 (16)–1.92 (18)	2.04 (16)–1.92 (18)
19–20	1.22–1.11	1.94	1.85 (20)–1.82 (19)
21–22	1.11–1.00	1.22 (22)–1.05 (21)	1.31 (21)–1.17 (22)
Chiasmata/cell (range)	43.47 (32–55)(N=27)	50.61 (43–60)(N=41)	51.91 (derived from bivalents from 297 cells)

Note: Figures in italics refer to specific chromosomes by their number.
[a]Jagiello et al. (1976).
[b]Hultén (1974).
[c]Ferguson-Smith (1976).

chiasma frequency per unit chromosome length than the longer ones (in keeping with the old observations of Darlington and Dark, 1932). For example, taking an average of 1.05 chiasmata for chromosome 21, with an average haploid relative length of 1.63%, chromosome 1 should have, pro rata, 5.84 chiasmata, whereas it has 3.90. McDermott (1973) had suggested, on statistical evidence, that bi-armed chromosomes in man might have two obligatory chiasmata, one per arm. Hultén also found evidence of chiasma interference, but it did not seem to extend across the centromere of bi-armed chromosomes. She estimated the maximum differential distance of chiasma position (Mather, 1938) at about 1.63% to 1.82% of the haploid relative autosomal length (a value of almost 2.0% would represent an "unconstrained differential distance"), and she assessed the interference distance at 4.16% by considering chromosome arms where well over one chiasma could fit. It should be noted that on the whole there is no evidence of an age effect on chiasma frequency in human males (Edwards, 1970; Lange et al., 1975).

Data for the human female tend to be much more anecdotal. Chiasma frequencies are decidedly lower and variation is greater (Yuncken, quoted by Edwards, 1970; Jagiello et al., 1976). This may seem to run counter to expectation if it is accepted that chiasmata can be equated with crossing over and recombination due to crossing over (Catcheside, 1977), and that recombination frequencies, in parallel with chiasma frequencies, differ in the two sexes, as was originally proposed by Crew and Koller (1932). Recombination frequencies tend overall to be greater in the homogametic sex generally, when suitable tests have been made (see Darlington, 1931a).

For mammals, there are good data on recombination in relation to sex in the house mouse. However, even in this case, and possibly more generally, there are marked deviations in favor of the male sex that run counter to the general Haldane-Huxley rule (Dunn and Bennett, 1967). Henderson and Edwards (1968) found a similar overall lower chiasma frequency in female compared with male mice, although the effect of age complicated matters. Nevertheless, they suggested that the reciprocal relationship between what is usually a higher recombination frequency and a lower chiasma frequency in the female, compared with the male, may be explained by differences in chiasma position in the two sexes (see also Henderson, 1970). However, there is also evidence on sex differences of chiasmata in the mouse in the other direction to that reported in man and found by Henderson and Edwards (1968) in some strains of mice. Kyslíková and Forejt (1972), Lyon (1976), and Polani and Jagiello (1976) found in other strains of mice values that range from 22 to 26 in the male and from 27 to 30 in the female, but undoubtedly in some strains, of the seven or so that have been tested, the difference is minimal (Speed, 1977). However, in the mouse, evidence suggests that chiasma count depends on the stage of the cells studied, as well as on the age of the animal (Polani and Jagiello, 1976), so that only comparisons between like stages can be valid, and allowance must be made for the different ages sampled. Furthermore, in males, total chiasma counts are done and expressed over 19 autosomal bivalents, whereas in females, 20 bivalents are scored, including the X pair. Therefore, for comparative purposes, it is preferable to express chiasmata as averages per bivalent rather than per cell (Polani and Jagiello, 1976).

With age, chiasma frequency increases, if anything, in the male mouse, but in the female it falls somewhat and the strength of the effect seems strain-dependent (Henderson and Edwards, 1968; Luthardt, Palmer, and Yu, 1973; Polani and Jagiello, 1976). Incidentally, these values are for laboratory mice. In male wild mice, for example, autosomal values of 21.09 and even lower (19.57) have been observed by the author and by Searle, Berry, and Beechey (1970).

Besides the number, the distribution of chiasmata is different in the male compared with the female mouse, and there is some evidence for chiasma localization rather than randomness (Polani, 1972). Differences in chiasma localization in the two sexes is seen in grasshoppers and various other species of animals and plants (Jones, Stamford, and Perrey, 1975), and Darlington (1931a) has pointed out that when crossing over differs in the sexes, chiasmata in the heterogametic sex must be localized. Lyon (1976) reviewed genetic evidence on clustering detected by recombination and interpreted the observations as the result of nonrandomness of crossing over along chromosomes. There are marked differences in recombination frequencies for some loci and alleles between males and females, for example, on chromosome 17 (Dunn and Bennett, 1967), which suggests differences in crossover position between the sexes. To support the idea of nonrandomness of crossovers, there are suggestive correlations between chiasma localization and gene clustering, for example, on chromosome 15 (Lyon, 1976; Polani, 1972). The gene stretch involved here is near the distal third of that chromosome and centers on the *Caracul (Ca)* locus, whereas the chiasmata are almost always single and distal in position. As for the correspondence between a cytological map based on chiasmata and a genetic recombination map, the female mouse is stated to show about 25% more crossing over when an average is taken over the autosomal map (Renwick and Schulze, 1964; although see Dunn and Bennett, 1967, and especially Wallace and Mallyon, 1972, whose findings relate to chromosome 15, around the *Ca* locus). According to Renwick, among others, there is a rough correspondence between map lengths estimated genetically and cytologically from chiasma frequencies. Slizynski (1955) attributed to the male mouse an autosomal chiasma map length of 1920 cMo (but see Slizynski, 1960) and Carter estimated a genetic map length of 1620±350 cMo (Ford, 1969). More recent data suggest lower chiasma counts than those found by Slizynski in males at diakinesis (Kyslíková and Forejt, 1972; Polani and Jagiello, 1976) and in females. By correcting Carter's estimates or by using information from the linkage map of the mouse (Mouse News Letter, 1977), a reasonable correspondence between genetic map length and map length calculated from chiasma counts can be obtained. Thus the genetic autosomal map length in males can be estimated to be 1263 cMo and the autosomal diakinesis chiasma map length to be 1380 cMo; in females, the genetic map can be estimated to be 1339 cMo in length versus 1353 cMo at metaphase I from chiasmata.

For man, it has been estimated that the ratio of crossovers for chromatid segments in human females to those of human males (the so-called susceptibility ratio) is 1.4, with 95% confidence limits of between 1.04 and 1.98, or a little narrower (Renwick, 1971). Thus, given a human map length of 25 Morgan in the male, corresponding to 50 chiasmata, the female map could measure about 35 Morgan, which would correspond to some 70 chiasmata if a straight proportional comparison existed between chiasmata and recombination generally in the two sexes.

It is clear that chiasmata in the human female at least requires further investigation and more information, but perhaps it is worth noting that although the method for obtaining meiotic chromosome preparations differs considerably between human males and females, the respective techniques used in the mouse are similar to those in man, so that an artifactual bias of chiasma counts between men and women seems unlikely in the light of the findings in male and female mice by some workers. Naturally, more data are wanted, in parallel, on genetically assessed crossover (recombination) differences.

NONDISJUNCTION AND TRISOMY IN MAN

Information on the parental source of the primary nondisjunction that leads to trisomy 21 has been circumstantial, but since the first delineation of the clinical syndrome it had been observed that Down syndrome children tended to appear late in families. By the 1930s the importance of maternal age, as opposed to the correlated effects of paternal age and of parity, had been established statistically and, except for an exiguous minority of cases that were attributed to a paternal age effect (although not one that caused primary trisomy), there the matter stood. The discovery of the autosomal primary trisomy of Down syndrome in 1959 led automatically to attributing its origin to nondisjunction at oogenesis while the centric fusion (or interchange) trisomy was shown to have an origin independent of maternal age (Polani et al., 1960). The topic concerning primary trisomy 21 was reopened by the statistical work of Stene and Stene (1977) and Stene et al. (1977), who claimed that a proportion of Down syndrome births were dependent on the age of the father and that the risk increased significantly after age 55. Erickson (1978), using a different statistical approach, concluded that a paternal age effect, independent of the age of his partner, was not demonstrable in his large sample. However, his statistical approach and sample have been criticized by Stene and Stene (1978). No evidence is to hand on age-related meiotic anomalies in the male mouse, at least (Leonard and Leonard, 1975). Since 1970, mitotic studies using banding techniques and exploiting the existing polymorphic heteromorphisms of human chromosomes have led to a direct and individual approach to the problem of chromosome source of the primary trisomic set—given some reasonable assumptions on the position of crossovers in chromosome 21. Thus, in 1973 two reports of the origin of trisomy 21 through paternal nondisjunction appeared (Sasaki and Hara, 1973; Uchida, 1973). Subsequent reports on a total of 55 informative matings attributed a paternal origin of the trisomy to 18 (or about one-third) and a maternal source to the rest (Bott, Sekhon, and Lubs, 1975; Hara and Sasaki, 1975; Mikkelsen, Hallberg, and Poulsen, 1976; Wagenbichler et al., 1976; and cases quoted by Erickson, 1978; Uchida, 1973), and there are other, more anecdotal, reports that follow the same trend. The data on 62 examples have been summarized by Langenbeck et al. (1976). The findings suggest that nondisjunctional errors are equally frequent at either meiotic division. However, these deductions are biased not only because informative families are relatively few and may not be representative of the total situation but because it is easier to obtain conclusive information from errors occurring at second meiotic division when only one parental chromosome 21 can be distinguished. Incidentally, a similar type of analysis was undertaken with trisomy 16 (Lauritsen and Friedrich, 1976); the results suggested errors mostly at first, but also at second, meiotic division, more often during oogenesis than spermatogenesis. Robinson (1977) used a different approach, based on fluorescence heteromorphism of chromosome 21 in Down syndrome subjects. Her results fit almost perfectly a model with a 100% first meiotic nondisjunction, but a second model of 50% at first and 50% at second division has only one-thirtieth of the probability of the first model.

Before considering the possible mechanisms relating primary nondisjunction of chromosome 21 to advancing maternal years, and more especially to errors of chromosome segregation at the first meiotic division, we should consider a fundamental question: whether all human chromosomes are equally prone to nondisjunction. Is there or is there not something special about the tendency to nondisjunction of chromosome 21? The best approach is to consider the different autosomal trisomies detected among spontaneously aborted embryos and fetuses. Because of selective mortality the data on survivors represent only the tip of the iceberg of human autosome, and some sex chromosome, anomalies. Even the data on abortuses are suspect and, unfortunately, scanty. They are suspect because we have to rely on cultured material and thus on the proliferative ability of chromosomally unbalanced cells that may be uneven, as between different autosomal trisomies, but more especially because we can only detect anomalies that are compatible with a relatively prolonged pregnancy, albeit short in absolute terms. For example, we think that the deficiencies of autosomal monosomies and of XYY triploidy may be accounted for from these sources of bias. The other problem is that there are few data, because only relatively recently has chromosome banding been applied to the identification of individual trisomies.

About 30% or more of spontaneously aborted fetuses are chromosomally abnormal, and over 50% of these are trisomic for an autosome more frequently than for a sex chromosome. Carr (1971) suggested that abortuses with autosomal trisomy of the smaller chromosomes were found more frequently than those of the larger ones. Evidence summarized by Creasy (1977) and by Boué and Boué (1978) confirms this but shows that many large autosomes may be found to be trisomic (Table 2). It suggests, in addition, that among the smaller autosomes there may be some oddities. First, trisomy of chromosome 16, a small but not very small autosome, is by far the most common of all trisomies, and yet trisomy of chromosome 17, of rather similar size, would appear to be exceptionally rare. Trisomy 16 may have an estimated frequency of between 0.9% and 1.5% of all conceptions. Second, all the acrocentrics are relatively frequently represented among the trisomics, but it seems that chromosome 21, the smallest autosome of man, takes the leading position in this set of autosomes—indeed, among all autosomes excluding 16. Trisomy 21 may have a frequency of 0.45% to 0.65% of all conceptions. Furthermore, it is these very acrocentric autosomes whose primary trisomies seem more strongly correlated with parental age—or maternal age, as evidence from primary trisomy 21 survivors would suggest.

Table 2.   Trisomies and double trisomies ($N = 318$)

Trisomic chromosome	%	Trisomic chromosome	%
1		14	7.2
2	4.0	15	8.2
3	0.6	16	29.6
4	2.2	17	
5	0.3	18	5.3
6	0.3	19	0.3
7	3.5	20	1.6
8	4.4	21	9.1
9	2.2	22	10.1
10	2.5	XXX	0.6
11	0.3	XXY	0.6
12	0.9	XXY + autosome	0.9
13	3.5	Double autosome	1.6

Adapted from Creasy (1977).

PRIMARY NONDISJUNCTION: ITS CAUSES AND MECHANISMS

Primary nondisjunction is mostly attributed to errors at first meiotic division, although we have seen that errors at second meiotic division seem to occur in man as they do in other species. Often, but not invariably, errors occur during oogenesis that are not infrequently related to advancing maternal age. A common mechanism for the first meiotic errors is chromosome asynapsis or desynapsis. Briefly, desynapsis may follow regular chiasma formation, but asynapsis is an achiasmate condition that results from failure of chiasma formation during the zygotene/pachytene stage when the primary event (crossing over between pairs of homologous chromosomes) occurs (see, e.g., Henderson, 1970). It should be recalled that diplonema had been suggested by Janssens (1909) as the stage when chiasma formation occurs. He subsequently (1924) suggested that it could happen between zygonema and diplonema. Darlington (1929a), after some hesitation, narrowed crossing over and chiasma formation to pachynema and, also, clearly identified the essential feature of partial chiasmatypy (1930a, 1931b).

Darlington (1929a) was the first to suggest, although perhaps not very explicitly, that homologous chromosomes must be tied together by chiasmata at diakinesis in order to segregate at first meiotic metaphase (the mechanical function of chiasmata; see also Darlington, 1930b; 1935). The point was made very clearly by Dobzhansky (1933) and Mather (1938). It is envisaged that the homologues of a bivalent need at least one chiasma for normal chromosome segregation and that this obligatory or compulsory chiasma (Darlington, 1939a; Mather, 1938) is an essential quality of chiasmate organisms, or sexes, or, at the very least, of most bivalents in a given chiasmate species.

Disregarding a genotypic origin of the achiasmate state (with or without asynapsis), as in some of the meiotic mutants described in animals and plants (Baker and Hall, 1976; Parker, 1975; Riley, 1966; Riley and Law, 1965), we turn to consider environmental effects responsible for asynapsis or desynapsis. Two main sets of environmental influences have received attention: age and temperature, the effects of which were noticed in the early days of *Drosophila* genetics. In both cases the influence of these environmental variables was observed genetically on recombination rather than cytologically on chiasmata. Aging resulted in a decline of crossing over in all chromosomes, in segments near the centromere (Bridges, 1927, in ad hoc experiments; Grell, 1966, during experiments on temperature effects), but there were cases when the situation was not necessarily as simple as this (Redfield, 1966). Bridges (1915), in the course of linkage and interference studies, first observed that in *Drosophila* females the frequency of crossing over declined with brood (i.e., age) within the first week of life, and it has been hypothesized that the change in recombination may correlate with hormonal changes during pupation (King, 1970). That effects of age on nondisjunction interact with temperature has been established, and these effects have pointed to involvement of the later stages of the meiotic prophase (Tokunaga, 1970a, b). Temperature by itself, either raised or lowered, could increase meiotic recombination in segments of some chromosomes (Grell, 1966; Plough, 1917, 1921). Henderson (1970), whose work is also relevant to this discussion, noticed that chiasma frequency fell in some of his temperature experiments with grasshoppers while univalents formed in proportion to the drop in chiasma frequency, and that the impaired chiasma formation tended to affect particularly the association of the smaller and medium-size rather than the larger chromosomes. Conversely, as chiasma frequency increased in some other experiments, it was especially the larger and at times the medium chromosomes that managed to fit in more chiasmata.

If we return now to man and take the data on abortuses at their face value, the findings suggest that it is the smaller autosomes that are more frequently found to be trisomic, although there is a small proportion of abortuses trisomic for the larger ones. Among all primary trisomies, it is especially the acrocentrics (both the shorter and the longer ones) that are often involved, and they seem to show the more striking maternal age effect; this, in turn, incriminates oogenesis. In a general outline it is possible to formulate two sets of hypotheses of the mechanism of maternal age-related nondisjunction:

I.   Chiasma frequency (and recombination) is unaffected by age but, with age:
   A.   Desynapsis is precocious
      1.   Progressive terminalization
      2.   Loss of "chiasma binder"
   B.   The nucleolar cycle is affected and interferes with disjunction
      1.   Metabolic effect
      2.   Virus infection
   C.   Organelles of chromosome movement are affected
II. Chiasma frequency (and recombination) is decreased with age:
   A.   Primary asynapsis
      1.   Cause unspecified
      2.   ?Abnormal nucleolar cycle and interference with synapsis
   B.   Normal synapsis, but desynapsis due to primary chiasma failure

Either nondisjunction in some way follows normal crossing over and recombination and, as most workers accept, corresponding chiasma formation, or it affects non-crossover chromosomes, i.e., homologues that from the beginning were not held together by chiasmata. In either case we may feel that some special explanation is required for the apparent, somewhat selective, proneness of the acrocentric chromosomes to nondisjunction—although, as we have seen, their susceptibility is only relative, and the evidence on it is far from solid. In line with the first type of hypothesis, the nondisjunctional fate of the smaller autosomes especially would result from a premature desynapsis (one that occurred before metaphase I but well after pachynema/diplonema) of homologues that had recombined normally. This type of desynapsis can be viewed as a failure of chiasmata to perform their function during the long postdiplotene, or dictyotene, period of female mammalian meiosis, and thus it is seen as a premature lapse of the mechanism that binds recombinant chromosomes during this time. Precocious desynapsis could result from environmental effects, connected with aging, that specifically did not affect synapsis and chiasma formation. Such a divided effect from the environment on chiasma formation or on maintenance is not improbable in that there is a dual genetic control for these two properties of chiasmata, the mechanical and the recombinational (Maguire, 1978). This type of desynaptic behavior is akin, but only in its ultimate effects, to a terminalization hypothesis—a suggestion put forward by Slizynski (1960) to explain maternal age-related nondisjunction. Views on terminalization, a variable phenomenon first stressed by Darlington (1929b, 1931b; Darlington and Janaki-Ammal, 1932), differ (see, e.g., White, 1959, 1973) and its importance has been questioned (Henderson, 1969); particularly, the general applicability of the phenomenon to all or even many species has been denied. Jones (1978) investigated this problem in pollen mother cells of rye meiotic chromosomes that, because they have Giemsa C-band-positive telomeres, looked promising for such a study. He concluded that contraction of telomeres and stretching of bivalents may lead to a terminal position of distal chiasmata, but that it is likely that no "real" terminalization occurs. He referred to this terminal position as pseudoterminalization, but it is difficult to know whether rye telomeres are a general or a special case and thus whether a general extrapolation to other organisms is valid. At any rate, for many writers, terminal chiasmata would generally not be the result of terminalization but instead would be the expression of a terminal localization ad initio. Furthermore, it has been generally held that in species with variably sized chromosomes and hence with meiotic bivalents, some of which have many, others few (or even only one) chiasmata, terminalization affects classically only the distal chiasma of multichiasmate bivalents or the only chiasma of the smallest bivalents of the set (Darlington, 1939b; Mather, 1938; White, 1973). Thus, if aging is to be construed as leading to a progressive failure of the function of chiasmata in tying together the elements of the chromosomal bivalents whose chromatids had originally recombined in a normal way, it might be appropriate to consider that aging promotes the decay of a "chiasma binder" (Maguire, 1974) rather than leading to a progressive terminalization. Such a view would also conform better than classical terminalization with the observed correlation of trisomy of the longer autosomes with maternal age, a correlation that seems not as strong as in the case of the acrocentric autosomes. It would be inappropriate to leave the topic of terminalization without special reference to the classical views on telomeres (Muller, 1938) and the recent renewed molecular interest in them. Cavalier-Smith (1974) has put forward evidence on a special organization of their DNA, and ideas on their special position in chromosome organization and function are being strengthened by considering their relevance to chromosome attachment to the nuclear membrane (Comings and Okada, 1970; Hughes-Schrader, 1943) and by the discovery of other features that point to their unusual makeup (Dancis and Holmquist, 1977; Dutrillaux et al., 1977). Thus it is worth considering whether terminalization may be a special property related to the telomeres as special chromosomal organelles.

It is characteristic of this first hypothesis on the mechanisms of nondisjunction that the nondisjunctional chromosomes are usually recombinant. A good example of this dissociation, namely, independence of nondisjunction from exchange, is when nondisjunction is induced by x-rays (for example, in the X chromosome of *Drosophila melanogaster;* Day and Grell, 1966), but it should be noted that following x-irradiation nondisjunction seems to occur at both meiotic divisions (Anderson, 1931). Yet radiation affects oocytes during early prophase (Kiriazis and Abrahamson, 1968; Traut, 1970). Thus the effect may be remote in time, especially because radiation may cause nondisjunction by disturbing the spindle apparatus (Alberman et al., 1972a; Traut, 1971) or by affecting a specific chromosome organelle (Grell, Muñoz, and Kirschbaum, 1966). At any rate, it is clear that the mechanism of nondisjunction following radiation does not depend mostly on failed synapsis or premature desynapsis. Nevertheless, radiation-induced nondisjunction seems important to the origin of trisomy, and it appears that low-dose radiation is an environmental cause of nondisjunction in man (Uchida and Curtis, 1961). Experiments in the mouse (Uchida and Freeman, 1977; Uchida and Lee, 1974) support this, and the studies suggest an interaction between radiation and maternal age in the origin of numerical chromosome anomalies (Alberman et al., 1972a, b). First, it must be stressed that our calculations, which are only rough approximations, suggest that radiation can only be a relatively rare cause of maternal age-related nondisjunction and, second, that not all surveys have detected a radiation effect (discussed in Alberman et al., 1972a, b). Equally instructive with respect to recombination is the nondisjunction (as opposed to chromosome loss) at first meiotic division (Davis, 1969) caused by *claret-nondisjunctional* in *Drosophila* or that caused at second meiotic division in both sexes by the meiotic mutant *mei S322a* (Davis, 1971; Lindsley et al., 1968; Sandler et al., 1968), in both of which recombination occurs normally in the nondisjunctional chromosomes.

The second general hypothesis is that nondisjunction related to aging results from the production of oocytes with reduced crossing over and with lower chiasma frequencies. As a result of the decrease in number of chiasmata, it is particularly the smaller autosomes of the set that would be expected to suffer. The average number of chiasmata in chromosomes 21 to 22 of the human female is between 1.00 and 1.11, and in the large acrocentrics it is between 1.45 and 1.55 (Jagiello et al., 1976; Table 1). Within this view of decreased chiasma frequencies between bivalents of oocytes of older women, there are two possible mechanisms to be considered: either a primary asynapsis of the chromosomes that will eventually be involved in nondisjunction at first meiotic division, or a normal synapsis to start with but desynapsis when chromosome attraction lapses because there are no chiasmata to keep the homologous chromosomes paired. This lapse of attraction is reported to take place at the end of pachynema. So here, in contrast with desynapsis in the first general hypothesis, the origin of desynapsis is in a primary achiasmate association of bivalents during early meiotic prophase and right to the end of pachynema. To distinguish between primary failure of chiasma formation (and crossing over) and some form of lapsed association of normally crossover chromosomes, genetic evidence is required. There is no direct evidence on whether trisomic chromosomes are recombinant in mammals, but it is suggested that recombination in some chromosomal segments of the female mouse may decrease with her age (Bodmer, 1961; Reid and Parsons, 1963), in obvious contrast to nondisjunction (Gosden, 1973; Yamamoto, Endo, and Watanabe, 1973). However, the evidence on recombination is conflicting, and some data have shown an age effect in the male (Fisher, 1949). Wallace, MacSwiney, and Edwards (1976) made a special study of recombination in relation to parental age in the mouse. Considering different linked genes in different chromosomes, they could find no consistent relationship between recombination and maternal age, although fluctuations of recombination occurred in old female, but not in old male, mice. Scanty human data have shown no change in the proportion of recombinant children with age of the mother (Elston, Lange, and Namboodiri, 1976), but they have hinted at change with age of the father. Data on color blindness and XXY Klinefelter syndrome had suggested to Stern (1959) a possible explanation for the frequency of color vision defects in these males. Assuming, in line with general experience of nondisjunction, that the origin of the error was at the first meiotic division of oogenesis (on the grounds of the maternal age effect on the origin of XXYs), the frequency of color blindness implied free recombination between the *deutan/protan* loci and the centromere of the X chromosomes. Thus, in this trisomy the nondisjunctional X chromosomes would be recombinant. On the other hand, mixed nondisjunction, both paternal and maternal, at first and second meiotic divisions, could fit the color blindness findings even if there were no recombination between the chromosomes at oogenesis in that proportion of XXYs who are of maternal first meiotic origin.

We have already noted that the meiotic prophase of female mammals is a long drawn out phase because it is generally accepted that in most cases its early stages up to diplotene occur in utero or very soon after birth (Ohno et al., 1961) and that subsequently the oocyte becomes dormant before completing its maturation and proceeding through the first meiotic division shortly before, and in readiness for, fertilization. This process follows the stocking up of the embryonic ovary with all its primordial germ cells (Zuckerman, 1951, 1956, 1960, 1965) of extra-embryonic origin (Mintz, 1959, 1960; Peters, 1970; Witschi, 1948). It is also generally agreed that crossing over occurs during zygonema/pachynema and therefore that chiasmata are established during intrauterine life or soon thereafter, in the early postnatal period. Thus another view is possible of asynapsis (or desynapsis) without chiasma formation if these facts are kept in mind. In contrast with the idea that nondisjunction, as related to aging of the female, may be the result of events that affect the primary oocyte during its long, dormant, postnatal phase, Henderson and Edwards (1968) put forward a complex "production line" hypothesis of mammalian oogenesis linking sequential oocyte production with differences in crossing over, chiasmata, and recombination. It is based on observations in mice that the frequency of chiasmata at first meiotic division drops with advancing age while the proportion of chromosome univalents increases, and on the facts about the meiotic prophase of female mammals, already summarized. The resulting asynaptic univalents (or desynaptic when, after pairing, the attraction forces lapse and there are no chiasmata to keep the bivalents as "dyads") allegedly would undergo random segregation at first meiotic division, producing often unbalanced secondary oocytes.

Henderson and Edwards further made the essential postulates that, first, oogonia that were committed to meiosis earlier in intrauterine life had more chiasmata than those that entered meiotic prophase later and, second, that compared with these, they were released from the ovary sooner after puberty. Because, theoretically, in utero chiasma frequency was lower in the oocytes destined for a release in later life, and because therefore univalents were more frequent in them, the net result to be expected was an increased frequency of trisomic zygotes produced in a manner positively correlated with the age of the female. Thus, whereas nondisjunction that follows aging in the standard, or first, hypothesis may well be independent of recombination, so that the nondisjunctional chromosomes are as often recombinant as are those that disjoin normally, the prenatal aging hypothesis hinges on a relationship between age of the mother and decreasing crossing over in those oocytes that are released at progressively advancing age. If the hypothesis is correct and assuming that the univalents are true univalents, subject to their customary abnormal behavior, it is anticipated that the errors of first meiotic division would be reflected in aneuploidy, detectable at second meiotic metaphase. However, experiments showed that the great majority of the univalents observed at first meiotic division in older female mice were not true univalents, although the reduction of chiasma frequency with age was confirmed (Polani and Jagiello, 1976). Nevertheless, these experiments are not a direct test of the "production line hypothesis," which at present still hinges on a decreased frequency of chiasmata in the oocytes of older females. Henderson and Edwards (1968) thought that chiasmata were not less easily discernible, nor that they were "terminalized," nor that they had otherwise decreased in frequency between the time of their perinatal formation in the primary oocytes and when the oocytes are about to be released in later life. Clearly, a test of the hypothesis is the detection of reduced chiasmata and increased univalents in diplotene cells arising later in utero compared with the earlier maturing ones.

Jagiello and Fang (1979) made important observations in their comparison of 16-day with 18-day fetal mouse diplotene cells, which confirmed the decrease in chiasma frequency in the later cells compared to those found earlier and the increased proportion of univalents. Cytological observations apart, there is some (albeit meager) support for the hypothesis from data on recombination, as we have seen. Although this information should, in principle, give unequivocal answers on changes of recombination frequencies, or their absences, in the progeny of animals derived from older mothers and should relate such changes to the decreased chiasma frequency with age, the observations on a reciprocal relationship, in some mouse strains, between chiasmata and recombination frequencies of males and females (Henderson, 1970; Speed, 1977) calls for caution if what is expected is a *strict* correspondence between a decrease of chiasmata and a drop in recombination frequency. Differential chiasma location in the two sexes (Lyon, 1976; Polani, 1972) and the change in location with age and with chiasma frequency in females (Speed, 1977) also must be kept in mind. The ideal way of arriving at a conclusion, in the experimental situation, on the strength of recombination data would be to study the influence of maternal age on recombination not in a saltatory fashion but along the whole length of more than one densely mapped mouse chromosome.

Returning to man, we have to consider the possibility that acrocentrics may be more commonly involved in nondisjunction, and in a seemingly more strongly age-related manner, than other chromosomes of similar length, and that this may happen for special reasons in addition to their basic low chiasma frequency. The additional feature of these chromosomes that ought to be considered is the presence of the nucleolar organizers in their short arms. It has been suggested, although unclearly, that either the presence of nucleolar remnants in the meiotic prophase may interfere with pairing and thus chiasma formation, especially between the smaller homologous acrocentrics, or that the persistence of the nucleolus during the long meiotic prophase may so alter the nucleolus as to prevent its breakdown, with consequent nondisjunction of the chromosomes it attaches to (Polani et al., 1960). It has further been suggested that nucleolar persistence with consequent nondisjunction of the acrocentric autosomes may be a virus-dependent phenomenon in some cases (Evans, 1967). Obviously, the nucleolus could only interfere with synapsis during zygonema/pachynema. Such an interference would have to be prenatal so that aging would of necessity have to involve a production line system of oogenesis. Furthermore, it is doubtful whether such interference could be a reality because human male pachynema analysis, when nucleoli are clearly visible and sometimes large, gives no evidence of interference with accurate synapsis as judged from the formation of normal synaptonemal complexes in the acrocentric autosomes (Holm and Rasmussen, 1977). By contrast, undue persistence of the nucleolus might conceivably be responsible for nondisjunction if persistence depended on age or on environmental influences that tended to accumulate with the passing of time (for example, radiation or virus infection). At any rate, any hypothesis involving the nucleolus must obviously revolve around the behavior of the nucleolus through female mammalian meiosis, details of which are as yet insufficiently unraveled (Stahl et al., 1975; Wolgemuth-Jarashow, Jagiello, and Henderson, 1977).

Finally, the observations of Henderson and Edwards (1968) and Speed (1977) on CBA mice could be very relevant to the human situation. If extrapolated to man, the suggestion would be that women who genetically tend to have low chiasma oocytes (chiasma frequency control being at least in part genetic) may end up by having even fewer at advanced ages, and thus would be more prone to nondisjunction. In this way there would also be an answer to the increased risk of nondisjunction in women with a previous trisomic pregnancy (Alberman, this volume). Carrying the analogy further, these women should also tend to have a reduced fertile life.

SUMMARY

Evidence in the literature suggests that in the human female the chiasma frequency of oocytes at first meiotic division is considerably lower than in the human male, and some data in mice suggest a similar trend that is strain-dependent. This contrasts with evidence, both in man and mouse, that females tend to have higher recombination frequencies than males. The problems of comparing different sexes, and possibly different cell stages, are discussed and data suggest, although not conclusively, that at least in some chromosomal stretches the frequency of recombination decreases with age of the female. This and other facts suggest that recombination is nonrandom along the length of chromosomes and that crossover positions differ in the sexes and, at least in females, may change with age.

Evidence from spontaneous abortion suggests that nondisjunction may affect all autosomes, although with variable frequencies. It seems that the acrocentric autosomes are more frequently involved than the other autosomes and their trisomy seems to be more strongly maternal age-dependent. Thus their nondisjunction must be attributed often to oogenesis. Recent data on trisomy 21 and trisomy 16 confirm that the source of nondisjunction is at first meiotic division of the mother, but they also show that there is a sizable contribution of nondisjunctional events from the father's side and that both meiotic divisions can be involved.

As for the mechanisms of maternal age-related nondisjunction, two sets of hypotheses hold the ground. In the first, nondisjunction is seen as an abnormality of meiosis caused by aging, postnatally, of the oocyte, with progressive terminalization of chiasmata and failure of chiasmata to hold the bivalents together to diakinesis, and involving especially the smaller bivalents; or desynapsis due to aging of a chiasma binder. Environmental effects may also impinge upon chromosome movement and their organelles. There are also other possibilities that stress involvement of all acrocentrics preferentially and would be related to age-dependent disruption of the nucleolar cycle. In these hypotheses, the nondisjunctional chromosomes should have normal gene recombination frequency. In the second set of hypotheses, on the other hand, the primary error would result from a relative failure of chiasma formation. This may lead to asynapsis at zygonema or desynapsis when the attraction between homologous chromosomes lapses, at diplonema. Because the meiotic prophase takes place in utero in most female mammals, including humans, the stage for nondisjunction should be set before birth. If it is, then the influence of maternal age on trisomy requires an explanation based inter alia on sequential oocyte release from the ovary after puberty and thus leads to a "production line" hypothesis, as postulated by Henderson and Edwards (1968). Such a hypothesis based on a relative deficiency of chiasmata could explain the preferential nondisjunction of the smaller autosomes and should be supported by good data on genetic recombination, which so far are inadequate, even in experimental mammals.

REFERENCES

Alberman, E., Polani, P. E., Fraser Roberts, J. A., Spicer, C. C., Elliott, M., and Armstrong, E. 1972a. Parental exposure to X-irradiation and Down's syndrome. Ann. Hum. Genet. 36:195–208.

Alberman, E., Polani, P. E., Fraser Roberts, J. A., Spicer, C. C., Elliott, M., Armstrong, E., and Dhadial, R. K. 1972b. Parental X-irradiation and chromosome constitution in their spontaneously aborted foetuses. Ann. Hum. Genet. 36:185–194.

Anderson, E. G. 1931. The constitution of the primary exceptions obtained after X-ray treatment of Drosophila. Genetics 16:386–396.

Baker, B. S., and Hall, J. C. 1976. Meiotic mutants: Genetic control of meiotic recombination and chromosome segregation. In M. Ashburner and E. Novitski (eds.), The Genetics and Biology of Drosophila, 1a, pp. 251–434. Academic Press, New York.

Bodmer, W. F. 1961. Effects of maternal age on the incidence of congenital abnormalities in mouse and man. Nature 190:1134–1135.

Bott, C. E., Sekhon, G. S., and Lubs, H. A. 1975. Unexpected high frequency of paternal origin of trisomy 21 (abstr.). Am. J. Hum. Genet. 27:20A.

Boué, A., and Boué, J. 1978. Chromosome anomalies associated with fetal malformations. In J. B. Scrimgeour (ed.), Towards the Prevention of Fetal Malformation, pp. 49–65. Edinburgh University Press, Edinburgh.

Bridges, C. B. 1915. A linkage variation in Drosophila. J. Exp. Zool. 19:1–21.

Bridges, C. B. 1927. The relation of the age of the female to crossing over in the third chromosome of Drosophila melanogaster. J. Gen. Physiol. 8:689–700.

Carr, D. H. 1971. Genetic basis of abortion. In H. L. Roman, L. M. Sandler, and A. Campbell (eds.), Annual Review of Genetics, Vol. 5, pp. 65–80. Annual Reviews, Palo Alto, Calif.

Catcheside, D. G. 1977. The genetics of recombination. In K. R. Lewis and B. John (eds.), Genetics—Principles and Perspectives: A Series of Texts, Vol. 2, pp. 89–91. Edward Arnold, London.

Cavalier-Smith, T. 1974. Palindromic base sequences and replication of eukaryote chromosome ends. Nature 250:467–470.

Comings, D. E., and Okada, T. A. 1970. Association of chromatin fibers with the annuli of the nuclear membrane. Exp. Cell Res. 62:293–302.

Creasy, M. R. 1977. The cytogenetics of early human fetuses. Doctoral thesis, University of London, London.

Crew, F. A. E., and Koller, P. C. 1932. The sex incidence of chiasma frequency and genetical crossing-over in the mouse. J. Genet. 26:359–383.

Dancis, B. M., and Holmquist, G. P. 1977. Fusion model of telomere replication and its implications for chromosomal rearrangements. In A. de la Chappelle and M. Sorsa (eds.), Chromosomes Today, Vol. 6, pp. 95–104. Proceedings of the Sixth International Chromosome Conference held in Helsinki, Finland, August 29–31, 1977. Elsevier/North-Holland Biomedical Press, Amsterdam.

Darlington, C. D. 1929a. Chromosome behaviour and structural hybridity in the Tradescantiae. J. Genet. 21:207–286.

Darlington, C. D. 1929b. II. Aneuploid hyacinths. J. Genet. 21:17–56.

Darlington, C. D. 1930a. A cytological demonstration of "genetic" crossing-over. Proc. Roy. Soc. B 107:50–59.

Darlington, C. D. 1930b. Chromosome studies in Fritillaria. III. Chiasma formation and chromosome pairing in Fritillaria imperialis. Cytologia 2:37–55.

Darlington, C. D. 1931a. Meiosis in diploid and tetraploid Primula sinensis. J. Genet. 24: 65–96.

Darlington, C. D. 1931b. Meiosis. Biol. Rev. 6:221–264.

Darlington, C. D. 1935. Crossing-over and chromosome disjunction. Nature 136:835.

Darlington, C. D. 1939a. Evolution of Genetic Systems. Oliver & Boyd, Edinburgh. p. 46.

Darlington, C. D. 1939b. Evolution of Genetic Systems. Oliver & Boyd, Edinburgh. p. 27.

Darlington, C. D., and Dark, S. O. S. 1932. The origin and behaviour of chiasmata. II. *Stenobothrus parallelus.* Cytologia 3:169–185.

Darlington, C. D., and Janaki-Ammal, E. K. 1932. The origin and behaviour of chiasmata. I. Diploid and tetraploid *Tulipa.* Botan. Gazette 93:296–312.

Davis, B. K. 1971. Genetic analysis of a meiotic mutant resulting in precocious sister-centromere separation in *Drosophila melanogaster.* Mol. Gen. Genet. 113:251–272.

Davis, D. G. 1969. Chromosome behaviour under the influence of claret-nondisjunctional in *Drosophila melanogaster.* Genetics 61:577–594.

Day, J. W., and Grell, R. F. 1966. Radiation-induced non-disjunction and loss of chromosomes in *Drosophila melanogaster* females. II. Effects of exchange and structural heterozygosity. Mutat. Res. 3:503–509.

Dobzhansky, T. 1933. Studies on chromosome conjugation. II. The relation between crossing-over and disjunction of chromosomes. Z. Indukt. Abstamm. Vererb. 64:269–309.

Dunn, L. C., and Bennett, D. 1967. Sex differences in recombination of linked genes in animals. Genet. Res. 9:211–220.

Dutrillaux, B., Aurias, A., Couturier, J., Croquette, M. F., and Viegas-Pequignot, E. 1977. Multiple telomeric fusions and chain configurations in human somatic chromosomes. In A. de la Chappelle and M. Sorsa (eds.), Chromosomes Today, Vol. 6, pp. 37–44. Proceedings of the Sixth International Chromosome Conference held in Helsinki, Finland, August 29–31, 1977. Elsevier/North-Holland Biomedical Press, Amsterdam.

Eberle, P. 1966. Die Chromosomenstruktur des Menschen in Mitosis und Meiosis. [Human chromosome structure in mitosis and meiosis.] Gustav Fischer Verlag, Stuttgart.

Edwards, J. H. 1970. The operation of selection. In P. A. Jacobs, W. H. Price, and P. Law (eds.), Human Population Cytogenetics, pp. 241–262. Pfizer Medical Monographs, Vol. 5. Edinburgh University Press, Edinburgh.

Elston, R. C., Lange, K., and Namboodiri, K. K. 1976. Age trends in human chiasma frequencies and recombination fractions. II. Method for analyzing recombination fractions and applications to the ABO: Nail-Patella linkage. Am. J. Hum. Genet. 28:69–76.

Erickson, J. D. 1978. Down syndrome, paternal age, maternal age and birth order. Ann. Hum. Genet. 41:289–298.

Evans, H. J. 1967. The nucleolus, virus infection, and trisomy in man. Nature 214:361–363.

Ferguson-Smith, M. A. 1976. Meiosis in the human male. In P. L. Pearson and K. R. Lewis (eds.), Chromosomes Today, Vol. 5, pp. 33–41. John Wiley & Sons, New York.

Fisher, R. A. 1949. A preliminary linkage test with *Agouti* and *undulated* mice. Heredity 3:229–241.

Ford, C. E. 1969. Meiosis in mammals. In K. Benirschke (ed.), Comparative Mammalian Cytogenetics, pp. 91–106. Proceedings of an International Conference at Dartmouth Medical School, Hanover, New Hampshire, July 29–August 2, 1968. Springer-Verlag, Berlin.

Ford, C. E., and Hamerton, J. L. 1956. The chromosomes of man. Nature 178:1020–1023.

Gosden, R. G. 1973. Chromosomal anomalies of preimplantation mouse embryos in relation to maternal age. J. Reprod. Fertil. 35:351–354.

Grell, R. F. 1966. The meiotic origin of temperature-induced crossovers in *Drosophila melanogaster* females. Genetics 54:411–421.

Grell, R. F., Muñoz, E. R., and Kirschbaum, W. F. 1966. Radiation-induced non-disjunction and loss of chromosomes in *Drosophila melanogaster* females. I. The effect of chromosome size. Mutat. Res. 3:494–502.

Hara, Y., and Sasaki, M. 1975. A note on the origin of extra chromosomes in trisomies 13 and 21. Proc. Jap. Acad. 51:293–299.

Henderson, S. A. 1969. Chromosome pairing, chiasmata and crossing-over. In A. Lima-de-Faria (ed.), Handbook of Molecular Cytology, pp. 326–357. North-Holland Research Monographs: Frontiers of Biology, Vol. 15. North-Holland Publishing Co., Amsterdam.

Henderson, S. A. 1970. The time and place of meiotic crossing-over. In H. L. Roman, L. M. Sandler, and A. Campbell (eds.), Annual Review of Genetics, Vol. 4, pp. 295–324. Annual Reviews, Palo Alto, Calif.

Henderson, S. A., and Edwards, R. G. 1968. Chiasma frequency and maternal age in mammals. Nature 218:22–28.

Holm, P. B., and Rasmussen, S. W. 1977. Human meiosis. I. The human pachytene karyotype analyzed by three dimensional reconstruction of the synaptonemal complex. Carlsberg Res. Commun. 42:283–324.

Hughes-Schrader, S. 1943. Polarization, kinetochore movements, and bivalent structure in the meiosis of male mantids. Biol. Bull. 85:265–300.

Hultén, M. 1974. Chiasma distribution at diakinesis in the normal human male. Hereditas 76:55–78.

Hultén, M., and Lindsten, J. 1970. The behavior of structural aberrations at male meiosis. Information from man. In P. A. Jacobs, W. H. Price, and P. Law (eds.), Human Population Cytogenetics, pp. 23–61. Pfizer Medical Monographs, Vol. 5. Edinburgh University Press, Edinburgh.

Jagiello, G., Ducayen, M., Fang, J.-S., and Graffeo, J. 1976. Cytogenetic observations in mammalian oocytes. In P. L. Pearson and K. R. Lewis (eds.), Chromosomes Today, Vol. 5, pp. 43–63. Proceedings of the Leiden Chromosome Conference, July 15–17, 1974. John Wiley & Sons, New York.

Jagiello, G., and Fang, J. S. 1979. Analyses of diplotene chiasma frequencies in mouse oocytes and spermatocytes in relation to ageing and sexual dimorphism. Cytogenet. Cell Genet. 23:53–60.

Janssens, F. A. 1909. La théorie de la chiasmatypie. [The chiasmatype theory.] Cellule 25:387–411.

Janssens, F. A. 1924. La chiasmatypie dans les insectes. Spermatogenèse. 1. Stethophyma grossum (L). 2. Chorthippus parallelus (Zetterstedt). [Chiasmatypy in insects. Spermatogenesis. 1. Stethophyma grossum (L). 2. Chorthippus parallelus (Zetterstedt).] Cellule 34:133–359.

Jones, G. H. 1978. Giemsa C-banding of rye meiotic chromosomes and the nature of "terminal" chiasmata. Chromosoma 66:45–47.

Jones, G. H., Stamford, W. K., and Perrey, P. E. 1975. Male and female meiosis in grasshoppers. II. Chorthippus brunneus. Chromosoma 51:381–389.

King, R. C. 1970. Ovarian Development in Drosophila melanogaster. Academic Press, New York.

Kiriazis, W. C., and Abrahamson, S. 1968. The effectiveness of varying doses of X rays in the production of X chromosome loss and non-disjunction in stage 14 oocytes of Drosophila melanogaster. Genetics 60:193. (Abstract of paper presented at the 1968 meetings of the Genetics Society of America.)

Kjessler, B. 1966. Karyotype, meiosis and spermatogenesis in a sample of men attending an infertility clinic. In Monographs in Human Genetics, Vol. 2. S. Karger AG, Basel.

Kyslíková, L., and Forejt, J. 1972. Chiasma frequency in three inbred strains of mice. Folia Biol. 18:216–218.

Lange, K., Page, B. M., and Elston, R. C. 1975. Age trends in human chiasma frequencies and recombination fractions. I. Chiasma frequencies. Am. J. Hum. Genet. 27:410–418.

Langenbeck, U., Hansmann, I., Hinney, B., and Hönig, V. 1976. On the origin of the supernumerary chromosome in autosomal trisomies—With special reference to Down's syndrome. A bias in tracing nondisjunction by chromosomal and biochemical polymorphisms. Hum. Genet. 33:89–102.

Lauritsen, J. G., and Friedrich, U. 1976. Origin of the extra chromosome in trisomy 16. Clin. Genet. 10:156–160.

Leonard, A., and Leonard, E. D. 1975. Ageing and chromosome aberrations in male mammalian germ cells. Exp. Gerontol. 10:309–311.

Lindsley, D. L., Sandler, L., Nicoletti, B., and Trippa, G. 1968. Genetic control of recombination in Drosophila. In W. J. Peacock and R. D. Brock (eds.), Replication and Recombination of Genetic Material, pp. 253–269. Australian Academy of Science, Canberra, Aust.

Luciani, J. M. 1970. Les chromosomes méiotiques de l'homme. I. La méiose normale. [The meiotic chromosomes of man. Normal Meiosis.] Ann. Genet. 13:101–111.

Luthardt, F. W., Palmer, C. G., and Yu, P.-L. 1973. Chiasma and univalent frequencies in aging female mice. Cytogenet. Cell Genet. 12:68–79.

Lyon, M. F. 1976. Distribution of crossing-over in mouse chromosomes. Genet. Res. 28:291–299.

McDermott, A. 1973. The frequency and distribution of chiasmata in man. Ann. Hum. Genet. 37:13–20.

McIlree, M. E., Tulloch, W. S., and Newsam, J. E. 1966. Studies on human meiotic chromosomes from testicular tissue. Lancet 1:679–682.

Maguire, M. P. 1974. The need for a chiasma binder. J. Theor. Biol. 48:485–487.

Maguire, M. P. 1978. Evidence for separate genetic control of crossing over and chiasma maintenance in maize. Chromosoma 65:173–183.

Mather, K. 1938. Crossing-over. Biol. Rev. 13:252–292.

Mikkelsen, M., Hallberg, A., and Poulsen, H. 1976. Maternal and paternal origin of extra chromosome in trisomy 21. Hum. Genet. 32:17–21.

Mintz, B. 1959. Continuity of the female germ cell line from embryo to adult. Arch. Anat. Micr. Morph. Exp. 48:155–172.

Mintz, B. 1960. Embryological phases of mammalian gametogenesis. J. Cell. Comp. Physiol. 56(suppl. 1):31–44.

Mouse News Letter. 1977. 57:6.

Muller, H. J. 1938. The remaking of chromosomes. Collect. Net 13:181–195, 198.

Ohno, S., Makino, S., Kaplan, W. D., and Kinosita, R. 1961. Female germ cells of man. Exp. Cell Res. 24:106–110.

Parker, J. S. 1975. Chromosome-specific control of chiasma formation. Chromosoma. 49:391–406.

Peters, H. 1970. Migration of gonocytes into the mammalian gonad and their differentiation. Phil. Trans. Roy. Soc. Lond. B 259:91–101.

Plough, H. H. 1917. The effect of temperature on crossing over in Drosophila. J. Exp. Zool. 24:147–209.

Plough, H. H. 1921. Further studies on the effect of temperature on crossing over. J. Exp. Zool. 32:187–202.

Polani, P. E. 1972. Centromere localization at meiosis and the position of chiasmata in the male and female mouse. Chromosoma 36:343–374.

Polani, P. E., Briggs, J. H., Ford, C. E., Clarke, C. M., and Berg, J. M. 1960. A mongol girl with 46 chromosomes. Lancet 1:721–724.

Polani, P. E., and Jagiello, G. M. 1976. Chiasmata, meiotic univalents, and age in relation to aneuploid imbalance in mice. Cytogenet. Cell Genet. 16:505–529.

Redfield, H. 1966. Delayed mating and the relationship of recombination to maternal age in Drosophila melanogaster. Genetics 53:593–607.

Reid, D. H., and Parsons, P. A. 1963. Sex of parents and variation of recombination with age in the mouse. Heredity 18:107–108.

Renwick, J. H. 1971. The mapping of human chromosomes. In H. L. Roman, L. M. Sandler, and A. Campbell (eds.), Annual Review of Genetics, Vol. 5, pp. 81–120. Annual Reviews, Palo Alto, Calif.

Renwick, J. H., and Schulze, J. 1964. An analysis of some data on the linkage between Xg and colorblindness in man. Am. J. Hum. Genet. 16:410–418.

Riley, R. 1966. Genetics and the regulation of meiotic chromosome behaviour. Sci. Progr. 54:193–207.

Riley, R., and Law, C. N. 1965. Genetic variation in chromosome pairing. In E. W. Caspari and J. M. Thoday (eds.), Advances in Genetics, Vol. 13, pp. 57–114. Academic Press, New York.

Robinson, J. A. 1977. Meiosis. I. Non-disjunction as the main cause of trisomy 21. Hum. Genet. 39:27–30.

Sandler, L., Lindsley, D. L., Nicoletti, B., and Trippa, G. 1968. Mutants affecting meiosis in natural populations of Drosophila melanogaster. Genetics 60:525–558.

Sasaki, M., and Hara, Y. 1973. Paternal origin of the extra chromosome in Down's syndrome. Lancet 2:1257–1258.

Searle, A. G., Berry, R. J., and Beechey, C. V. 1970. Cytogenetic radiosensitivity and chiasma frequency in wild-living male mice. Mutat. Res. 9:137–140.

Skakkebaek, N. E., Bryant, J. I., and Philip, J. 1973. Studies on meiotic chromosomes in infertile men and controls with normal karyotypes. J. Reprod. Fertil. 35:23–36.

Slizynski, B. M. 1955. Chiasmata in the male mouse. J. Genet. 53:597–605.

Slizynski, B. M. 1960. Sexual dimorphism in mouse gametogenesis. Genet. Res. 1:477–486.

Speed, R. M. 1977. The effects of ageing on the meiotic chromosomes of male and female mice. Chromosoma 64:241–254.

Stahl, A., Luciani, J. M., Devictor, M., Capodano, A. M., and Gagné, R. 1975. Constitutive heterochromatin and micronuclei in the human oocyte at the diplotene stage. Humangenetik 26:315–327.

Stene, J., Fischer, G., Stene, E., Mikkelsen, M., and Petersen, E. 1977. Paternal age effect in Down's syndrome. Ann. Hum. Genet. 40:299–306.

Stene, J., and Stene, E. 1977. Statistical methods for detecting a moderate paternal age effect on incidence of disorders when a maternal one is present. Ann. Hum. Genet. 40:343–353.

Stene, J., and Stene, E. 1978. On data and methods in investigations on parental-age effects. Comments on a paper by J. D. Erickson. Ann. Hum. Genet. 41:465–468.

Stern, C. 1959. Colour-blindness in Klinefelter's syndrome. Nature 183:1452–1453.

Tokunaga, C. 1970a. The effects of low temperature and aging on nondisjunction in Drosophila. Genetics 65:75–94.

Tokunaga, C. 1970b. Aspects of low-temperature-induced meiotic nondisjunction in Drosophila females. Genetics 66:653–661.

Traut, H. 1970. The resistance of mature oocytes of Drosophila melanogaster to the induction of non-disjunction by X-rays. Mutat. Res. 10:156–158.

Traut, H. 1971. The influence of the temporal distribution of the X-ray dose on the induction of X-chromosomal nondisjunction and X-chromosome loss in oocytes of Drosophila melanogaster. Mutat. Res. 12:321–327.

Uchida, I. A. 1973. Paternal origin of the extra chromosome in Down's syndrome. Lancet 2:1258.

Uchida, I. A., and Curtis, E. J. 1961. A possible association between maternal radiation and mongolism. Lancet 2:848–850.

Uchida, I. A., and Freeman, C. P. V. 1977. Radiation-induced nondisjunction in oocytes of aged mice. Nature 265:186–187.

Uchida, I. A., and Lee, C. P. V. 1974. Radiation-induced nondisjunction in mouse oocytes. Nature 250:601–602.

Wagenbichler, P., Killian, W., Rett, A., and Schnedl, W. 1976. Origin of the extra chromosome no. 21 in Down's syndrome. Hum. Genet. 32:13–16.

Wallace, M. E., MacSwiney, F. J., and Edwards, R. G. 1976. Parental age and recombination frequency in the house mouse. Genet. Res. 28:241–251.

Wallace, M. E., and Mallyon, S. A. 1972. Unusual recombination values and the mapping of the lethal miniature in the house mouse. Genet. Res. 20:257–262.

White, M. J. D. 1959. Telomeres and Terminal Chiasmata—A Reinterpretation. University of Texas Publications, No. 5914. pp. 107–111.

White, M. J. D. 1973. Animal Cytology and Evolution. 3rd Ed. Cambridge University Press, Cambridge, England.

Witschi, E. 1948. Migration of the germ cells of human embryos from the yolk sac to the primitive gonadal folds. Contr. Embryol. Carneg. Inst. 32:69–80.

Wolgemuth-Jarashow, D. J., Jagiello, G. M., and Henderson, A. S. 1977. The localization of rDNA in small nucleolus-like structures in human diplotene oocyte nuclei. Hum. Genet. 36:63–68.

Yamamoto, M., Endo, A., and Watanabe, G. 1973. Maternal age dependence of chromosome anomalies. Nature New Biol. 241:141–142.

Zuckerman, S. 1951. The number of oocytes in the mature ovary. In G. Pincus (ed.), Recent Progress in Hormone Research, Vol. 6, pp. 63–109. Academic Press, New York.

Zuckerman, S. 1956. The regenerative capacity of ovarian tissue. In G. E. W. Wolstenholme and E. C. P. Miller (eds.), Ageing in Transient Tissues, pp. 31–54. Ciba Foundation Colloquia on Ageing, Vol. 2. J. & A. Churchill, London.

Zuckerman, S. 1960. Origin and development of oocytes in foetal and mature mammals. In C. R. Austin (ed.), Memoirs. Society for Endocrinology No. 7, Sex Differentiation and Development, pp. 63–70. Proceedings of a symposium held at the Royal Society of Medicine, Wimpole Street, London, April 10–11, 1958. Cambridge University Press, Cambridge, England.

Zuckerman, S. 1965. The natural history of an enquiry. Lecture delivered during the Annual General Meeting of the Royal College of Surgeons of England, Birmingham, December 5, 1964. Ann. Roy. Coll. Surg. Engl. 37:133–149.

The Synaptonemal Complex in Mammalian Meiosis

Montrose J. Moses

The perturbation of normal disjunction that gives rise to such chromosomal abnormalities as trisomy 21 (Robinson, 1977) may well have its origin in a malfunction of the synaptic processes leading to the reduction division at meiosis. The synaptic events of meiotic prophase (homologous recognition and collocation, pairing, synaptic register, crossing over, desynapsis, chiasma formation, and chiasma terminalization) are probably among the best-known in cell biology, but they are also the most poorly understood. The latter is partly due to the physical nature of the chromosomes at these particular stages and to the limitations of conventional microscopical techniques for studying them, both of which have contributed to the intractability of these stages to cytological study.

Although there is no promise that understanding these events will reveal directly how aneuploid gametes are produced, it is a necessary step toward achieving that goal. Using a new technique that is simple and rapid, we have begun to lay down new information about chromosome behavior and its control in meiosis, taking advantage of the fact that the synaptonemal complex (SC) provides a simplified representation of the chromosomes in meiotic prophase (Moses, 1977).

The SC, backbone of the bivalent, comprises the paired filamentous axes (lateral elements) of two homologous chromosomes, held together by a central filamentous element and accessory material (Figure 1). It is present in animals and plants, females and males—wherever crossing over occurs, and sometimes where it does not—and seems to be a prerequisite, although not the only one, for the recombinational event. How this proteinaceous structure functions is not clearly understood. However, it is reasonable to assume that as the agent of meiotic synapsis, the SC serves to hold sister chromatids together so they function as one, to hold homologous chromosomes together in side-by-side register for crossing over to occur, and to aid in positioning of

Research described in this paper was supported at various times by grants from the NSF (GB-40562, PCM-76-00440) and the NIH (GM-23047, HD-12225, 4-S01-RR-05405, and CA-14236).

131

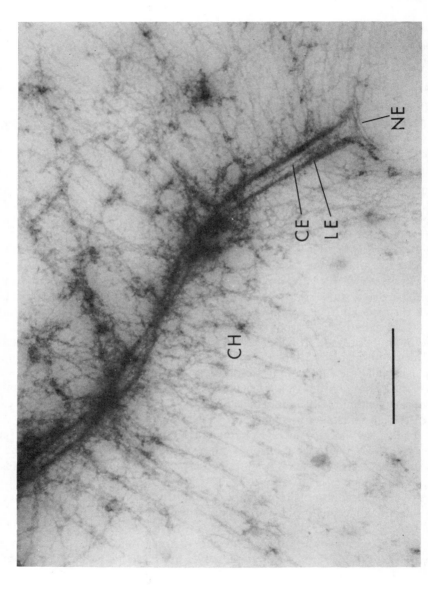

Figure 1. Electron micrograph of an autosomal bivalent from a Syrian hamster pachytene spermatocyte spread on 0.45% NaCl, stabilized with uranyl acetate, and protected dried from 0.5% polyvinyl pyrrolidone. Chromatin fibrils (CH) radiate as collapsed loops from the lateral elements (LE) of the prominent synaptonemal complex, which is straight and thick near its termination on the nuclear envelope (NE) and is twisted elsewhere. Central elements (CE) and transverse filaments are also visible. Magnification bar = 1 μm. (Reprinted with permission from Moses and Solari, 1976, *Journal of Ultrastructure Research 54*, p. 109.)

kinetochores for subsequent coorientation on the spindle. All of these conditions are likely to play determining roles in disjunction.

The defect leading to trisomy 21 may occur in the testis as well as in the ovary (Magenis et al., 1977; Mikkelsen, Hallberg, and Poulsen, 1976). Recent studies from our laboratory on the SC in mammalian spermatocytes (Moses, 1977a, d) bear on synapsis, desynapsis, and disjunction and thus may provide a background for understanding the origin of trisomy. Our results have been obtained using a technique introduced by Counce and Meyer (1973) and adapted by us to mammalian spermatocytes (e.g., Moses, Counce, and Paulson, 1975). It provides complete complements of SCs, selectively stained and displayed in their entirety (Figure 2). The kinetochore components of the lateral elements of the SC (chromosome axes) and the plaques by which SC ends are attached to the nuclear envelope are also stained. The X and Y chromosomes are clearly distinct from the autosomes (Moses, 1977b, c; Moses et al., 1975). Although the SC is visible by light microscopy (Moses, 1977b), definitive details depend on electron microscopy.

Studies were initially undertaken to develop the double potential of the method for establishing the behavior of the SC in synapsis and desynapsis (Moses, 1977b) and for constructing pachytene karyotypes from SC length and arm ratios (Moses et al., 1977). The technique is most effective for exactly those stages, leptotene through early diplotene, that are ordinarily difficult to analyze with the light microscope, particularly in mammals.

SC BEHAVIOR IN MEIOTIC PROPHASE

Rules of behavior of the axes during synapsis and desynapsis have been established. In particular, the nuclear envelope has emerged as a key structure in synapsis, being the site for initiation of axis assembly and SC formation, and for movement of chromosome ends, as shown schematically in Figure 3. Usually the homologues show no evidence of prior synapsis or pairing. Shortly after the axes begin to form, and often before they have completely assembled, homologous ends move together and zygotene begins by formation of an SC starting at the nuclear envelope. A central element forms between the two axes, and synapsis progresses toward the kinetochores, which are usually the last regions to pair. When the kinetochores are terminal, as in the mouse, initiation may either be interstitial or at the ends. This suggests that not only is there homologous recognition at the ends of the chromosomes but that it also may occur interstitially.

Pachytene is the stage at which all SCs have formed, as a consequence of which the two homologues are pulled together along their lengths; it is also the stage at which crossing over presumably occurs.

Desynapsis at diplotene is, at least superficially, a reverse process to zygotene. Desynapsis may initiate either interstitially or at the ends; there appears to be no specific pattern to the process. There are occasional regions in which short lengths of SC persist, and there is some evidence that such residual structures may represent chiasma sites (Solari, 1970b). The axes disassemble and disappear just before or during diplotene (e.g., Chinese hamster and mouse, respectively).

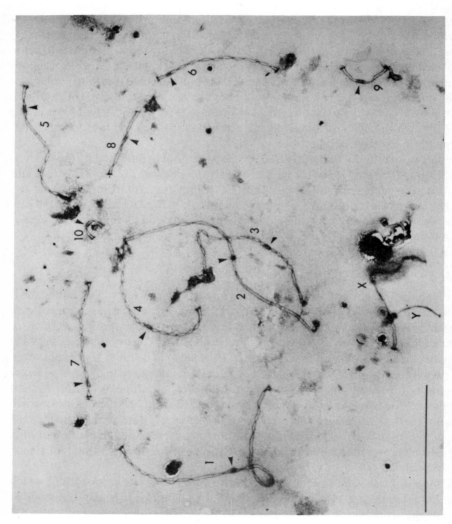

Figure 2.   Complete set of SCs from a Chinese hamster spermatocyte: Counce-Meyer preparation. Autosomal SCs are numbered according to ranked length as measured from one terminal to the other. Differentiation of the XY pair indicates the stage to be mid-late pachytene. Kinetochores (arrowheads) distinguish long and short arms for measurement. Magnification bar = 10μm. (Reprinted with permission from Moses et al., 1977, *Chromosoma 60*, pp. 345–375.)

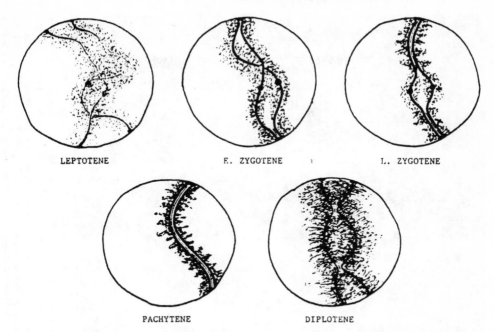

LEPTOTENE   E. ZYGOTENE   L. ZYGOTENE

PACHYTENE   DIPLOTENE

Figure 3.   Schematic diagram of autosomal synapsis and desynapsis in meiosis based on studies of spread preparations from five mammals. The essential structural components are shown: nuclear envelope, axial elements (chromosome axes), SC (with lateral and central elements), chromatin extending from the lateral (axial) elements, kinetochores on lateral (axial) elements, and terminal plaques by which axial and lateral elements are anchored to the inner face of the nuclear envelope. (Reprinted with permission from Moses, 1977d, in R. S. Sparkes, D. Comings, and C. Fox (eds.), *Molecular Human Cytogenetics,* Academic Press, New York.)

SC KARYOTYPES

Each SC is characterized at pachytene by its length between attachments to the nuclear envelope and by the position of its kinetochore (Figure 4). In Figure 4c, these features can be seen in an acrocentric human bivalent, measurement of which indicates it to be number 21 or 22; the presence of a nucleolus attached at the end of the short arm supports this identification. In Figure 5 are two mouse autosomal SCs, with nuclear envelope attachment plaques at their ends and the kinetochores terminal. Here there is no evidence of a short arm, in contrast to the acrocentric in the previous figure. The SC twists along its length; the central element is often not visible. Recombination nodules (Carpenter, 1975) are occasionally present.

From complete complements of SCs from the Chinese hamster (Figures 2, 6), measurements were made of total length and arm ratio (Moses et al., 1977). Analyses showed that each chromosome can be characterized by its relative length (i.e., measured length of the complex divided by the sum of the lengths of all of the autosomal complexes) and by the arm ratio (Figure 7). The demonstration that autosomal SC relative lengths and arm ratios are constant despite changes in absolute lengths during pachytene shows, first, the absence of significant length distortions during prepara-

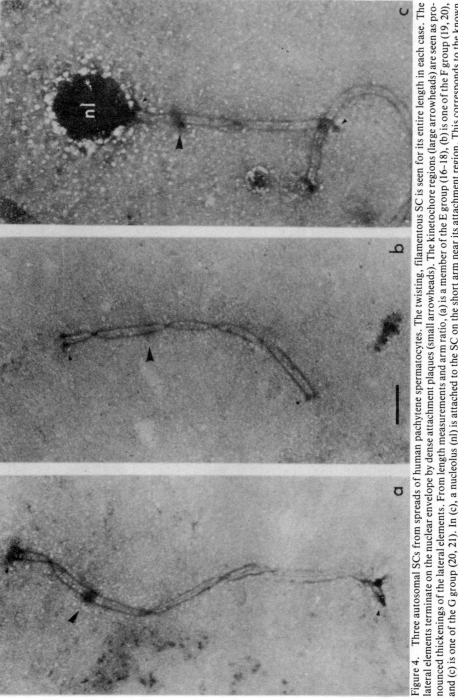

Figure 4.   Three autosomal SCs from spreads of human pachytene spermatocytes. The twisting, filamentous SC is seen for its entire length in each case. The lateral elements terminate on the nuclear envelope by dense attachment plaques (small arrowheads). The kinetochore regions (large arrowheads) are seen as pronounced thickenings of the lateral elements. From length measurements and arm ratio, (a) is a member of the E group (16–18), (b) is one of the F group (19, 20), and (c) is one of the G group (20, 21). In (c), a nucleolus (nl) is attached to the SC on the short arm near its attachment region. This corresponds to the known position of the nucleolus organizer region in chromosomes 21 and 22 (another autosomal SC crosses the long arm attachment region). Magnification bar = 1μm. (Reprinted with permission from Moses et al., 1975, *Science 187*, pp. 363–365. Copyright 1975 by the American Association for the Advancement of Science.)

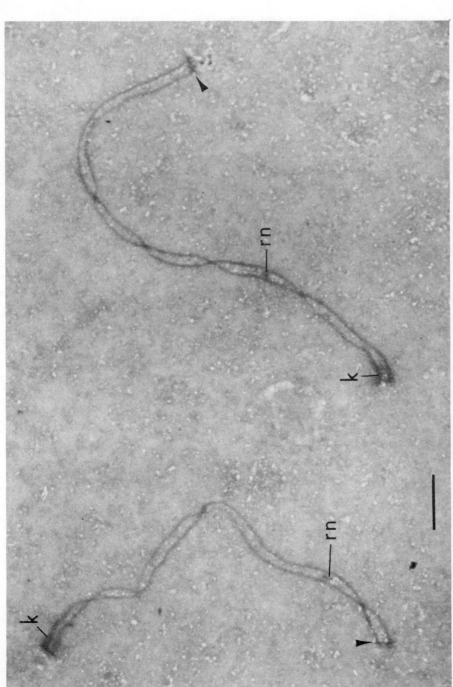

Figure 5. Electron micrograph of two mouse spermatocyte SCs prepared by the Counce-Meyer microspreading procedure. k, Kinetochore (terminal); rn, "recombination nodule" of Carpenter (1975); other SCs of this complement also show nodules. Magnification bar = 1 µm. (Reprinted with permission from Moses, 1977a, *Chromosomes Today 6*, pp. 71–82.)

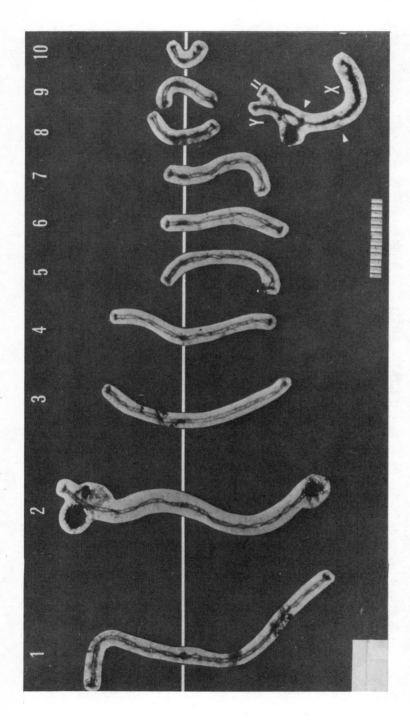

Figure 6. SC karyotype of the Chinese hamster. This full complement of 10 autosomal SCs and XY pair from a single primary spermatocyte nucleus prepared by microspreading (Counce-Meyer procedure), has been cut out from an electron micrograph; the SCs are ranked and numbered according to length and aligned by kinetochores, with short arms above and long arms below the line. All autosomal SCs are submetacentric except 5, 6, and 7, which are acrocentric, corresponding to the karyotype known from light-microscopic preparations of somatic metaphase. As in most mammals studied, the X and Y pair to form a short length of SC (=); the unpaired axes thicken and undergo structural differentiations. Ten divisions on the magnification scale = 4.64 μm. (Reprinted with permission from Moses et al., 1977, *Chromosoma 60*, pp. 345–375.)

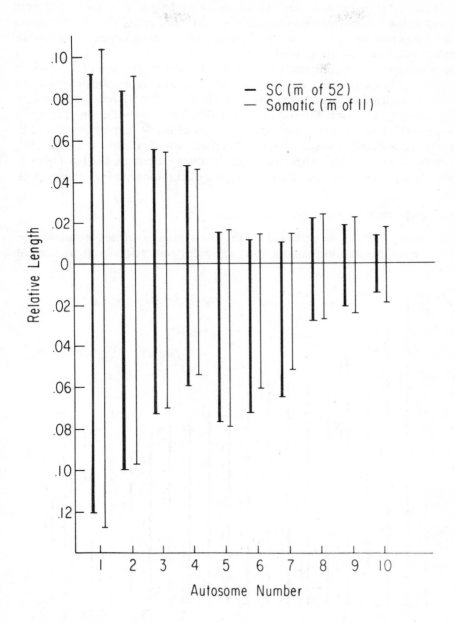

Figure 7.   Idiogram of Chinese hamster autosomal SCs, constructed from relative length measurements and arm ratios of 52 pachytene spermatocytes (thick bars) compared with similar data from 11 sets of mitotic autosomes (thin bars). From data in Moses et al. (1977).

tion, and, second, a regular, proportional control of SC length. The equivalence of pachytene SC karyotype data to similar measurements of mitotic metaphase autosomes indicates that similar controls of autosome length must operate in both meiosis and mitosis. Pachytene karyotypes have now been established for a number of species, using this method (Moses and Counce, 1976); all agree with their mitotic counterparts and reaffirm the validity of the method.

The situation is more complicated in the mouse, where, because the autosomes are telocentric (Figure 5), only relative length (and in some cases, the presence of a nucleolus) can be used to characterize the SCs. Here, relative SC length is also constant and directly proportional to relative length of mitotic chromosomes (Figure 8). However, the difference between adjacent members of the SC karyotype ranked by relative length is generally too small to permit certain identification of individual SCs by this means alone. On the other hand, the results substantiate the feasibility of intrachromosomal measurements and the mapping of chromosomal rearrangements.

SYNAPSIS AND DISJUNCTION OF THE X AND Y

Before discussing some of the pertinent results of our studies on chromosomal rearrangements, a few observations on the sex chromosomes are relevant. In most mam-

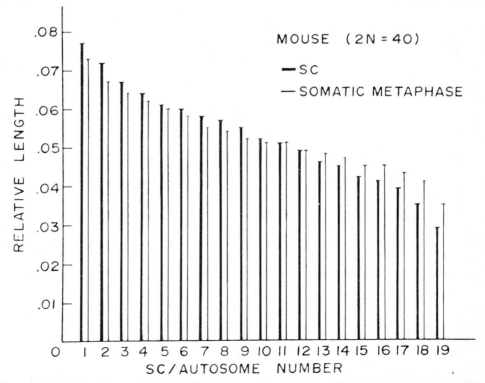

Figure 8.   Idiogram of mouse autosomal karyotype constructed from relative length measurements of eight full SC complements (thick bars), compared with somatic metaphase karyotype (thin bars). (Reprinted with permission from Moses, 1977a, *Chromosomes Today 6,* pp. 71–82.)

mals, the X and Y chromosomes pair and form an SC for part of their lengths (Solari, 1974) along regions that are thus thought to be homologous. The SC, which always ends in an attachment plaque, is generally indistinguishable from autosomal SCs, while the unpaired axial cores thicken and undergo a variety of differentiations that appear to be species-specific (e.g., Moses, 1977c; Moses et al., 1975; Moses, Russell, and Cacheiro, 1977; Tres, 1977). Synapsis and desynapsis of the sex pair are on a separate time schedule from the autosomes. In the human (Moses et al., 1975) and mouse (Moses, Russell, and Cacheiro, 1977, Solari, 1970a; Tres, 1977), XY synapsis is apt to occur late in the autosomal synapsing period, whereas desynapsis is precocious, beginning in midpachytene (c.f. Chinese hamster XY (Moses, 1977c), where desynapsis does not begin until late pachytene). In the mouse, the maximal synaptic segment occupies about 80%–90% of the distal portion of the Y (Figure 9a) and is reduced for much of pachytene to a short length (about 20% of the Y) (Figure 9b). At desynapsis the ends of the pairing segment remain together, and the opposite ends also tend to associate. In the Egyptian sand rat (Solari and Ashley, 1977) there is no synapsis of the X and Y, but the ends nevertheless associate. Thus, if XY disjunction, which is normal in this case, depends in some way upon chromosome association at pachytene, it must be through end-to-end contacts rather than synapsis and SC formation. Some recent studies on mice with high incidences of sex chromosome nondisjunction tend to support this notion (Ashley, Cumming, Sotomayor, and Moses, unpublished observations).

Association of the X with the Y, upon which disjunction apparently depends, may be inhibited by interference with the pairing region as a consequence of a chromosomal rearrangement. This conclusion comes from analyses of SCs in mice heterozygous for two different X-autosome translocations (Moses, Russell, and Cacheiro, 1977). The SC configurations observed accord precisely with those predicted from classical cytogenetic theory (Figures 10, 11). Breakpoints are distinguishable by the sharp differences in thickness between autosomal and sex chromosomal axes. Their positions, as calculated from length measurements of the SC figures, agree well with those determined by mitotic chromosome banding. In one case [T(X;7)6Rℓ], the breakpoint falls in the pairing region of the X (Figure 10). The Y, probably as a consequence, does not associate with the X; neither SCs nor end attachments are formed. From the foregoing, this is a condition that could lead to nondisjunction. By contrast, in another translocation, [T(X;7)2Rℓ], the breakpoint is proximal to the pairing region (Figure 11), and synapsis and SC formation between the X and Y do occur and presumably disjunction could follow. Unfortunately, information about disjunction is not available because spermatogenesis ceases after pachytene in all mouse T(X; autosome)s.

THE SC AND DISJUNCTION IN HETEROMORPHIC TRIVALENTS

One of the possible functions of the SC in disjunction is as an accessory in the establishment and maintenance of the coorientation of the kinetochores that is necessary for correct disjunction and distribution of chromosomes subsequently at anaphase I. Evidence consistent with this idea comes from observations on Robertsonian fusion heterozygotes.

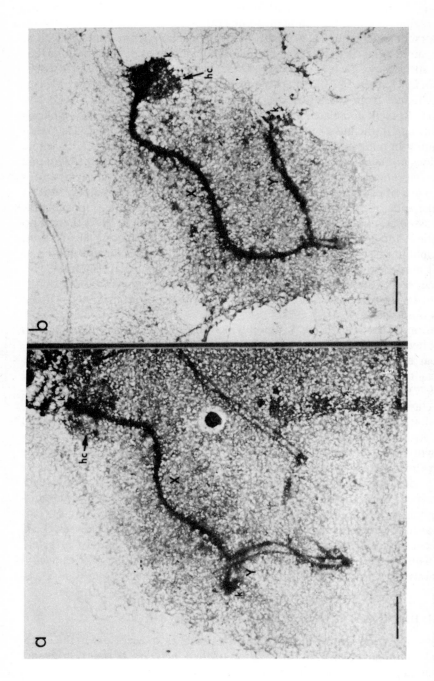

Figure 9. Mouse XY pair. a, Early pachytene: most of the Y axis has paired distally with the distal end of the X to form an SC. b, At mid pachytene the X and Y axes have desynapsed precociously, leaving a short length of SC at their distal ends. Unpaired axes are thicker and denser, and in places appear double. k, kinetochore region; hk, heterochromatic knob. Magnification bars = 1 μm. (a, Reprinted with permission from Moses, 1977d, in R. S. Sparkes, D. Comings, and C. Fox (eds.), *Molecular Human Cytogenetics*, Academic Press, New York. b, Reprinted with permission from Moses et al., 1977, *Science 196*, pp. 892–894. Copyright 1977 by the American Association for the Advancement of Science.)

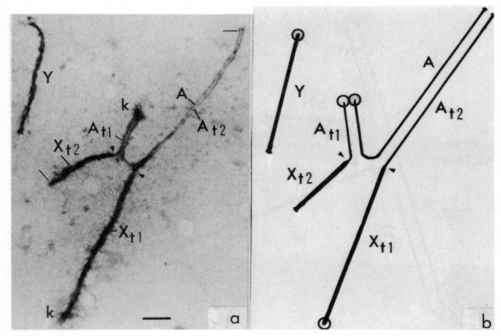

Figure 10.   Pairing figure of mouse X-autosome translocation heterozygote [T(X;7)6R*l*]. Compare the electron micrograph (a) with the schematic diagram (b). A, nontranslocated autosomal axis; A_{t1} and A_{t2}, axes of translocated portions of autosome; X_{t1} and X_{t2}, translocated portions of X axis; k, kinetochore region; Y, Y axis; (−), distal attachment plaque; arrowheads, translocation breakpoints. The thicker X axes are distinct from the autosome axes to which they are translocated. Normally, most of the Y chromosomes pair with the distal portion of the X chromosome at early pachytene to form an SC (see Figure 9a). Here, in the smaller translocation product, $A_{t1}X_{t2}$, the distal (X_{t2}) segment is shorter than the full pairing region of the X chromosome. The Y chromosome is unpaired, possibly as a consequence of interruption of the X chromosome pairing region. Magnification bar = 1 μm. (Reprinted with permission from Moses et al., 1977, *Science 196*, pp. 892–894. Copyright 1977 by the American Association for the Advancement of Science.)

Hybrid offspring from interspecies mating of lemurs [*Lemur fulvus* ($2n = 60$) × *L. macaco* ($2n = 44$)] are both viable and fertile (Hamilton and Moses, 1979). They have been shown by chromosome banding to contain acrocentrics from the *L. fulvus* parent that match the arms of the Robertsonian metacentrics from the *L. macaco* lar acrocentric/metacentric fertile hybrid produced by crossing *L. fulvus* ($2n = 60$) with *L. f. collaris* ($2n = 51$) showed a highly regular orientation of the three kinetochores in each trivalent (Figure 12). The two kinetochores of the acrocentrics are always in the cis configuration with respect to the kinetochore of the metacentric, implying predetermined pairing faces on the homologues. This kinetochore configuration may be essential to subsequent coorientation and proper disjunction leading to the production of balanced gametes, as inferred from the fertility of the hybrids.

SYNAPSIS AND HOMOLOGY

The diagrammatic explicitness of the electron microscopic images of the axial elements (lateral elements of the SC) provides a valuable new way of detecting and iden-

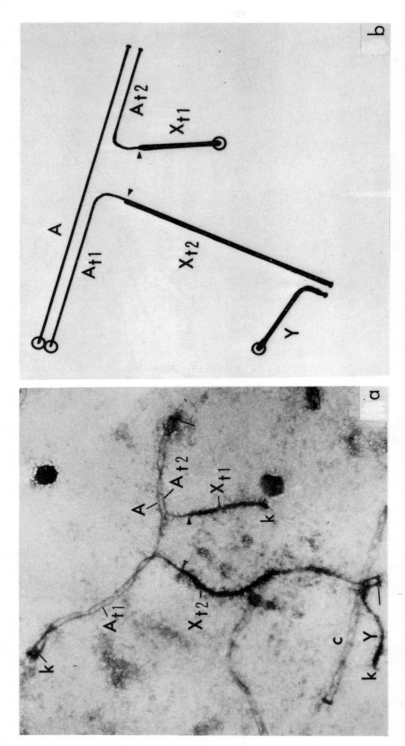

Figure 11. a, Translocation quadrivalent from a male mouse heterozygous for a different X-autosome translocation [T(X;7)2Rℓ]; compare with schematic in (b). Symbols as in Figure 10. In the long translocation product, $A_{t1}X_{t2}$, the X_{t2} portion consists of the distal three-quarters of the X. The breakpoint occurs proximally to the pairing region and the X and Y are terminally synapsed via a short segment of SC (compare with Figure 9b). An autosomal SC (c) accidentally crosses the XY pair. Autosomal portions of the two translocated axes have either failed to pair with, or have stripped away from, the nontranslocated (A) axis for a short distance near the translocation breakpoints. Magnification bar = 1 μm. (Reprinted with permission from Moses et al., 1977, *Science 196*, pp. 892–894. Copyright 1977 by the American Association for the Advancement of Science.)

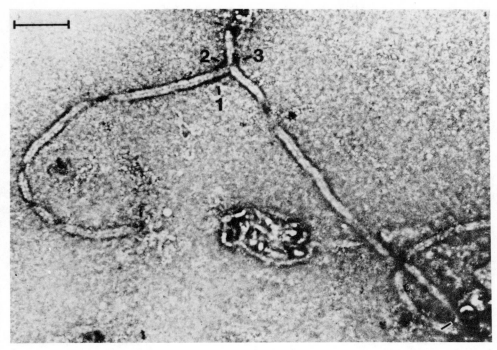

Figure 12.   SC of one of five heteromorphic trivalents from a spermatocyte of a *Lemur fulvus* × *L. f. collaris* hybrid with $2n = 55$. Two acrocentrics (from the *L. fulvus* parent), known from banding studies to be homologous with the arms of the metacentric from the other parent (*L. f. collaris*), have paired with the latter to form the SC of the trivalent. The three kinetochores are adjacent and nearly equidistant from one another; that of the metacentric is numbered 1, those of the two acrocentrics are 2 and 3. The short arms of the acrocentrics have also paired to form an SC side arm. Dashes mark the plaques attaching the SCs of the nuclear envelope. Magnification bar = 1 μm. (Reprinted with permission from Moses et al., 1979, *Chromosoma 70*, pp. 141-160.)

tifying chromosomal rearrangements at a stage of meiotic prophase that has hitherto been resistant to cytological analysis with the light microscope. Furthermore, the good correspondence among independent SC measurements, mitotic chromosome banding, and genetic analysis found in the studies of the mouse translocations (Moses, Russell, and Cacheiro, 1977) has also been encountered in a tandem duplication (Moses et al., 1977) and in two paracentric inversions (Moses et al., 1978), and has led to a new and practical approach to analyzing and mapping structural irregularities in meiotic chromosomes.

The studies of chromosomal rearrangements in mouse have been doubly informative: not only have they validated an independent and sensitive method for cytogenetic analysis of chromosomal irregularities but they have provided a new and unanticipated biological insight into the relationship between synapsis and homology in meiotic prophase.

Two different paracentric inversions have been examined in collaboration with T. H. Roderick and M. T. Davisson of the Jackson Laboratory (Moses et al., 1978). In both cases, classical inversion loops are formed by the SC in mice heterozygous for

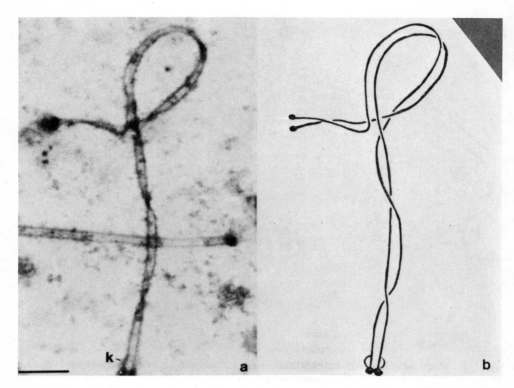

Figure 13. a, Early pachytene SC inversion loop from a mouse heterozygote; Roderick and Davisson's [In(2)5Rk]. b, Schematic tracing of (a). k, kinetochore. Magnification bar = 1 μm. (Reprinted with permission from Moses, 1977a, *Chromosomes Today 6*, pp. 71–82.)

the rearrangements (Figure 13). Measurements of loop (inversion) lengths and break-points accord well with chromosome banding and genetic data.

The inversion loops are structural contortions by which homologous synapsis is accommodated. It would appear not only that the chromosomes are inhibited from synapsing nonhomologously but that the drive for them to synapse homologously is sufficient to produce the contortion. Thus, homologous recognition and control are active forces during this period of synapsis (zygotene).

On the other hand, inversion loops do not answer the question of whether synapsis involves initial homologous register at one or a few points, with progressive synapsis bringing homologous regions into register mechanically, or whether homology is required at each step of the synaptic way. The answer to the question has come from analysis of a tandem duplication heterozygote in collaboration with L. B. Russell and N. L. Cacheiro, Oak Ridge National Laboratory (Moses et al., 1978). Again, the identification of the rearrangement, its length, and its position agree with chromosome banding and genetic data. The duplication-bearing chromosome is longer than the normal, and a buckle is formed at synapsis (Figure 14). The position of the buckle varies within sharply defined limits, implying that while synapsis may progress from

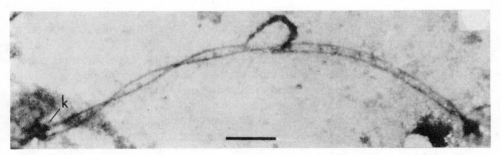

Figure 14.   Tandem duplication (from L. B. Russell and N. L. A. Cacheiro) in a mouse heterozygote; an unpaired duplication loop is seen at early pachytene. Axis lengths differ by 15%, reflecting the length of the duplicated segment. Magnification scale = 1 μm. (Reprinted with permission from Moses, 1977a, *Chromosomes Today 6*, pp. 71–82.)

either direction, it will not proceed beyond the point at which homology ends and nonhomology, occasioned by the duplication, begins. Thus, the progress of synapsis must be under the continuous control of homologous recognition along the length of the pairing regions.

SYNAPTIC ADJUSTMENT

A surprising observation has revealed a second phase of synapsis in pachytene (Moses, 1977a; Moses et al., 1978). The duplication buckle as well as the loops of all of the four inversions examined so far are replaced at late pachytene by normal-appearing SCs whose relative lengths are indistinguishable from those of controls. Intermediate stages of buckle and loop reductions during pachytene show that limited desynapsis of the SC occurs, followed by resynapsis between nonhomologous regions of the axes to form normal-appearing SCs. In the case of the duplication, the long axis shortens to equal the short axis. In the inversion loop, a switch of axial element pairing partners occurs. The author has termed the process of desynapsis and resynapsis to give nonhomologous SC formation *synaptic adjustment*. It is evidently part of a second, nonhomologous pairing phase in pachytene that follows and replaces the primary, homology-controlled pairing phase of zygotene. The nonhomologous pairing phase probably accounts for known instances of synapsis and SC formation between nonhomologous chromosomes (e.g., McClintock, 1933; Gillies, 1974; Rasmussen, 1977).

It is not clear why the chromosomes, having taken pains to accommodate homology, should then reject (or be released from) its control, undo the structural accommodations, and revert to a topologically simpler structure. While the nonhomologous pairing phase may well play a role in disjunction, particularly of nonhomologous chromosomes (Grell, 1965), that role is only hypothetical at the moment.

CONCLUSION

It should not be taken from the comments herein that the SC is a requirement for disjunction of homologues in the first meiotic division. A well-known case in point is that of male *Drosophila,* in which neither chromosome axis nor SC (nor crossing over, for that matter) occurs, and yet normal disjunction is the rule. On the other hand, a role, although not an exclusive one, is to be seen for the SC, when it is present, in predisposing for proper disjunction through providing for at least three conditions that must be met: sister chromatid cohesion, association of homologues, and orientation of kinetochores. The observations presented here only suggest the parts that the SC may play in this determination.

In any case, as paradigms of the chromosomes, the axial elements of the homologues (lateral elements of the SCs) allow us to see and to analyze synaptic events in meiosis that would otherwise remain obscure. The stage is now set for an examination of the behavior of the SC in fathers identified as being the sources of the nondisjunction leading to trisomy 21 offspring.

ACKNOWLEDGMENTS

It is a pleasure to acknowledge the capable assistance of Mr. T. Gambling, Ms. N. Staddon, and Ms. M. Johnson. I am also grateful for valuable discussions with Drs. S. J. Counce and T. Ashley, and the collaboration of Mr. M. Dresser and Ms. P. Poorman.

Shortly after preparation of this chapter, M. Dresser in our laboratory introduced the demonstration of SCs and nucleoli by both light and electron microscopy using silver staining of mammalian spermatocytes, microspread as described herein (Dresser and Moses, 1979). The correlated LM-EM study showed that although light microscopy has the advantages of easily prepared, large samples of clearly stained cells for rapid examination, the information obtainable is limited; the added resolution of the electron microscope is necessary for obtaining essential details unequivocally. Thus, light microscopy of silver-stained spreads now provides a rapid, practical method for preliminary scanning of the kind of material discussed in this chapter, the definitive details following from an EM examination of the same material. The correlated LM-EM approach makes SC analysis more accessible for clinical as well as experimental use.

REFERENCES

Carpenter, A. T. C. 1975. Proc. Nat. Acad. Sci. 72:2186–2189.
Counce, S. J., and Meyer, G. F. 1973. Chromosoma 44:231–253.
Dresser, M., and Moses, M. J. 1979. Exp. Cell Res. 121:416–419.
Gillies, C. B. 1974. Chromosoma 48:441–453.
Grell, R. F. 1965. Nat. Cancer Inst. Monogr. 18:215–242.
Hamilton, A. E., and Moses, M. J. 1979. Am. J. Phys. Anthropol. 50:445–446.
McClintock, B. 1933. Z.f. Zellforsch. Mikr. Anat. 19:192–237.
Magenis, R. E., Overton, K. M., Chamberlin, J., Brady, T., and Lovrien, E. 1977. Hum. Genet. 37:7–16.
Mikkelsen, M., Hallberg, A., and Poulsen, H. 1976. Hum. Genet. 32:17–21.
Moses, M. J. 1977a. Chrom. Today 6:71–82.
Moses, M. J. 1977b. Chromosoma 60:99–125.
Moses, M. J. 1977c. Chromosoma 60:127–137.
Moses, M. J. 1977d. In R. S. Sparkes, D. Comings, and C. Fox (eds.), Molecular Human Cytogenetics, pp. 101–125. Academic Press, New York.
Moses, M. J., and Counce, S. J. 1976. J. Cell Biol. 70:131a.
Moses, M. J., Counce, S. J., and Paulson, D. F. 1975. Science 187:363–365.

Moses, M. J., Karatsis, P. A., and Hamilton, A. E. 1979. Chromosoma 70:141–160.
Moses, M. J., Poorman, P. A., Russell, L. B., Cacheiro, N. L., Roderick. T. H., and Davisson, M. T. 1978. J. Cell Biol. 79:123a.
Moses, M. J., Poorman, P. A., Russell, L. B., Cacheiro, N. L., and Solari, A. J. 1977. J. Cell Biol. 75:135a.
Moses, M. J., Russell, L. B., and Cacheiro, N. L. 1977. Science 196:892–894.
Moses, M. J., Slatton, G., Gambling, T., and Starmer, F. 1977. Chromosoma 60:345–375.
Moses, M. J., and Solari, A. J. 1976. J. Ultrastruct. Res. 54:109–114.
Rasmussen, S. W. 1977. Carlsberg Res. Commun. 42:163–197.
Robinson, J. A. 1977. Hum. Genet. 39:27–30.
Solari, A. J. 1970a. Chromosoma 29:217–236.
Solari, A. J. 1970b. Chromosoma 31:217–230.
Solari, A. J. 1974. Int. Rev. Cytol. 38:273–317.
Solari, A. J., and Ashley, T. 1977. Chromosoma 62:319–336.
Tres, L. L. 1977. J. Cell Sci. 25:1–15.

Reproduction in Down Syndrome

Georgiana Jagiello

This presentation of some aspects of reproductive function in subjects with Down syndrome was prompted by a practical clinical need, as well as by theoretical genetical interests. The life expectancy of those with Down syndrome has increased greatly in recent years, and problems of the management of these young adults in their reproductive years have arisen. Discussions of contraception would ideally be based on data that reflect accurately their potential fertility and the risk of abnormal offspring. Theoretically, the examination of the endocrine status and gametogenesis of subjects with Down syndrome should yield useful clues to the original nondisjunctional event(s) that produced the patient.

This discussion of the reproductive performance of patients with Down syndrome is limited to trisomy 21 and mosaic trisomy 21 people, thus setting aside data for translocation and familial Down cases. Many of the data in the literature are anecdotal. Stated briefly, it is generally accepted that females with "pure 21" are relatively infertile, and the males more so. The evidence related to these generalizations is presented in three sections: 1) a discussion of descriptive aspects of the reproductive anatomy and physiology of Down syndrome, 2) data on oogenesis and spermatogenesis, and 3) a review of the reproductive histories in the literature of female and male Down and mosaic Down patients.

REPRODUCTIVE ANATOMY AND PHYSIOLOGY

Trisomy 21 Females

Benda (1969) wrote the classical description of the genitalia of female subjects with Down syndrome, noting that "some babies have gonads in the normal range." Subsequently, however, in the adult Down subjects in his series, the ovaries were found to be small and hypoplastic, never normal size. Histologically, they were noted to: 1) have no activity of the germinal epithelium, with a few, often degenerate, follicles and an increase in fibrous stroma, 2) be hypoplastic, with numerous large follicular cysts in a diminished ovarian cortex with very few primordial follicles, or 3) hypoplastic, with no evidence of mature follicles in ovaries in which the entire stroma was filled with atretic corpora lutea. The internal genitalia were not well described by Benda or any other authors. The external genitalia were characterized by Beidelman (1945) as showing full labia majora, tiny or absent labia minora, and a large clitoris.

Features of reproductive physiology in the female patients described by Benda (1969), Stearns, Droulard, and Sahhar (1960), and Versteeg (1956) have been delayed menarche, delayed breast development, and absent areolar glands, and (Smith, Warren, and Turner, 1963) diminished or absent axillary hair. Occasional facial hirsutism has been noted. Beidelman (1945) further stated that 50% of the females never menstruate. However, Stearns et al. (1960), in a small series of 54 females (23 over the age of 12 years), noted that menstrual periods, once established, seemed to be regular and of approximately normal duration. Øster (1953) studied the menses of 121 Down females 15 years of age or older and found that 109 menstruated regularly. No instance of amenorrhea was seen by Masterson et al. (1970) in 75 females between 15 and 36 years.

The suggestion of regular menses was extended in 1964 by Tricomi, Valenti, and Hall (1964), who reported in 12 women, ages 19–41, that ovulation as detected by serial vaginal smears was seen in 5 of 13 cases, possible ovulation in 4, and the remainder did not ovulate in the 2 months studied. Endocrine data of hFSH, hLH cycles, or serum estrogen and progesterone values as measured with contemporary techniques are thus far lacking for the female Down population.

Trisomy 21 Males

As with the female Down subject, the basic descriptions of trisomy 21 males are those of Benda (1969). He characterized the gonads in 26 subjects, ranging in age from 2.5 months to 31 years. As with the ovaries, the testes of some in the under-2 years age group were shown to contain normal Sertoli cells and a few spermatogonia. The remainder were a-spermatogenic and described as "Sertoli cell only." An older group of eight subjects between 4 and 15 years had small testes with small tubules containing only Sertoli cells. Another group of nine patients between 6 and 31 years revealed either moderate testicular size, with some spermatogenic and Sertoli cells but no mature sperm, or small testes, with Sertoli cells only. Interstitial cells in most instances were not described as normal. Benda noted a 50% incidence of undescended testes in his subjects. Corroboration of decreased testicular size was found by Sylvester and Rundle (1962), but they did not agree with the increased incidence of cryptorchidism. Scrotums and penises were considered underdeveloped. Bearding was noted by Swersie, Hueckel, and Paulsen (1978, personal communication) to be normal. Voice pitch was described as normal by Michel and Carney (1964) in young males. Pubic hair was reported as nonandrogenized in character and distribution (Beidelman, 1945; Smith et al., 1963).

Quantitative histological examination of seminiferous epithelium in eight subjects with Down syndrome by Skakkebaek, Hultén, and Philip (1973) was correlated with testis size, secondary sex characteristics, and fertility. No sperm counts were noted. The subjects showed either complete Sertoli cell-only syndrome or "partial Sertoli cell only," with a reduction in germ cell number. No paternity was annotated. Schröder, Lydecken, and de la Chapelle (1971) described three young trisomic males in whom abundant, normal, and complete spermatogenesis was found in tubules adjacent to other tubules containing relative lack of spermatogenesis.

Swersie et al. (1978, personal communication) studied six adult institutionalized males with Down syndrome, ages 25–45, for detailed evaluation of the pituitary-testicular axis. The subjects had no acute or chronic illnesses that might have affected the measurements. Testicular size was normal in three men, with mild atrophy in the others. Serum testosterone levels were normal in all subjects except one, in whom it was marginal. Serum LH was elevated in five subjects and serum FSH levels were normal in four of six and elevated in the remaining two.

Detailed reproductive, anatomical, or endocrinological data like these for pure trisomy 21 were not available for normal 21 mosaic persons. New or sophisticated techniques might have to be used to detect variations from the abnormal in this population.

With these basic descriptions in mind, meiosis in these patients is presented. The general predictive aspects of secondary nondisjunction are well known and are not detailed.

GAMETOGENESIS IN PURE TRISOMY 21 FEMALE AND MALE DOWN PATIENTS

Oogenesis

The principal report of fetal oogenesis in trisomy 21 cases is that of Luciani et al. (1976). They presented partial pachytene analyses of oocytes originating from 18-, 20-, and 22-week-old fetuses diagnosed by amniocentesis. Maternal ages were 43, 39, and 41 years, respectively. It was found that the "milestones" of oogenesis in these fetuses were comparable to control 46,XX female fetuses of the same gestational age. The numbers of oocytes and the degree of atresia were stated to be normal. Of all oocytes observed (number not stated), 42 were found to be abnormal. In the 42 diagnosed, 14 contained a clear trivalent, 13 contained a trivalent with an asynaptic region in the long arm below the q21 band, and in 15 oocytes, a bivalent and a univalent were seen side by side. The asynapsis was at variance with Hungerford et al.'s (1970) report on male trisomy 21 pachytene cells. The chromomere patterns were stated to be in agreement with those of Hungerford et al. with the exception that in oocytes, the centromere, short arm (p11), secondary constriction (p12), and satellite (p13) were very clear. In contrast, these regions were condensed into a single large chromomere in trisomy 21 spermatocytes (Hungerford et al., 1970). Fourteen subbands were diagnosed. The chromomere patterns were felt to correspond with G-band mitotic metaphase bands of chromosome 21.

Spermatogenesis

More work with meiotic analysis has been done with male Down patients. No pachytene analyses are available, but many reports of later meiotic stages exist. In 1952, Mittwoch interpreted a meiotic testis preparation from a male Down as "normal." In a subsequent study in 1960, Miller, Mittwoch, and Penrose reported four cases of male trisomy 21. They saw cells that contained 22, 23, or 24 bodies; usually 23 and

Table 1. Testicular chromosomal data in trisomy 21 Down males: Mitotic and meiotic

Author	Age (Years)	Spermatogonia				Bodies		Meiosis		21 configuration		
		46	47	48	Total	23 XY	24 XY	24 X+Y	25 X+Y	I	III	?
Sasaki (1965)	45	–	3	–	3	10	1	5	–	1	15	–
Finch et al. (1966)	21	–	–	–	–	–	+	–	–	+	0	–
Hultén and Lindsten (1970)	16	0	3	2	5	16	39	3	5	44	19	25
Kjessler and de la Chapelle (1971)[a]	27	–	–	–	–	4	3	0	1	4	0	–
	28	–	–	–	–	7	2	2	1	3	0	–
Schröder et al. (1971)[b]	30	2	2	–	4	16	10	1	–	10(6)[b]	7	10
	24	1	–	–	1	4	2	1	1	3	–	5
	25	1	2	–	3	6	4	1	1	5	3	4
Giraud et al. (1971)	52	–	2	–	2	+	+	–	–	+	+	–

[a]Case "K" was reported in part by Schröder et al. (1971).

[b]Case "K" was reported in part by Kjessler and de la Chapelle (1971).

154

trivalents, univalents, and multivalents were diagnosed. Other, more recent representative studies are presented in Table 1, which summarizes the information available on spermatogonial metaphase complements and diakinesis/metaphase I analyses. The last column describes the configuration of the chromosome 21s as stated by the authors. A diagnosis of a univalent was made in 70 cells and of a trivalent in 44 cells out of a total observed of 158. However, in 44 cells of the 158, a diagnosis could not be made. Quite possibly a contracted trivalent may have existed in this category, but a univalent would have been detected. Giraud et al.'s (1971) report was of particular interest in that it described a 52-year-old Down subject with diabetes. The analysis of the testis biopsy revealed two spermatogonia with 47 chromosomes and a nonspecified number of diakinesis cells with trivalents or a bivalent plus a univalent. This report contained the only data on second metaphase cells, which were stated to contain only 23 X or 23 Y chromosomes.

GAMETOGENESIS IN MOSAIC, NONDISJUNCTIVE TRISOMY 21 MALE AND FEMALE DOWN PATIENTS

Oogenesis

Very few data are available concerning meiotic behavior of oocytes from mosaic trisomy 21 mothers. One case has been reported in part from the Paediatric Research Unit of Guy's Hospital (London). The propositus was born to a 30-year-old mosaic mother who had 4% trisomy 21 cells in blood and 14% in skin cultures. Ovarian cultures yielded 69% and 78% cells with trisomy 21. One oocyte at diakinesis/meiosis I that was recovered after hormone treatment had 22 bivalents and one trivalent (Figure 1).

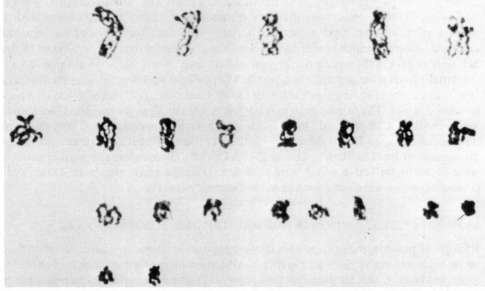

Figure 1. Oocyte at diakinesis/metaphase I from a mosaic female Down patient. Note 21 trivalent.

Spermatogenesis

Hungerford et al. (1970) reported the only available meiotic analyses in a mosaic male patient who was 23 years old. Oligospermia was present. Normal chromosome 21 pachytene bivalents were seen, as well as trivalents. The short arms of the trivalent were unassociated, or two of the three constituent elements were paired. The long arms of all three chromosomes were closely associated, with few asynaptic regions. Meiosis in a mosaic male studied by Hsu et al. (1971) revealed that 10% of spermatogonia studied contained 47 chromosomes. Twenty-one diakinesis/metaphase I cells were studied. Eighteen had 23 bivalents and 3 had 24 bodies, including a univalent G.

REPRODUCTIVE PERFORMANCE IN "PURE TRISOMY 21" PATIENTS

Data on trisomy 21 females were difficult to clarify because some reports were duplications. Twenty-four female trisomy 21 Down syndrome patients and their progeny have been reported. Table 2, taken from Smith and Berg (1976), describes 22 of these mothers and their progeny; 9 had Down syndrome, 2 were retarded, 10 were normal, and 3 were stillborn. Mean maternal age of Down mothers at the birth of their affected children was 22 years, although their own mothers averaged 36 years. Other points of interest in these data that reveal the products of several kinds of matings include: 1) A normal female in Sawyer's case (1949; Sawyer and Shafter, 1957) was born from a mating with the propositus's father; 2) Schlaug's (1957) case may represent a female with "partial trisomy 21 syndrome" resulting from a mating with the patient's father; 3) Hanhart's (1960) cases, a female and a male with Down syndrome, were the products of matings with the patient's older brother, an "imbecile"; 4) Moric-Petrovic and Garzicic (1970) reported on a normal son born to a trisomy 21 mother and a normal father; and 5) Reiss, Lovrien, and Hecht (1971) reported on a father who had a reported IQ of 70 but to whom a "normal" child was born. Walker and Ising's (1969) report was the only instance of a stated mosaic parent with a mosaic offspring. No clear pattern of progeny resulting from various matings has emerged. Two additional cases have been reported briefly that are not in the table. Scharrer et al. (1975) reported a 21-year-old trisomy 21 mother who gave birth to a "normal" male who had aplasia of the left fifth finger and dermatoglyphic features felt by the authors to be consonant with Down syndrome, but the child was chromosomally normal. The other case was reported in 1976 by Francesconi and Guaschino, who described a 28-year-old Down mother with a trisomic daughter. Thus, the total number of reported Down syndrome mothers at this writing is 24. The ratio of chromosomally normal to trisomy 21 was 15/10. Of these chromosomally normal cases, 2 were mentally defective and 3 were stillborn. Data on confirmed male Down syndrome paternity were not detected in the literature search.

REPRODUCTIVE FUNCTION IN NORMAL/TRISOMY 21 (MOSAIC) PATIENTS

Reports of parental mosaicism with Down propositi were not frequent, but they may be an underestimate, since all parents of all Down offspring have not had chromosome analyses. Considerations of grandparental age and several other ideas emerge from the available data as tabulated in Table 3. To date, 36 mosaic parents have been

Table 2. Offspring of fully affected Down syndrome (D.S.) females

Description of child	Age of D.S. mother at birth of her child (years)	Maternal age at birth of D.S. mother (years)	Karyotype		Authors
			D.S. mother	Child	
Normal female	25				Sawyer (1949); Sawyer and Shafter (1957)
D.S. male	30	42			Lelong et al. (1949)
D.S. female	19	19	Trisomy 21	Trisomy 21	Rehn and Thomas (1957); Stiles (1958); Stiles and Goodman (1961); Johnston and Jaslow (1963)
Retarded male	30	42	Trisomy 21	Normal	Forssman and Thysell (1957); Forssman, Lehman, and Thysell (1961)
Retarded female	29	39			Schlaug (1957)
Normal male	22	22	Trisomy 21	Normal	Levan and Hsu (1959, 1960)
Normal male	23	44			Mullins, Estrada, and Gready (1960)
D.S. male	21	44	Trisomy 21		Hanhart (1960)
D.S. female			Trisomy 21	Trisomy 21	Hanhart, Delhanty, and Penrose (1961)
Stillborn male twins	14	34	Trisomy 21	Normal (both twins)	Priest et al. (1963); Thuline and Priest (1961)
Normal male	21	40			Thompson (1961)
Stillborn female	20	22	Trisomy 21		Thompson (1961, 1962)
D.S. male	22	22	Trisomy 21	Trisomy 21	Thompson (1961, 1962)
Normal female	18	46	Trisomy 21	Normal	Foxton et al. (1965)
Normal female	27	35	Trisomy 21	Normal	Tagher and Reisman (1966)
D.S. female	18	43	Trisomy 21	Trisomy 21	Finley et al. (1968)
D.S. male	17	37	Trisomy 21	Trisomy 21	Friedman et al. (1970)
Normal female	19	39	Trisomy 21	Normal	Masterson et al. (1970)
Normal female	30	42	Trisomy 21	Normal	Masterson et al. (1970)
Normal male	16		Trisomy 21	Normal	Morić Petrović and Garzicic (1970)
D.S. female	23	40	Trisomy 21	Trisomy 21	Rethoré et al. (1970)
Normal female	25	40	Trisomy 21	Normal	Reiss, Lovrien, and Hecht (1971)
D.S. male	20		Trisomy 21	Trisomy 21	Fuchs-Mecke and Passarge (1972)

Reprinted with permission from Smith and Berg, 1976, *Down's Anomaly* (2nd ed.), Churchill & Livingstone, London.

Table 3. Data from 36 mosaic parents

Sex	Maternal age at birth of mosaic parent	Age of mosaic parent at birth of Down infant	% trisomic cells in blood	% trisomic cells in skin	Comments	Source
F	40	28	15.0	23.0		Blank et al. (1962)
F	39	18, 19	27.0	75.0		Smith et al. (1962)
F	39	17	20.0	2.2		Weinstein and Warkany (1963)
F	34	30	10.0	24.0	Two blood cultures	Verresen et al. (1964)
M	27	25	25.0	20.0		Ferrier (1964)
F		20		44.0	Pooled	Turner et al. (1966)
F	38	33	4.3			Taylor (personal communication)
F	37	45	7.0			Taylor (1967, personal communication)
M	30	35	21.5			Massimo et al. (1967)
F	32	25	5.3			Pfeiffer (personal communication)
F		22	8.5			Gloor (personal communication)
F	39	22, 24	5.0		Two Down	Aarskog (1969)
F		27	18.0			Izaković and Getlik (1969)
M			23.0			Walker and Ising (1969)
F	22	20, 29	2.3	13.8	Different father	Mikkelsen (1970)
F	22	27	10.0			Timson et al. (1971)
M	35	24, 26	0	7.5	Testis 4%	Hsu et al. (1971)
M	30	21	6.0			Hsu et al. (1971)
M		30	4.0	4.0		Hsu et al. (1971)
F		33	10.0			Krmpotic and Hardin (1971)
F			7.0			Sutherland et al. (1972)
M		23	6.0		Three Down	Mehés (1973)
F	44	24, 26	2.6	2.0	Two blood cultures	Richards (1974)
F	27		25.5	22.0	Three blood cultures	Richards (1974)
M	31	26	6.7			Richards (1974)
F			2.0		195 cells	Richards (1974)
F	30	27	21.5			Richards (1974)
F		32	4.6			Richards (1974)
F	37	35	22.5	28.6		Richards (1974)
F	18	32, 34	2.2			Richards (1974)
F	19	25, 29	7.8			Richards (1974)
M	33	30	6.0			Papp et al. (1974)
M		24	11.0		Testis 0%	Domány and Métneki (1976)
M		27	15.0		Testis 0%	Domány and Métneki (1976)
M			4.0	0	Testis 0%	Paediatric Research Unit (Guy's Hospital)
F	24	30	4.0	14.0	Ovary R = 78% L = 69%	Published in part

documented, 12 of whom were male and 24 of whom were female. The mean grand-parental age at the time of birth of the mosaic parent was 31.6 years. The mean age of the mosaic parent at the time of birth of the Down progeny was 26.9 years. These data were in agreement with Papp, Varadi, and Szabo (1977), who reported a study of 262 children with trisomy 21. In these data, if the mother was under 30, the mean maternal and paternal grandmaternal age was higher than controls. However, analyses were not done of all parents to confirm their mosaic state. Nevertheless the total cumulative data seem to support the concept that mosaic parents have been born to a mother who was older than mothers bearing normal infants. Grandpaternal age has not been reported.

The detection of mosaicism may have been more successful in skin fibroblasts (18.2% average) than in lymphocytes (10.6%). Testicular cultures in these cases were of low yield, but in one case, ovarian cultures yielded 69% and 78% trisomic cells.

Of the cases where data were given, 38 Down and 12 chromosomally normal infants were born to mosaic parents in a total of 50 progeny, quite different from the distribution for the progeny of pure trisomy 21 patients.

SUMMARY

Pure trisomy 21 female Down syndrome patients are capable of reproduction. Twenty-four patients have produced 15 chromosomally normal and 10 trisomy 21 offspring.

No report exists of a bona fide male trisomy 21 parent.

Twelve mosaic (nondisjunctive trisomy 21) fathers and 24 mothers have produced 38 chromosomally abnormal and 12 normal offspring in 50 progeny. Mean grandparental age at the birth of the mosaic parent was 31.6 years in these cases, and the mean of the mosaic patient's ages at the birth of the Down infant was 26.9 years.

Many more studies are needed of pure and mosaic trisomy patients, particularly of reproductive anatomy and physiology, as well as detailed analyses of meiosis.

REFERENCES

Aarskog, D. 1969. Down's syndrome transmitted through maternal mosaicism. Acta Paediatr. Scand. 58:609.

Beidelman, B. 1945. Mongolism: A selective review. Am. J. Ment. Defic. 50:35.

Benda, C. E. 1969. Endocrine and general pathology. In C. E. Benda, Down's Syndrome: Mongolism and Its Management, pp. 183–190. Rev. ed. Grune & Stratton, New York.

Blank, C. E., Gemmell, E., Casey, M. D., and Lord, M. 1962. Mosaicism in a mother with a mongol child. Br. Med. J. 2:378.

Domány, Z., and Métneki, J. 1976. Mosaik-Trisomie bei den vätern von zwei kindern mit Down-Syndrom. Acta Paediatr. Acad. Sci. Hung. 17(3):177.

Ferrier, S. 1964. Enfant mongolien-parent mosaique. Etude de deux familles. [Mongoloid infant-mosaic parent. Study of two families.] J. Genet. Hum. 13:315.

Finch, R. A., Böök, J. A., Finley, W. H., Finley, S. C., and Tucker, C. C. 1966. Meiosis in trisomic Down's syndrome. Ala. J. Med. Sci. 3:117.

Finley, W. H., Finley, S. C., Hardy, J. P., and McKinnon, T. 1968. Down's syndrome in mother and child. Obstet. Gynecol. 32:200.

Forsmann, H., Lehman, O., and Thysell, T. 1961. Reproduction in mongolism. Chromosome studies and re-examination of a child. Am. J. Ment. Defic. 65:495.

Forsmann, H., and Thysell, T. 1957. A woman with mongolism and her child. Am. J. Ment. Defic. 62:500.

Foxton, J. R. V., Pitt, D., Wiener, S., Brasch, J., and Ferguson, J. 1965. Reproduction in a female with Down's syndrome. Aust. Paediatr. J. 1:176.

Francesconi, D., and Guaschino, S. 1976. Trisomy 21 in mother and daughter. Clin. Genet. 9:346.

Friedman, J. M., Sternberg, W. H., Varela, M., and Barclay, D. L. 1970. Trisomy-21 in mother and child. Obstet. Gynecol. 36:731.

Fuchs-Mecke, S., and Passarge, E. 1972. Kinder von muttern mit Down syndrome (Mongolismus). Deutsch. Med. Wschr. 97:338.

Giraud, F., Luciani, J. M., Mattei, J.-F., Galinier, L., Stahl, A., and Gascard, E. 1971. Etude clinique, mitotique et méiotique d'une trisomie 21 avec diabète chez un homme de 52 ans. [Clinical, mitotic and meiotic study with a 52-year-old man with diabetes.] Marseille Med. 1:31.

Hanhart, E. 1960. Mongoloide idiotie bei mutter und swei kindern aus inzesten. Acta Genet. Med. 9:112.

Hanhart, E., Delhanty, J. D. A., and Penrose, L. S. 1961. Trisomy in mother and child. Lancet 1:403.

Hsu, L. Y. F., Gertner, M., Leiter, E., and Hirchhorn, K. 1971. Paternal trisomy 21 mosaicism and Down's syndrome. Am. J. Hum. Genet. 23:592.

Hultén, M., and Lindsten, J. 1970. The behaviour of structural aberrations at male meiosis. In P. A. Jacobs, W. H. Price, and P. Law (eds.), Human Population Cytogenetics, pp. 24–61. Pfizer Medical Monographs 5. Edinburgh University Press, Edinburgh.

Hungerford, D. A., Mellman, W. J., Balaban, G. B., LaBadie, G. U., Messatzzia, L. R., and Haller, G. 1970. Chromosome structure and function in man. III. Pachytene analysis and identification of the supernumerary chromosome in a case of Down's syndrome (mongolism). PNAS 67:221.

Izakovič, V., and Getlík, A. 1969. Mozaika 46,XX/47,XX,G+ U Matky dieťaťa s Downovým syndrómom—Trizómiou G_1. Cesk. Pediatr. 24:698.

Johnston, A. W., and Jaslow, R. I. 1963. Children of mothers with Down's syndrome. New Engl. J. Med. 269:439.

Kjessler, B., and de la Chapelle, A. 1971. Meiosis and spermatogenesis in two postpubertal males with Down's syndrome: 47,XY,G+. Clin. Genet. 11:50.

Krmpotic, E., and Hardin, M. B. 1971. Secondary nondisjunction causing regular trisomy 21 in the offspring of a mosaic trisomy 21 mother. Am. J. Obstet. Gynecol. 110:589.

Lelong, M., Borniche, P., Kreisler, L., and Baundy, R. 1949. Arch. Franc. Pediatr. 6:231.

Levan, A., and Hsu, T. C. 1959. The human idiogram. Hereditas 45:665–674.

Levan, A., and Hsu, T. C. 1960. The chromosomes of a mongoloid female, mother of a normal boy. Hereditas 46:770–772.

Luciani, J. M., Devictor, M., Morazzani, M. R., and Stahl, A. 1976. Meiosis of trisomy 21 in the human pachytene oocyte. Chromosoma 57:155.

Massimo, L., Borrone, C., Vianello, M. G., and Dagna-Bricarelli, F. 1967. Familial immune defects. Lancet 1:108.

Masterson, J. G., Law, E. M., Power, M. M., Stokes, B. M., and Murphy, D. 1970. Reproduction in two females with Down's syndrome. Ann. Genet. 13:38.

Mehés, K. 1973. Paternal trisomy 21 mosaicism and Down's anomaly. Humangenetik 17:297.

Melnyk, J. 1972. Meiosis in the male. In S. Wright, B. Crandell, and L. Boyer (eds.), Perspectives in Cytogenetics: The Next Decade, p. 25. Charles C Thomas Publisher, Springfield, Ill.

Michel, J. F., and Carney, R. J. 1964. Pitch characteristics of mongoloid boys. J. Speech Dis. 29:121.

Mikkelsen, M. 1970. A Danish survey of patients with Down's syndrome born to young mothers. Ann. N.Y. Acad. Sci. 171:370.

Miller, O. J., Mittwoch, U., and Penrose, L. S. 1960. Spermatogenesis in man with special reference to aneuploidy. Heredity 14:456.

Mittwoch, U. 1952. The chromosome complement in a mongolian imbecile. Ann. Eugen. 17:37.

Moric-Petrovic, S., and Garzicic, B. 1970. Mother with Down's syndrome and her child. J. Ment. Defic. Res. 14:68.

Mullins, D. H., Estrada, W. R., and Gready, T. G. 1960. Pregnancy in an adult mongoloid female. Obstet. Gynecol. 15:781.

Øster, J. 1953. Mongolism. Danish Science Press, Copenhagen.

Papp, Z., Csecsfi, K., Skapinyecz, J., and Dolhay, B. 1974. Paternal normal/trisomy 21 mosaicism as an indication for amniocentesis. Clin. Genet. 6:192.

Papp, Z., Váradi, E., and Szabó, Z. 1977. Grandmaternal age at birth of parents of children with trisomy 21. Hum. Genet. 39:221.

Priest, J. H., Thuline, H. C., Norby, D. E., and La Veck, G. D. 1963. Reproduction in human autosomal trisomics—Chromosome studies of a mongol mother, her nonmongol twins, and her family. Am. J. Dis. Child 105:31.

Rehn, A. T., and Thomas, E. 1957. Family history of a mongolian girl who bore a mongolian child. Am. J. Ment. Defic. 62:496.

Reiss, J. A., Lovrien, E. W., and Hecht, F. 1971. A mother with Down's syndrome and her chromosomally normal infant. Ann. Genet. 14:225.

Rethoré, M., Lafourcade, J., Prieur, M., Caille, B., Cruveillier, J., Tanzy, M., and Lejeune, J. 1970. Mere et fille trisomiques 21 libres. [Mother and daughter with trisomy 21.] Ann. Genet. 13:42.

Richards, B. W. 1974. Investigation of 142 mosaic mongols and mosaic parents of mongols; cytogenetic analysis and maternal age at birth. J. Ment. Defic. Res. 18:199.

Sasaki, M. 1965. Meiosis in a male with Down's syndrome. Chromosoma 16:652.

Sawyer, G. M. 1949. Case report: Reproduction in a mongoloid. Am. J. Ment. Defic. 54:204.

Sawyer, G. M., and Shafter, A. J. 1957. Reproduction in a mongoloid: A follow-up. Am. J. Ment. Defic. 61:793.

Scharrer, S., Stengel-Rutkowski, S., Rodewald-Rudescu, A., Erdlen, E., and Zang, K. D. 1975. Reproduction in a female patient with Down's syndrome. Humangenetik 26:207.

Schlaug, R. 1957. A mongolian mother and her child. A case report. Acta Genet. 7:533.

Schröder, J., Lydecken, K., and de la Chapelle, A. 1971. Meiosis and spermatogenesis in G-trisomic males. Humangenetik 13:15.

Skakkebaek, N. E., Hultén, M., and Philip, J. 1973. Quantification of human seminiferous epithelium. IV. Histological studies in 17 men with numerical and structural autosomal aberrations. Acta Pathol. Microbiol. Scand. 81:112.

Smith, D. W., Therman, E. M., Patau, K. A., and Inhorn, S. L. 1962. Mosaicism in mother of two mongoloids. Am. J. Dis. Child. 104:534.

Smith, G. S., Warren, S. A., and Turner, D. R. 1963. Hair characteristics in mongolism (Down's syndrome). Am. J. Ment. Defic. 68:362.

Smith, G. F., and Berg, J. 1976. Down's Anomaly. 2nd Ed. Churchill Livingstone, London.

Stearns, P. E., Droulard, K. E., and Sahhar, F. H. 1960. Studies bearing on fertility of male and female mongoloids. Am. J. Ment. Defic. 65:37.

Stiles, K. A. 1958. Reproduction in a mongoloid imbecile. Proc. 10th Int. Cong. Genet. Montreal 2:276.

Stiles, K. A., and Goodman, H. O. 1961. Reproduction in a mongoloid. Acta Genet. Med. 50:457.

Sutherland, G. R., Fitzgerald, M. G., and Danks, D. M. 1972. Difficulty in showing mosaicism in the mother of three mongols. Arch. Dis. Child. 47:970.

Sylvester, P. E., and Rundle, A. T. 1962. Endocrinological aspects of mental deficiency. II. Maturational status of adult males. J. Ment. Defic. Res. 6:87.

Tagher, P., and Reisman, C. E. 1966. Reproduction in Down's syndrome (mongolism): Chromosomal study of mother and normal child. Obstet. Gynecol. 27:182.

Thompson, M. W. 1961. Reproduction in two female mongols. Can. J. Genet. Cytol. 3:351.

Thompson, M. W. 1962. 21-Trisomy in a fertile female mongol. Can. J. Genet. Cytol. 4:352.

Thuline, H. C., and Priest, J. H. 1961. Pregnancy in a 14-year-old mongoloid. Lancet 1:1115.

Timson, J., Harris, R., Gadd, R. L., Ferguson-Smith, M. E., and Ferguson-Smith, M. A. 1971. Down's syndrome due to maternal mosaicism, and the value of antenatal diagnosis. Lancet 1:549.

Tricomi, V., Valenti, C., and Hall, J. E. 1964. Ovulatory patterns in Down's syndrome. Am. J. Obstet. Gynecol. 89:651.

Turner, J. H., Kaplan, S., and Tomley, J. 1966. Mosaicism and mongoloid stigmata in the mother of a Down's syndrome child. Hum. Chrom. News. 20:31.

Verresen, H., van den Berghe, H., and Creemers, J. 1964. Mosaic trisomy in phenotypically normal mother of mongol. Lancet 1:526.

Versteeg, J. M. 1956. Onderzoek naar de functie der eierstokken bij oliogophrenen. Doctoral thesis, Leiden.

Walker, F. A., and Ising, R. 1969. Mosaic Down's syndrome in a father and daughter. Lancet 1:374.

Weinstein, I. D., and Warkany, J. 1963. Maternal mosaicism and Down's syndrome (Mongolism). J. Pediatr. 63:599.

Role of the Nucleolus Organizer in the Etiology of Down Syndrome

Orlando J. Miller

Down syndrome is almost always caused by the presence of an entire extra copy of chromosome 21 (trisomy 21: 94% of cases) or to the presence of an extra copy of the long arm of chromosome 21 due to aberrant segregation of a Robertsonian translocation (about 4% of cases). Darlington (1935), working with plants, suggested that the nucleolus might predispose to nondisjunction because its presence could interfere with pairing of homologous chromosomes in meiotic prophase and thus prevent formation of chiasmata between the chromosome(s) carrying a nucleolus organizer (NO). Without chiasmata to hold the two homologous chromosomes together as a paired bivalent, the homologues would remain as unpaired univalents and pass at random to one or the other daughter cell at anaphase, resulting in a high incidence of nondisjunction, with both copies of the NO chromosome going to the same daughter cell.

Although no evidence in support of this hypothesis has ever been reported, and no comparable data on mitotic chromosomes exist, there is evidence in mice that chiasma frequencies decline with advancing maternal age (Polani and Jagiello, 1976). Since pairing of homologous chromosomes occurs early in first meiotic prophase, before the prolonged dictyotene stage, which begins before birth and continues until shortly before ovulation 10–50 years later, it is unclear how a maternal age effect on nondisjunction could be due to nucleolar interference with homologous pairing or chiasma formation. Nucleolar persistence, however, might interfere with separation of homologous NO chromosomes.

Polani et al. (1960) suggested that persistence of a nucleolus may play a role in the nondisjunction leading to trisomy 21 and in the centric fusion leading to Robertsonian translocation. Although this hypothesis has received relatively little attention,

This work was supported, in part, by the National Foundation—March of Dimes.

163

it appears to be worth considering in the light of existing knowledge about Down syndrome. Any hypothesis concerning the origin of nondisjunctional gametes in trisomy 21 in particular must take account of these characteristic features of trisomy 21:

The maternal age effect
Origin more often maternal than paternal
Origin usually at meiosis I rather than meiosis II
A probable increase following gonadal ionizing irradiation of either parent
A possible role of virus infection

We believe that all these features can be explained if the nucleolus plays a role in nondisjunction. Let us therefore briefly review the evidence for each of these features and then examine the role of the nucleolus and the nucleolus organizer regions (NORs).

MATERNAL AGE EFFECT

The most clearly established predisposing factor in trisomy 21 is advanced maternal age. The incidence of trisomy 21 is strongly related to maternal age, rising exponentially with increasing age from about 1 in 2000 live births in women under age 20 to about 1 in 40 live births in women over age 45 (Hook and Hamerton, 1977; Trimble and Baird, 1978). The true incidence may be somewhat higher than these figures indicate, because of difficulty in ascertaining all cases in newborns and selective postnatal mortality. Data from prenatal diagnostic studies on cultured amniotic fluid cells suggest that the incidence of trisomy 21 at midtrimester of pregnancy is much higher: about 2% in women over 35 and at least 10% in women over 45 (Alberman, this volume). In view of such figures, more and more older pregnant women are seeking prenatal diagnosis and requesting selective termination of pregnancy to prevent the birth of a child with Down syndrome.

PREDISPOSING FACTORS IN YOUNG MOTHERS

Despite the great importance of maternal age as an indicator of the relative risk of a trisomic birth, well over 50% of such births occur to women under age 35. As more older women resort to prenatal diagnosis and selective termination of pregnancy, this proportion seems likely to grow. It is therefore important to seek means of detecting young women who are at increased risk of having trisomy 21 births. It is clear that among women under 35 the risk of having a trisomic child is not evenly distributed. For example, couples who have had a trisomic child are at increased risk of having another affected child (Smith and Berg, 1976). This has been attributed in a minority of cases to chromosomal mosaicism in one of the parents; Penrose (1967) estimated, from quantitative analysis of dermatoglyphic features, that 10% of the mothers of trisomy 21 offspring were 46,XX/47,XX, + 21 mosaics. However, in most cases of trisomy 21, such mosaicism has not been demonstrated by chromosome studies in either parent, and quantitative dermatoglyphic analysis has not become an established means of detecting such presumptive high risk couples. Whether or not dermatoglyphic studies become more widespread in their application, it seems important to look for predisposing factors other than chromosomal mosaicism.

SOURCE OF THE EXTRA CHROMOSOME

Polymorphism of heterochromatin on chromosome 21 is very common, so the parental source of the extra chromosome in trisomy 21 can be determined in at least a third of the cases by following the inheritance of chromosome markers (Langenbeck et al., 1976; Magenis et al., 1977). Assuming these provide an unbiased estimate of the relative frequencies of maternal and paternal nondisjunction, one can conclude that more than 75% of trisomy 21 progeny result from maternal nondisjunction. Furthermore, these studies have shown that the two chromosomes 21 contributed by the nondisjunctional parent have dissimilar short arm polymorphisms in most cases, indicating, if one assumes no crossing over in the very short short arm, that most cases of trisomy 21 arise by nondisjunction at the first meiotic division rather than at the second meiotic division.

IONIZING RADIATION

Radiation has been implicated in the etiology of trisomy 21. The incidence of trisomy 21 may be higher in couples where either spouse has received gonadal ionizing radiation as a result of medical procedures (Uchida, 1977) or as a result of high background radiation, as in the Indian state Kerala (Kochupillai et al., 1976). Treatment of cultured human somatic cells (or the serum or plasma in which they are grown) with 50 rads led to a fourfold increase in hyperdiploid cells, usually involving chromosome 21 or the X (Uchida, this volume). Animal data also support the idea that ionizing radiation increases the frequency of meiotic nondisjunction, the effect being particularly marked in older female mice (Uchida and Freeman, 1977).

VIRUS INFECTION

Viruses are another type of agent that may play a role in nondisjunction. Clustering of cases of Down syndrome has been related to a specific hepatitis epidemic in Australia (Stoller and Collmann, 1965), although this has not been confirmed in other countries. Although the evidence is weak, viral infections cannot be entirely ruled out as significant predisposing factors in trisomy 21 (Evans, 1967). Meiotic aneuploidy with a four-fold increase in the frequency of second division cells with chromosomes 19 or 21 has been observed in a mouse strain with a latent ectromelia virus infection (Schröder, Halkka, and Brummer-Korvenkontio, 1970).

NORs, rRNA GENES, AND NUCLEOLI

Each NOR is the chromosomal site of a cluster of rRNA genes, rDNA (Henderson, Warburton, and Atwood, 1972). This site may be visible in metaphase chromosomes as an achromatic gap or secondary constriction (Ferguson-Smith and Handmaker,

1963). Electron microscopy shows this not to be a constriction in the chromosome but a highly specialized region with a different nucleoprotein structure than that of the rest of the chromosome (Goessens and Lepoint, 1974; Hsu, Brinkley, and Arrighi, 1967). This difference is reflected in the differential staining of this region by silver-staining methods (Howell, Denton, and Diamond, 1975) similar to those used for many years to stain the nucleolus selectively (Fernández-Gòmez et al., 1972). The close correspondence of the silver-stained regions (AgNOR) to the sites of rDNA has been demonstrated by correlated studies on metaphase chromosomes of nine mammalian species (Goodpasture and Bloom, 1975; Hsu, Spirito, and Pardue, 1975) and by studies throughout the mitotic cell cycle and during meiosis (Schwarzacher, Mikelsaar, and Schnedl, 1978).

In the human, as in many other organisms, NORs are present at multiple sites, which can sometimes be detected by the presence of a secondary constriction (Ferguson-Smith and Handmaker, 1963), by in situ hybridization with radioactive rRNA (Henderson et al., 1972), or by the presence of silver staining. The amount of silver staining of a particular NOR is generally inherited in simple Mendelian fashion (Markovic, Worton, and Berg, 1978) and is usually proportional to the size of the nucleolus (Lau and Arrighi, 1976). Studies in interspecific hybrid cells have shown that silver staining is restricted to NORs whose rRNA genes have been actively transcribed (Croce et al., 1977; D. A. Miller et al., 1976; O. J. Miller et al., 1976).

Activity of rRNA genes is accompanied by the appearance of nucleoli. Each nucleolus is the site of rRNA synthesis. This can be visualized by spreading gently lysed nuclei or nucleoli on water and observing the resultant spreads with an electron microscope (O. L. Miller and Hamkalo, 1972). Each nucleolus contains a large number (e.g., 20–200) of small, fir tree-like assemblies in tandem array, each consisting of an rDNA axis with a series of closely spaced and progressively longer nascent rRNA precursor molecules attached to the axis and, attached to the RNA, proteins that are involved in processing the precursor into 28S, 18S, and 5.8S pieces that become structural components of the ribosomes. That is, the transcription and processing involved in the synthesis of rRNA take place on rDNA templates in the nucleolus (Perry, 1976).

Some of the characteristics of nucleoli that are important in analyzing the role of the nucleolus in the etiology of Down syndrome are listed below:

> Absent in meiosis II
> In meiosis I, larger in females
> Size proportional to rDNA transcriptional activity
> Size proportional to AgNOR size
> Tendency to fuse, proportional to size

A consideration of these leads to some of the predictions on frequency of nondisjunction (see p. 170). Nucleoli are present during the first meiotic division but not the second (McClintock, 1934; Schmid et al., 1977). If the nucleolus and NORs play an important role in meiotic nondisjunction, this event should occur predominantly at meiosis I rather than mieosis II. This appears to be the case. In one series of 24 cases of trisomy 21 of maternal origin, 23 were meiosis I events and only one a meiosis II event (Magenis et al., 1977). In the same series, of the seven cases of paternal origin, five were meiosis I and two were meiosis II.

Nucleolar size is a reflection of the level of rRNA gene activity. The nucleoli are larger in first meiotic division oocytes than in spermatocytes at the corresponding stage (Luciani and Stahl, 1971), perhaps reflecting the greater metabolic activity required to stock the cytoplasm of a larger ovum than that of a tiny sperm. The human ovum does not store the large quantity of material found in amphibian eggs, and one would not expect much, if any, increase in the number of ribosomal RNA genes in the human, whereas there is a thousandfold amplification of these genes in *Xenopus laevis* (Brown and Dawid, 1968). However, the presence of multiple micronucleoli in addition to two to three large nucleoli in human oocyte indicates that some degree of rRNA gene amplification has occurred (Stahl et al., 1975) and provides a basis for the observed increase in nucleolar material in oocytes in comparison to spermatocytes.

Ribosomal RNA synthesis is quite restricted in spermatocytes during meiosis I (Galdieri and Monesi, 1974; Kierzenbaum and Tres, 1974; Schwarzacher et al., 1978). Whatever the mechanism, the end result is a decided difference in size of nucleoli. Thus, if nucleoli and NORs play a role, nondisjunction should be more frequent in female meiosis than in male meiosis. These predictions match the observations made on trisomy 21 (Magenis et al., 1977).

Ionizing radiation has multiple effects, some of which involve the nucleolus. X-rays produce an increase in the size of nucleoli, with an increased RNA content (Scherer, Ringleb, and Ventzke, 1953) and an increase in nucleolar vacuolation (Peters, 1956). DNA virus infections also affect the nucleolus (Granboulan et al., 1963), and may increase the persistence of nucleoli into metaphase (reviewed by Evans, 1967). Since both ionizing radiation and viruses affect the nucleolus, the hypothesis that the nucleolus plays a role in nondisjunction would provide a mechanism by which these factors could increase the incidence of trisomy 21.

NUCLEOLAR FUSION

Nucleoli first appear in late telophase and increase in size as interphase progresses (Dearing, 1934). In telophase the number of nucleoli equals the number of chromosomes with NORs. However, nucleoli tend to fuse, so that many cells have only one or two nucleoli (Dearing, 1934; McClintock, 1934). Numerous factors influence nucleolar fusion: cell cycle, nucleolar size, rDNA cluster size, AgNOR size, and (perhaps) age. The average number of nucleoli is tissue-specific (Shea and Leblond, 1966) and in highly inbred mice is strain-specific (Flaherty, Bennett, and Graef, 1972; Ivanyi, 1971), suggesting the importance of genetic factors in nucleolar function as well as structure. There is a marked difference between the modal number of nucleoli in cultured fibroblasts from the laboratory mouse (five in the NMRI outbred stock) and those from the tobacco mouse (two) (Natarajan and Gropp, 1972), with F_1 hybrids closely resembling their tobacco mouse parent. In cultured fibroblasts from humans of various ages, one to eight nucleoli (modal number three) have been observed (Peterson and Therkelsen, 1962), whereas in similar embryonal cultures, one to 10 nucleoli have been observed (Anastassova-Kristeva, 1977), the greater maximal number perhaps reflecting the higher rate of rRNA synthesis in embryonal cells. This is supported by the much higher number of nucleoli in 6-day blastocysts (usually four to five, but up to seven) than in 20-day embryos (usually one, sometimes two) in the rabbit (Hancock, 1964) and by the higher rate of rRNA synthesis found in *Xenopus* cells with two nucleoli than in those with a single-fused nucleolus (Kurata et al., 1978). There is a decrease in rRNA synthesis in aging human fibroblast cultures (Bowman, Meek, and Daniel, 1976). It is unclear whether this is correlated with an increase in nucleolar fusion or whether this can happen in human oocytes as well.

Some of the effects of nucleolar fusion are: the association of NOR chromosomes, with both rDNA and protein connectives, and possible 1° and 2° nondisjunction and Robertsonian translocation.

SATELLITE ASSOCIATION

The short arms of the human acrocentric chromosomes tend to lie close together in metaphase spreads, in one or more clusters of acrocentric chromosomes. These satellite associations, which occur in mitotic (Ferguson-Smith and Handmaker, 1963) and meiotic I cells (Ferguson-Smith, 1964), are the result of fusion of the nucleoli organized by the NORs of the associated chromosomes. This is supported by the finding of both rDNA connectives (Henderson, Warburton, and Atwood, 1973) and Ag-stainable nucleoprotein connectives (D. A. Miller et al., 1977) between the NORs of acrocentric chromosomes in satellite associations. The presence of DNA and nucleoprotein connectives between NOR chromosomes could play a role in nondisjunction.

Nankin (1970) found the frequency of satellite association to be positively correlated with the extent of nucleolar persistence into early metaphase. Mattei et al. (1976) demonstrated a small increase in satellite association with age, and also noted (Mattei et al., 1974), as did Rosenkranz and Holzer (1972), a slight increase in satellite association in parents of trisomy 21 offspring. Hansson and Mikkelsen (1974) found the increased satellite association in parents of trisomics to be limited to chromosome 21, and to the mothers. This could not be confirmed by Taysi (1975). Increased satellite association in a woman thus may not be an indication that she has an increased risk of having a trisomy 21 birth.

The presence of a structural abnormality of an NOR (probably involving an increase in rDNA) is accompanied by an increase in satellite association (de Capoa, Rocchi, and Gigliani, 1973; Henderson and Atwood, 1976). It may not be fortuitous that one of the small number of people known to have had a double satellite on chromosome 14 had a child with Down syndrome (de Capoa et al., 1973). Even in persons who lack such a structurally abnormal NOR, the probability of involvement in satellite association is not randomly distributed among the NOR chromosomes but is a highly individual characteristic for each acrocentric chromosome, varying between homologues as well as among chromosomes (Mattei et al., 1976; D. A. Miller et al., 1977; Schmid, Krone, and Vogel, 1974). The probability of association for a given acrocentric chromosome is usually proportional to the number of rRNA genes in the NOR (Warburton, Atwood, and Henderson, 1976). It is even more closely correlated with the amount of silver staining of the NOR (D. A. Miller et al., 1977). Silver staining of NORs is a reflection of earlier rRNA gene activity (D. A. Miller et al., 1976), as is satellite association.

NUCLEOLAR PERSISTENCE

Nucleoli usually regress during prophase, with the cessation of rRNA synthesis. In some circumstances, nucleoli persist into prometaphase or throughout metaphase. Polani et al. (1960) suggested that persistence of a nucleolus into metaphase during human female meiosis might lead to nondisjunction and trisomy, and that persistence of nucleoli might be enhanced in older women, thus accounting for the well-known maternal age effect in trisomy 21. At that time, the idea seemed natural, because two of the three known human trisomies involved chromosomes with secondary constrictions that were presumed and later demonstrated to be nucleolus organizer regions (Hungerford, LaBadie, and Balaban, 1971; Hungerford et al., 1971).

The studies of spontaneous abortions by Boué, Boué, and Lazar (1975), Carr and Gedeon (1977), Creasy, Crolla, and Alberman (1976), Hassold et al. (1978), and Kajii et al., (1973) established that trisomies of every chromosome can occur, not just those of NOR chromosomes. This appears to rule out a major direct role for the nucleolus or NORs in the etiology of nondisjunction. However, closer examination of the relative frequencies of trisomy for the various chromosomes (Hook and Hamerton, 1977) has led us to reconsider this idea. It is true that trisomy 16 is by far the most common, accounting for over 30% of all trisomic abortuses. Except for trisomy 16, however, the most common trisomies are those of the D and G group (NOR) chromosomes, which make up about 40% of all trisomic abortuses, with trisomy 21 responsible for 25% of these. Thus trisomy of NOR chromosomes is about three times as common as trisomy for other autosomes, with the exception of chromosome 16. The differences in frequency could be entirely due to differential viability of trisomic zygotes, but there is no compelling evidence for this view. There may, in fact, be highly significant differences in the frequencies of nondisjunction of the various chromosomes, with the nucleolus (including nucleolar fusion and nucleolar persistence) playing an important predisposing role.

A number of factors are known to influence the extent of nucleolar persistence:

1. Species
    Chinese hamster > human > mouse
2. Age
    High during embryogenesis
    Decreases with age?
3. Environmental agents
    Cobalt salts
    4-Nitroquinoline-1-derivatives
    Time in culture

There are species differences, with persistence extremely frequent in Chinese hamster cell lines (63%–98%), less frequent in human cell lines (18%), and uncommon (4%) in mouse cells (Hsu et al., 1965). Persistence of nucleoli is more likely to occur in rapidly growing cells, such as during embryogenesis (Newman, Hoffner, and DiBerardino, 1977), and probably reflects a higher rate of rRNA synthesis. One wonders whether nucleolar persistence might be more common in oocytes, with their high metabolic demands. Nucleolar material is more abundant throughout prophase in fetal human oocytes than in the corresponding stage in human spermatocytes (Luciani and Stahl, 1971).

Exogenous agents have been implicated in the persistence of nucleoli; for example, nontoxic levels of cobalt salts (but not nickel, zinc, chromium, manganese, iron, or beryllium) markedly enhance the persistence of nucleoli, even into telophase, in chick embryo cultures (Heath, 1954). The effect is maximal at 10–14 hr. Both carcinogenic and noncarcinogenic derivatives of 4-nitroquinolin-1-oxide produce a similar effect on cultured rat sarcoma cells, with a maximal effect at 24 hr in metaphase cells (Isaka et al., 1977). The carcinogenic 4-nitroquinoline-n-oxide produced multiple effects on the nucleoli of human cells, including fusion (Reynolds, Montgomery, and Karney, 1963). It can transform diploid, contact-inhibited Syrian hamster cells into noncontact-inhibited cells that differ from most transformed lines in that some cells show few but highly specific chromosome changes: trisomy B7 and monosomy B10 (Popescu and diPaolo, 1972). Although it is tempting to conclude that nucleolar persistence may have played a role in these nondisjunctional events, this is rendered less likely because B7 and B10 are not NOR chromosomes (Bigger and Savage, 1976). Predictions regarding frequency of nondisjunction, if NORs play a role, include:

Meiosis I > meiosis II
Maternal > paternal
No maternal age effect
Proportional to size of AgNOR
Proportional to size of rDNA cluster
Chinese hamster > human > mouse

ROBERTSONIAN TRANSLOCATIONS

McClintock (1941) noted that breakage can occur frequently in the NOR in *Zea mays*. Polani et al. (1960) proposed this as a mechanism of production of Robertsonian translocations in the human, with fusion of nucleoli bringing the NORs of different acrocentric chromosomes into proximity, and breakage, followed by nonrestitutional rejoining, leading to centric fusion. This could occur during one of the mitotic divisions that occur in the germ line before meiosis, or during meiosis itself, before metaphase of meiosis I. In the former case, centric fusions would be more likely to occur in the male germ line, which has so many more mitotic divisions than the female germ line. If centric fusions occur during meiosis, most should occur in the female, because of the very long duration of oocyte meiosis I and therefore greater change of chromosome breakage and translocation. There are few data on the sex of origin of human Robertsonian translocations, although it is known that they can be both paternal and maternal, with some examples of each reported (see, e.g., Mikkelsen, Hansson, and Jacobsen, 1975) and that there is no maternal or paternal age effect on their incidence (Jacobs, Frackiewicz, and Law, 1972).

It may appear obvious that nucleolar fusion is important in the origin of Robertsonian translocations, but this has not been proved. In the mouse, whose 20 pairs of chromosomes are acrocentric, all 19 autosomes have participated in Robertsonian translocations (O. J. Miller and Miller, 1975). NORs, on the other hand, are found in only three to five pairs of chromosomes in a given strain (Dev et al., 1977). A mouse model for the study of the role of the nucleolus and nucleolar fusion could thus be developed:

Advantages
All chromosomes acrocentric
Multiple NOR chromosomes
Each NOR near centromere
Nucleolar fusion common
Many Rb translocations available

Disadvantages
Satellite DNA on all chromosomes
Each NOR on long arm of chromosome
Low level of nucleolar persistence
Low level of NOR association at metaphase

Such a model would have still other advantages. There are multiple NOR chromosomes (as in man). Each NOR is near a centromere with much polymorphism in AgNOR size (Dev et al., 1977); nucleolar fusion is common (Flaherty et al., 1972; Ivanyi, 1971), just as in the human; and many Robertsonian translocation stocks are available. There are also some disadvantages. Identical satellite DNA sequences are present in the centromeric heterochromatin of all (or nearly all) the chromosomes, and this may play a part in the frequent association of the centromeric ends of nonhomologous chromosomes and the occurrence of quasi-linkage (Stockert, Boyse, and Sato, 1976). Each NOR is on the long arm of a chromosome, which is different from the human situation and may restrict opportunities for Robertsonian translocation. There appears to be a lower level of nucleolar persistence than in the human, and a lower level of NOR association at metaphase. Since satellite DNA is nucleolus-associated in the mouse (Schildkraut and Maio, 1968), the nucleolus-organizing chromosomes should be commonly involved in Robertsonian translocations. However, nuclear fusion is probably relatively unimportant because nucleoli do not persist and the NOR chromosomes are no longer associated at metaphase. These expectations are fairly well borne out by the existing data on Robertsonian translocations in the mouse. In all four sporadic, naturally occurring Robertsonian translocations, a single NOR chromosome is present, whereas in one-half of the more numerous Robertsonian translocations found in cultured cell lines, a single NOR chromosome is found twice as often as expected by chance; Robertsonian translocation involving two NOR chromosomes is an unusual event. Thus, in the mouse, the nucleolus is very important, but nucleolar fusion plays a relatively minor role (O. J. Miller et al., 1978), perhaps because the presence of satellite DNA in all centromeric regions enhances the general probability of Robertsonian translocation.

SECONDARY NONDISJUNCTION

Nondisjunction occurs with an increased frequency in heterozygous carriers of a Robertsonian (or other type of) translocation. This can apparently involve any chromosome in the complement, but the case of special interest and greatest frequency is that involving one of the acrocentric chromosomes homologous to one arm of the translocation chromosome. Could this be influenced by the nucleolus? In this case, nondisjunction arises by aberrant segregation of the chromosomes at meiosis I, and a role for nucleolus organizer activity is therefore conceivable. It is difficult to envision how nucleolar fusion could be involved, since the NORs tend to be lost in the translocation (Buys et al., 1978). On the other hand, if NORs are involved, we can make certain predictions similar to those for primary nondisjunction:

Maternal > paternal
No parental age effect
Proportional to size of AgNOR
Proportional to size of rDNA cluster
Chinese hamster > human > mouse?

Aberrant segregation should occur more frequently in female (because of the larger meiotic nucleoli in females) than in male translocation heterozygotes, and this is what is found in the human (Hamerton, 1968) and in the mouse (Gropp, Kolbus, and Giers, 1975; White et al., 1974). There should be no parental age effect, and there is none (Jacobs et al., 1972).

CONCLUSION

Although conclusive evidence is not available, the information reviewed in this chapter suggests that the nucleolus and nucleolus organizer regions may play a significant role in the origin of primary and secondary nondisjunction and Robertsonian translocation. The presence of an increased number of rRNA genes on chromosome 21 may make that chromosome more likely to be involved in such events, especially if the genes are active. The amount of silver staining of NORs is a simple measure of the level of activity of these genes. Consequently, a comparison of the size of AgNORs on chromosomes 21 might provide a measure of the relative risk a person has of producing a child with Down syndrome. Studies with parents of trisomy 21 and controls could provide a simple test of this hypothesis.

REFERENCES

Anastassova-Kristeva, M. 1977. The nucleolar cycle in man. J. Cell Sci. 25:103–110.
Bigger, T. R. L., and Savage, J. R. K. 1976. Location of nucleolar organizing regions on the chromosomes of the Syrian hamster (*Mesocricetus aureus*) and the Djungarian hamster (*Phodopus sungorus*). Cytogenet. Cell Genet. 16:495–504.
Boué, J., Boué, A., and Lazar, P. 1975. Retrospective and prospective epidemiological studies of 1500 karyotyped spontaneous human abortions. Teratology 12:11–26.
Bowman, P. D., Meek, R. L., and Daniel, C. W. 1976. Decreased synthesis of nucleolar RNA in aging human cells in vitro. Exp. Cell Res. 101:434–437.
Brown, D. D., and Dawid, I. B. 1968. Specific gene amplification in oocytes. Oocyte nuclei contain extrachromosomal replicas of the genes for ribosomal RNA. Science 160:272–280.
Buys, C. H. C. M., Osinga, J., Gouw, W. L., and Anders, G. J. P. A. 1978. Rapid identification of chromosomes carrying silver-stained nucleolus-organizing regions. Application to a case of 21/21 Robertsonian translocation. Hum. Genet. 44:173–181.

Carr, D. H., and Gedeon, M. 1977. Population cytogenetics of human abortuses. In E. B. Hook and I. H. Porter (eds.), Population Cytogenetics: Studies in Humans, pp. 1–9. Academic Press, New York.

Creasy, M. R., Crolla, J. A., and Alberman, E. D. 1976. A cytogenetic study of human spontaneous abortions using banding techniques. Hum. Genet. 31:177–196.

Croce, C. M., Talavera, A., Basilico, C., and Miller, O. J. 1977. Suppression of production of mouse 28S ribosomal RNA in mouse-human hybrids segregating mouse chromosomes. Proc. Nat. Acad. Sci. 74:694–697.

Darlington, C. D. 1935. The internal mechanics of the chromosomes. II. Prophase pairing at meiosis in Fritillaria. Proc. Roy. Soc. Lond. B 118:59–73.

Dearing, W. H., Jr. 1934. The material continuity and individuality of the somatic chromosomes of Ambystoma tigrinum, with special reference to the nucleolus as a chromosomal component. J. Morphol. 56:157–179.

de Capoa, A., Rocchi, A., and Gigliani, F. 1973. Frequency of satellite association in individuals with structural abnormalities of nucleolus organizer region. Humangenetik 18:111–115.

Dev, V. G., Tantravahi, R., Miller, D. A., and Miller, O. J. 1977. Distribution of nucleolus organizers in Mus musculus subspecies and in the RAG mouse cell line. Genetics 86:389–398.

Evans, H. J. 1967. The nucleolus, virus infection and trisomy in man. Nature 214:361–363.

Ferguson-Smith, M. A. 1964. The sites of nucleolus formation in human pachytene chromosomes. Cytogenetics 3:124–134.

Ferguson-Smith, M. A., and Handmaker, S. D. 1963. The association of satellited chromosomes with specific chromosomal regions in cultured human somatic cells. Ann. Hum. Genet. 27:143–156.

Fernández-Gómez, M. E., Risueño, M. C., Giménez-Martín, G., and Stockert, J. C. 1972. Cytochemical and ultrastructural studies on normal and segregated nucleoli in meristematic cells. Protoplasma 74:103–112.

Flaherty, L., Bennett, D., and Graef, S. 1972. Genetic control of nucleolar number in mouse. Exp. Cell Res. 70:13–16.

Galdieri, M., and Monesi, V. 1974. Ribosomal RNA in mouse spermatocytes. Exp. Cell Res. 85:287–295.

Goessens, G., and Lepoint, A. 1974. The fine structure of the nucleolus during interphase and mitosis in Ehrlich tumor cells cultured in vitro. Exp. Cell Res. 87:63–72.

Goodpasture, C., and Bloom, S. E. 1975. Visualization of nucleolar organizer regions in mammalian chromosomes using silver staining. Chromosoma 53:37–50.

Granboulan, N., Tournier, P., Wicker, R., and Bernhard, W. 1963. An electron microscope study of the development of SV40 virus. J. Cell Biol. 17:423–441.

Gropp, A., Kolbus, U., and Giers, D. 1975. Systematic approach to the study of trisomy in the mouse. II. Cytogenet. Cell Genet. 14:42–62.

Hamerton, J. L. 1968. Robertsonian translocation in man: Evidence for prezygotic selection. Cytogenetics 7:260–276.

Hancock, R. L. 1964. Nucleolar organizers of blastocyst nuclei. Growth 28:251–256.

Hansson, A., and Mikkelsen, M. 1974. An increased tendency to satellite association of human chromosome 21: A factor in the aetiology of Down's syndrome. ICRS 2:1617.

Hassold, T. J., Matsuyama, A., Newlands, I. M., Matsuura, J. S., Jacobs, P. A., Manuel, B., and Tsuei, J. 1978. A cytogenetic study of spontaneous abortions in Hawaii. Ann. Hum. Genet. 41:443–454.

Heath, J. C. 1954. The effect of cobalt on mitosis in tissue culture. Exp. Cell Res. 6:311–320.

Henderson, A. S., and Atwood, K. C. 1976. Satellite-association frequency and rDNA content of a double-satellited chromosome. Hum. Genet. 31:113–115.

Henderson, A. S., Warburton, D., and Atwood, K. C. 1972. Location of ribosomal DNA in the human chromosome complement. Proc. Nat. Acad. Sci. 69:3394–3398.

Henderson, A. S., Warburton, D., and Atwood, K. C. 1973. Ribosomal DNA connectives between human acrocentric chromosomes. Nature 245:95–97.

Hook, E. B., and Hamerton, J. L. 1977. The frequency of chromosome abnormalities detected in consecutive newborn studies—Differences between studies—Results by sex and severity of phenotypic involvement. In E. B. Hook and I. H. Porter (eds.), Population Cytogenetics: Studies in Humans, pp. 63–80. Academic Press, New York.

Howell, W. M., Denton, T. E., and Diamond, J. R. 1975. Differential staining of the satellite regions of human acrocentric chromosomes. Experientia 31:260–262.

Hsu, T. C., Arrighi, F. E., Klevecz, R. R., and Brinkley, B. R. 1965. The nucleoli in mitotic divisions of mammalian cells *in vitro*. J. Cell Biol. 26:539–553.

Hsu, T. C., Brinkley, B. R., and Arrighi, F. E. 1967. The structure and behavior of the nucleolus organizers in mammalian cells. Chromosoma 23:137–153.

Hsu, T. C., Spirito, S. E., and Pardue, M. L. 1975. Distribution of 18 + 28S ribosomal genes in mammalian genomes. Chromosoma 53:25–36.

Hungerford, D. A., LaBadie, G. U., and Balaban, G. B. 1971. Chromosome structure and function in man. II. Provisional maps of the two smallest autosomes (chromosomes 21 and 22) at pachytene in the male. Cytogenetics 10:33–37.

Hungerford, D. A., LaBadie, G. U., Balaban, G. B., Messatzzia, L. R., Haller, G., and Miller, A. F. 1971. Chromosome structure and function in man. IV. Provisional maps of the three long acrocentric autosomes (chromosomes 13, 14, and 15) at pachytene in the male. Ann. Genet. 14:256–260.

Isaka, H., Koura, S., Koura, M., and Hattammann, K. 1977. Persistent nucleoli in cultured Yoshida sarcoma cells exposed to a series of carcinogenic and non-carcinogenic derivative of 4-nitroquinoline-1-oxide. Gann 68:251–252.

Ivanyi, D. 1971. Genetic studies on mouse nucleoli. Exp. Cell Res. 64:240–242.

Jacobs, P. A., Frackiewicz, A., and Law, P. 1972. Incidence and mutation rates of structural rearrangement of the autosomes in man. Ann. Hum. Genet. 35:301–319.

Kajii, T., Ohama, K., Niihawa, N., Ferrier, A., and Avirachan, S. 1973. Banding analysis of abnormal karyotypes in spontaneous abortion. Am. J. Hum. Genet. 25:539–547.

Kierszenbaum, A. L., and Tres, L. L. 1974. Nucleolar and perichromosomal RNA synthesis during meiotic prophase in the mouse testis. J. Cell Biol. 60:39–53.

Kochupillai, N., Verma, I. C., Grewal, M. S., and Ramalingaswami, V. 1976. Down's syndrome and related abnormalities in an area of high background radiation in coastal Kerala. Nature 262:60–61.

Kurata, S., Misumi, Y., Sakaguchi, B., Shiokawa, K., and Yamana, K. 1978. Does the rate of ribosomal RNA synthesis vary depending on the number of nucleoli in a nucleus? Exp. Cell Res. 115:415–419.

Langenbeck, U., Hansmann, I., Hinney, B., and Honig, U. 1976. On the origin of the supernumerary chromosome in autosomal trisomies—With special reference to Down's syndrome. A bias in tracing nondisjunction by chromosomal and biochemical polymorphisms. Hum. Genet. 33:89–102.

Lau, Y.-F., and Arrighi, F. E. 1976. Studies of the squirrel monkey, *Saimiri sciureus*, genome. I. Cytological characterizations of chromosomal heterozygosity. Cytogenet. Cell Genet. 17:51–60.

Luciani, J.-M., and Stahl, A. 1971. Rapports des nucléolus avec les chromosomes méiotiques de l'ovocyte fetal humain. [Relationships of nucleoli to meiotic chromosomes in the human fetal oocyte.] C. R. Acad. Sci. Paris 273:521–524.

McClintock, B. 1934. The relation of a particular chromosomal element to the development of the nucleoli in *Zea mays*. Z. Zellforsch. Mikr. Anat. 21:294–328.

McClintock, B. 1941. Spontaneous alterations in chromosome size and form in *Zea mays*. Cold. Spr. Harb. Symp. Quant. Biol. 9:72–81.

Magenis, R. E., Overton, K. M., Chamberlin, J., Brady, T., and Lovrien, E. 1977. Parental origin of the extra chromosome in Down's syndrome. Hum. Genet. 37:7–14.

Markovic, V. D., Worton, R. G., and Berg, J. M. 1978. Evidence for the inheritance of silver-stained nucleolus organizer regions. Hum. Genet. 41:181–187.

Mattei, J.-F., Ayme, S., Mattei, M. G., Gouvernet, J., and Giraud, F. 1976. Quantitative and qualitative study of acrocentric associations in 109 normal subjects. Hum. Genet. 34:185–194.

Mattei, J.-F., Mattei, M. G., Ayme, S., and Giraud, F. 1974. Etude chromosomique chez les parents d'enfants trisomiques 21. Associations entre chromosomes acrocentriques. [Chromosome study with parents of trisomy 21 infants. Associations among acrocentric chromosomes.] Humangenetik 25:29–48.

Mikkelsen, M., Hansson, A., and Jacobsen, P. 1975. Translocation (13q21q). Four generation family study with analysis of satellite associations, fluorescent markers, and prenatal diagnosis. Humangenetik 27:303–307.

Miller, D. A., Dev, V. G., Tantravahi, R., and Miller, O. J. 1976. Suppression of human nucleolus organizer-activity in mouse-human somatic hybrid cells. Exp. Cell Res. 101:235–243.

Miller, D. A., Tantravahi, R., Dev, V. G., and Miller, O. J. 1977. Frequency of satellite association of human chromosomes is correlated with amount of Ag-staining of the nucleolus organizer region. Am. J. Hum. Genet. 29:490–502.

Miller, O. J., and Miller, D. A. 1975. Cytogenetics of the mouse. Annu. Rev. Genet. 9: 285–303.

Miller, O. J., Miller, D. A., Dev, V. G., Tantravahi, R., and Croce, C. M. 1976. Expression of human and suppression of mouse nucleolus organizer activity in mouse-human somatic cell hybrids. Proc. Nat. Acad. Sci. 73:4531–4535.

Miller, O. J., Miller, D. A., Tantravahi, R., and Dev, V. G. 1978. Nucleolus organizer activity and the origin of Robertsonian translocations. Cytogenet. Cell Genet. 20:40–50.

Miller, O. L., Jr., and Hamkalo, B. A. 1972. Visualization of RNA synthesis on chromosomes. Int. Rev. Cytol. 33:1–25.

Nankin, H. R. 1970. In vitro alteration of satellite association and nucleolar persistence in mitotic human lymphocytes. Cytogenetics 9:42–51.

Natarajan, A. T., and Gropp, A. 1972. A fluorescence study of heterochromatin and nucleolar organization in the laboratory and tobacco mouse. Exp. Cell Res. 74:245–250.

Newman, G. R., Hoffner, N., and DiBerardino, M. A. 1977. The nucleolar chromosome in embryos of *Rana pipiens*. Experientia 33:430–432.

Penrose, L. S. 1967. Studies on mosaicism in Down's anomaly. In G. A. Jervis (ed.), Mental Retardation, pp. 1–16. Charles C Thomas Publisher, Springfield, Ill.

Perry, R. P. 1976. Processing of RNA. Annu. Rev. Biochem. 45:605–629.

Peters, K. 1956. Variationsstatistiche Untersuchungen über das Auftreten von Vakuolen in den Nukleolen von Hühnerherzfibroblasten in vitro nach den Einwirkung von Röntgenstrahlen, Megaphen und Kälte. [Statistical studies on the development of vacuoles in the nucleoli of chick heart fibroblasts in vitro after the action of X-rays, Megaphen and cold.] Z. Zellforsch. 44:14–26.

Peterson, G. B., and Therkelsen, A. J. 1962. Number of nucleoli in female and male human cells in tissue culture. Exp. Cell Res. 28:590–592.

Polani, P. E., Briggs, J. H., Ford, C. E., Clarke, C. M., and Berg, J. M. 1960. A mongol girl with 46 chromosomes. Lancet 1:721–724.

Polani, P. E., and Jagiello, G. M. 1976. Chiasmata, meiotic univalents, and age in relation to aneuploid imbalance in mice. Cytogenet. Cell Genet. 16:505–529.

Popescu, N. C., and diPaolo, J. A. 1972. Identification of Syrian hamster chromosomes by acetic-saline-Giemsa (ASG) and trypsin techniques. Cytogenetics 11:500–507.

Reynolds, R. C., Montgomery, P. O. B., and Karney, D. H. 1963. Nucleolar "caps"—A morphologic entity produced by the carcinogen 4-nitroquinoline-N-oxide. Cancer Res. 23:535–538.

Rosenkranz, W., and Holzer, S. 1972. Satellite association. A possible cause of chromosome aberrations. Humangenetik 16:147–150.

Scherer, E., Ringleb, D., and Ventzke, L. E. 1953. Über den Einfluss der Röntgenstrahlen auf den Nucleolar-Apparat der Zellen (Beobachtungen am Milz, Knochenmark und Ascitestumor). [On the influence of X-rays on the nucleolar apparatus of cells (observations on spleen, bone marrow and ascites tumor).] Strahlentherapie 90:41–52.

Schildkraut, C. L., and Maio, J. J. 1968. Studies on the intranuclear distribution and properties of mouse satellite DNA. Biochim. Biophys. Acta 161:76–93.

Schmid, M., Hofgärtner, F. J., Zenzes, M. T., and Engel, W. 1977. Evidence for postmeiotic expression of ribosomal RNA genes during male gametogenesis. Hum. Genet. 38:279–284.

Schmid, M., Krone, W., and Vogel, U. 1974. On the relationship between the frequency of association and the nucleolar constriction of individual acrocentric chromosomes. Human-genetik 23:267–277.

Schröder, J., Halkka, O., and Brummer-Korvenkontio, M. 1970. Meiotic aneuploidy in a mouse strain with latent ectromelia infection. Hereditas 65:297–300.

Schwarzacher, H. G., Mikelssar, A. V., and Schnedl, W. 1978. The nature of the Ag-staining of nucleolus organizer regions: Electron- and light-microscopic studies on human cells in interphase, mitosis, and meiosis. Cytogenet. Cell Genet. 20:24–39.

Shea, J. R., Jr., and Leblond, C. P. 1966. Number of nucleoli in various cell types of the mouse. J. Morphol. 119:425–434.

Smith, G. F., and Berg, J. M. 1976. Down's Anomaly. 2nd Ed. Churchill Livingstone, London.

Stahl, A., Luciani, J. M., Devictor, M., Capodano, A. M., and Gagné, R. 1975. Constitutive heterochromatin and micronucleoli in the human oocyte at the diplotene stage. Human-genetik 26:315–327.

Stockert, E., Boyse, E. A., and Sato, H. 1976. Heredity of the GIX thymocyte antigen associated with murine leukemia virus: Segregation data simulating genetic linkage. Proc. Nat. Acad. Sci. 73:2077–2081.

Stoller, A., and Collmann, R. D. 1965. Incidence of infective hepatitis followed by Down's syndrome nine months later. Lancet 2:1221.

Taysi, K. 1975. Satellite association: Giemsa banding studies in parents of Down's syndrome patients. Clin. Genet. 8:313–323.

Trimble, B. K., and Baird, P. A. 1978. Maternal age and Down syndrome: Age-specific incidence rates by single-year intervals. Am. J. Med. Genet. 2:1–5.

Uchida, I. A. 1977. Maternal radiation and trisomy 21. In E. B. Hook and I. H. Porter (eds.), Population Cytogenetics: Studies in Humans, pp. 285–299. Academic Press, New York.

Uchida, I. A., and Freeman, C. P. V. 1977. Radiation-induced nondisjunction in oocytes of aged mice. Nature 265:186–187.

Warburton, D., Atwood, K. C., and Henderson, A. S. 1976. Variation in the number of genes for rRNA among human acrocentric chromosomes: Correlation with frequency of satellite association. Cytogenet. Cell Genet. 17:221–230.

White, B. J., Tjio, J. H., Van de Water, L. C., and Crandall, C. 1974. Trisomy 19 in the laboratory mouse. I. Frequency in different crosses at specific developmental stages and relationship of trisomy to cleft palate. Cytogenet. Cell Genet. 13:217–231.

The Organizational Structure of Human Genes on Chromosome 21

Roy Schmickel and Golder Wilson

Down syndrome is a condition characterized by abnormal mental and physical development, which is associated with a disturbance in the expression of many genes. It is not known how these genes interact or how they are organized. It would be reasonable to assume that the expression of the genes is related to their structural organization at a level below that of the entire chromosome. This chapter concerns the structural organization of a set of genes located on chromosome 21 and explores the possibility that the structural organization of the genes may influence both homologous and nonhomologous recombination and indirectly cause nondisjunction. The techniques employed to dissect the molecular anatomy of a gene are also described.

QUANTITATION

There is no way to say how many genes are involved in the causation of Down syndrome because there may be many important interchromosomal interactions. A chromosome 21 represents almost 1% of the genetic material. Since the entire human genome has sufficient DNA to code for about 6 million genes, the DNA of chromosome 21 could accommodate 60,000 genes. (Perhaps only 30% of the DNA is used for unique genes, and the actual number may be closer to 20,000 (Britten and Kohne, 1968).) This is much too large for a reasonable hope of analysis. Our strategy for the analysis of genes is to reduce the number of the genes studied and to amplify a particular segment for direct analysis. The group of genes on chromosome 21 that we have chosen to study are the genes for rRNA.

First, we can quantitate the genes for rRNA by RNA/DNA hybridization (Schmickel, 1973). When labeled rRNA is purified and mixed with single stranded DNA, the rRNA will bind to its specific template. With an excess of rRNA and a small amount of DNA fixed to nitrocellulose discs, the template becomes saturated. Increasing amounts of rRNA above the saturation point does not increase the hybridization (Figure 1). If we calculate the amount of rRNA bound to a fixed amount of DNA at saturation, we know the relative concentration of ribosomal genes in the genome. Saturation occurs at 0.014%. Knowing that a human genome contains 5.5×10^{12} daltons of DNA, we can then calculate the daltons of rRNA bound per human genome. By dividing that number by the molecular weight of rRNA (2.4×10^6), we arrive at the number of ribosomal genes per cell – 320:

a.   Percentage of genome that binds rRNA (daltons of DNA per genome) = daltons of rDNA per genome: 0.014% $(5.5 \times 10^{12}) = 7.7 \times 10^8$ daltons per genome.
b.   Daltons of rDNA per genome/molecular weight of rRNA = copies of rRNA template per genome: $7.7 \times 10^8 \div 2.4 \times 10^6 = 320$ copies per cell.

This means that there is a moderately high level of redundancy for this gene.

Since there are 320 rRNA genes per cell, it is possible to look for them on chromosomes. This is accomplished by in situ hybridization. The same technique is used as in hybridization to nitrocellulose discs, but this time the rRNA is hybridized to the

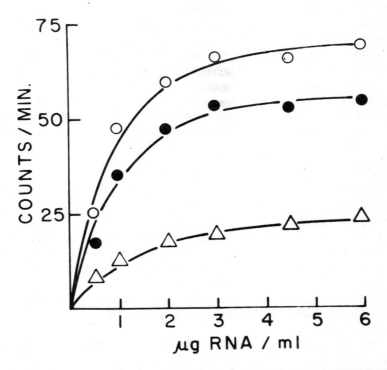

Figure 1.   Hybridization of human DNA with [3H] rRNA (18,000 cpm/μg). Hybridization was performed on nitrocellulose discs by the method of Gillespie and Spiegelman (1965) in 0.3 M NaCl at 65° for 12 hr; 30 μg of DNA were fixed to each nitrocellulose disc. At saturation the ratio of RNA bound to the discs to the DNA on the discs was 1.4×10^{-3}.

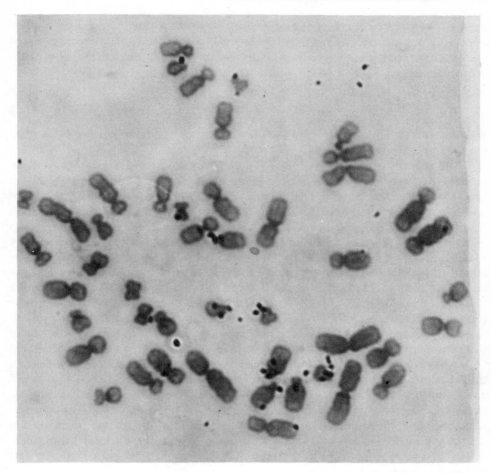

Figure 2.   Autoradiograph of a normal karyotype hybridized with rRNA. The chromosomes were denatured with 0.07 M NaOH and hybridized with 50 μl [^{3}H] rRNA (0.2μg/ml). The slides were dipped in emulsion and incubated for 60 days before development. Twenty-seven grains are over the short arms of acrocentric chromosomes, whereas four grains are scattered randomly over the other chromosomes (Schmickel and Knoller, 1977).

DNA of denatured chromosome preparations. As seen in Figure 2, the genes are clustered on the acrocentric chromosomes. They are roughly evenly divided among the five acrocentric chromosomes (numbers 13, 14, 15, 21, 22). This would mean that each chromosome contains about 30 genes.

RESTRICTION ANALYSIS

Further understanding of structure and organization is possible with endonuclease restriction fragment analysis of total human DNA (Smith and Nathans, 1973). These nucleases recognize palindromes (sequences that spell the same thing in both directions) that occur randomly in DNA. There are over 50 different endonucleases, and each nuclease recognizes a specific palindrome. In double-stranded DNA, the palindrome recognized by the enzyme EcoRI is:

$$G^|A\ A\ T\ T\ C$$
$$C\ T\ T\ A\ A_|G$$

Starting with G, both strands read the same. The restriction endonuclease cuts after the G to give a staggered break.

The size of the DNA fragments generated by a restriction endonuclease are determined by the distance between its specific palindromic sites. Each gene should generate a characteristic set of restriction fragments after cleavage with a given endonuclease. In the case of repeated genes, the genes should have identical restriction fragments if the genes are identical (i.e., if all ribosomal genes are alike).

Restriction fragments can be analyzed by gel electrophoresis, DNA transfer (Southern blot), and hybridization (Southern, 1975). In an agarose gel, fragments migrate a distance inversely proportional to the square of their molecular weight, giving us the ability to assign molecular weights to the fragments. The fragments are visualized by using the Southern method of transfer of DNA and autoradiography (Figure 3). When separated, DNA is transferred to nitrocellulose and then hybridized to a radioisotope-labeled probe. The radioisotope permits us to locate the fragment by exposure of an overlying x-ray film. This allows us to assign a size to the separated fragment. For instance, EcoRI endonuclease digestion of human rDNA generates three fragments. The 4.8 megadalton fragment hybridizes to 28S rRNA and the 3.8 and 13 megadalton fragments to 18S rRNA (Figure 4). By digesting with several enzymes we can gradually see how the gene fits together. However, two things must be remembered: 1) the fragments are only visible by hybridization so that fragments that do not hybridize to rRNA will not be visible, and 2) since there are 320 genes, there may be several fragments for each section. (This would be analogous to mixing several puzzles together.)

One way to study gene arrangement further is by digesting with more than one enzyme. This permits us to assign a fragment's position in relationship to another. Figure 4 also shows the results of digestion with combinations of two enzymes, which permitted us to fashion the map given in Figure 5.

As we digest with more enzymes, we can become more certain of the gene structure. The following features have emerged:

1. The gene only requires 5 million daltons for the final RNA products, yet it is about 17 million daltons in size.
2. There is a space between the transcribed genes.
3. The gene arrangement can best be explained by assuming that the genes are identical and repeated tandemly.

A further feature of the ribosomal genes is becoming more apparent. That is, there is a limited variability of the restriction sites. For instance, Bam HI 28S fragments are over 20 million daltons (Table 1). The only way to account for this large size is to postulate that several fragments are located at the same position in the gene. Figure 5 demonstrates this arrangement to show that there are some genes that can vary within the individual. In comparing one individual with another, there are also distinct differences in patterns.

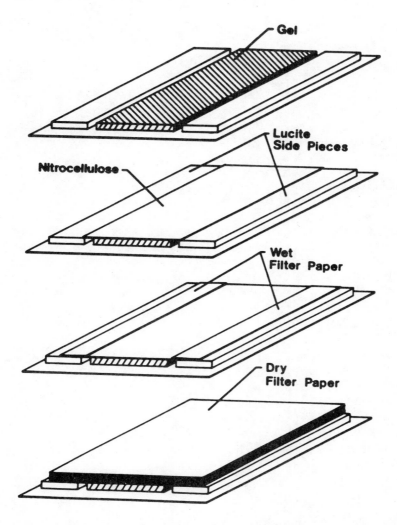

Figure 3.   The method for transfer of single-stranded DNA from a gel to nitrocellulose (Southern, 1975). From top to bottom: An agarose gel with denatured DNA fragments is placed on a glass with Lucite spacers of equal thickness; the gel is overlaid with nitrocellulose, wet filter paper, and finally dry filter paper. The DNA moves from the gel and binds to the nitrocellulose as moisture is absorbed into the dry filter paper from the gel. The nitrocellulose paper with the bound DNA is hybridized with radioactive rRNA to locate those fragments with a rRNA template.

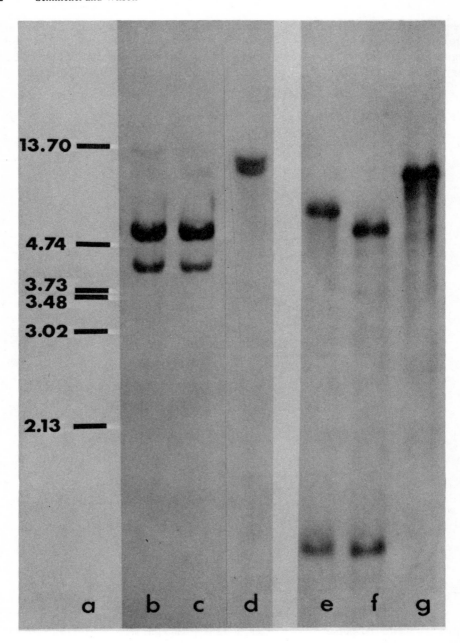

Figure 4.   Autoradiography of a hybridization of [125]I rRNA to DNA. Whole human DNA has been digested with the restriction nuclease indicated and transferred to nitrocellulose by the Southern technique, shown in Figure 3, hybridized with labeled rRNA, and exposed to x-ray film. The digestions with human DNA: a) standard-size fragments of lambda phage, given in megadaltons; b) EcoRI; c) EcoRI and Hind III; d) Hind III; e) Hind III and Sal I; f) EcoRI and Sal I; g) Sal I.

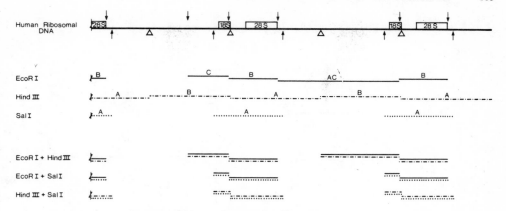

Figure 5.   A diagram of the arrangement of fragments generated by the endonuclease digestions depicted in Figure 4. The top figure is the arrangement of genes 18S and 28S and the sites of the nuclease targets: ⏐ EcoRI, ↑ Sal I, and △ Hind III. The single digests of Figure 4b, 4d, and 4g are depicted in the next three lines and the double digests of Figure 4c, 4e, and 4f in the last three lines.

RECOMBINANT DNA TECHNIQUES

The restriction analysis led us to the direct analysis of these genes with the technique of recombinant technology (Wilson et al., 1978). Figure 6 summarizes the steps of that technique: 1) enrichment of DNA for ribosomal genes, 2) digestion of human DNA by the restriction nuclease EcoRI, 3) ligation of human DNA with a lambda vector, 4) selection of the human rDNA/lambda recombinant, and 5) purification for further study.

Table 1.   Summary of rDNA restriction fragments

Restriction enzyme	Measurements	Visible fragments	Size	Hybridizes with	Variable sites
EcoRI	35	3	4.6	28 + 18	1
			3.8	18	
			> 13	18	
Hind III	38	2	8.3	18	0
			9.2	28	
Sal	20	1	7.2	28 + 18	?1
Bam	22	7	4.8	28	4
			4.5	28	
			4.3	28	
			3.9	28	
			3.6	28 + 18	
			1.4	18	
			0.8	28	
Hind II	16	4	3.7	28 + 18	
			3.5	28	
			2.8	28	2
			1.1	28	

MOLECULAR DISSECTION OF HUMAN DNA

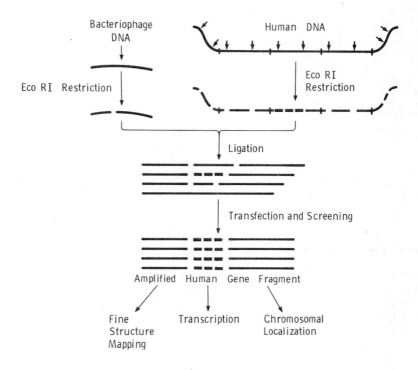

Figure 6.   Schematic description of the recombinant technique for inserting rDNA in a lambda phage vector. The bacteriophage is Blattner et al.'s (1977) Charon 16A. The dashed insert represents the human rDNA insert in a stable recombinant phage. The cloning experiments were carried out in a certified P3 biohazard laboratory.

We have screened several thousand phage plaques by the technique shown in Figure 7. Plaques containing human DNA lose their ability to metabolize the lactose analogue (Blattner et al., 1977). These recombinants are then tested for their ability to hybridize with rRNA. Plaques that cannot metabolize lactose and hybridize with radioactive rRNA are presumed to contain the ribosomal gene.

We selected 11 clones to study in detail. At this point, we had achieved a gene enrichment of 5000-fold and an amplification of 10^{12}ml. This permitted us to examine a human gene directly. Figure 8 shows the comparison of 11 different rDNA genes. They are all identical at this level of analysis.

What are some of the implications of identical gene structure on separate chromosomes? It indicates that there may be a mechanism responsible for the maintenance of homogeneity. For instance, the ribosomal genes have been separated on different chromosomes since before the divergence of higher apes. There are differences in gene organization of rDNA between primates that are not present between chro-

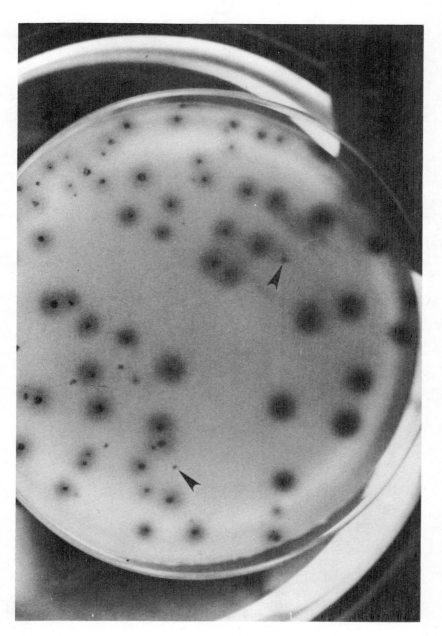

Figure 7. A petri dish containing parental and recombinant lambda phages. Two of the recombinant phages are indicated by arrows. They are not surrounded by dye as are the nearby parental phages. The recombinant molecules have DNA inserted into the lactose gene of the phages. This insertion inactivates the gene. The lack of dye around the recombinant phage plaque results from the inability of the phage to metabolize the chromogenic lactose analogue.

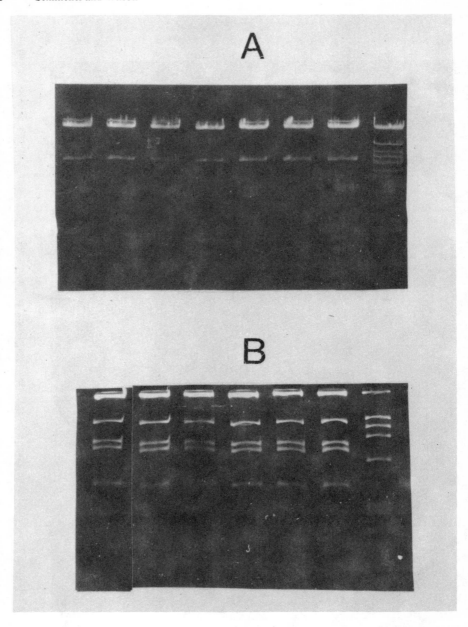

Figure 8.   Electrophoretic analysis of DNA restriction products of seven separate 18S rDNA recombinants. A, Electrophoretic analysis on a 1% agarose gel of 1 μg of seven separate clones digested with EcoRI. B, The same clones in 4% agarose digested with Bam HI and Sal I. The far right lanes are lambda standards. These digestions show that there are no detectable differences between clones by this restriction analysis.

mosomes. Could the maintenance of homogeneity be due to exchange between non-homologous chromosomes? If this is true, the exchange may also lead to abnormal events. For instance, in situ hybridization indicates that this type of interaction can cause the loss of a set of ribosomal genes or the transfer of ribosomal genes to other chromosomes. It is not unreasonable to assume that the divergence of chromosomes and the duplication of chromosomes in higher animal evolution have some abnormal consequences. One such consequence may be that it encourages exchange between nonhomologous chromosomes, and this exchange can lead to nondisjunction. This possibility was discussed by Dr. Miller in the preceding chapter.

In summary, the development of techniques to directly examine human genes has permitted us to explore the question of gene organization and its variation. Our early observations indicate that there is some variability of the repeated genes yet a surprising amount of similarity and conservation of nontranscribed sections of the gene. Second, direct observation permits us to observe interchromosomal exchanges and interaction. Third, the stability of hereditary material that does not have the constraints of a unique structural gene can also be examined in detail to determine the mechanisms necessary for ensuring the stability of our inheritance.

We believe that the direct examination of the organization of genes and establishment of normal variations in human DNA will reveal important clues to understanding the basis for alterations of gene organization in conditions like Down syndrome.

REFERENCES

Blattner, F. R., Williams, B. G., Blechl, A. E., Dennison-Thompson, K., Faber, H. E., Fuilery, L., Grunwald, D. J., Kiefer, D. O., Moore, D. D., Schumm, J. W., Sheldon, E. L., and Smithies, O. 1977. Science 196:161.

Britten, R., and Kohne, D. 1968. Science 161:529.

Gillespie, D., and Spiegelman, S. 1965. J. Mol. Biol. 12:829.

Schmickel, R. 1973. Pediatr. Res. 7:5.

Schmickel, R. D., and Knoller, M. 1977. Pediatr. Res. 11:929.

Smith, H. O., and Nathans, D. 1973. J. Mol. Biol. 81:419.

Southern, E. M. 1975. J. Mol. Biol. 98:503.

Wilson, G. N., Hollar, B. A., Waterson, J. R., and Schmickel, R. D. 1978. Proc. Nat. Acad. Sci. 75:5367.

The Meiotic Nondisjunction of Homologous Chromosomes in *Drosophila* Females

L. Sandler

The case of sex determination serves as a constant (and humbling) reminder of the danger of applying genetic conclusions from *Drosophila* directly to apparently similar situations in humans. On the other hand, it is foolish not to recognize the considerable generality of many genetic phenomena and therefore to at least notice possible analogs in *Drosophila* when attempting to elucidate the genetic basis of human disease. This is especially true in the case of a condition like Down syndrome, where the etiology involves a perturbation in the evolutionarily very conservative process of meiosis. It is, therefore, to expose such possibly fruitful analogies that the basic cytogenetic properties of meiotic nondisjunction as they have been developed in *Drosophila* are reviewed here.

In 1916, C. B. Bridges exhibited three different modes of meiotic nondisjunction of the X chromosome in females, all three modes resulting in the production of diplo-X- and nullo-X-bearing eggs. The first of these, *primary nondisjunction,* resulted from the occasional failure of two nonrecombinant, homologous X chromosomes to disjoin; these were interpreted as owing to rare anomalous first meiotic divisions that had been followed by normal meioses II. The second mode, *equational nondisjunction,* was even more rare than primary nondisjunction and involved the failure to separate of a recombinant and a nonrecombinant X chromosome; these were interpreted as instances of anomalous second meiotic divisions that had been preceded by normal meioses I (this sequence of events is diagrammed in Figure 1).

The third type of meiotic nondisjunction, *secondary nondisjunction,* is not discussed here because it offers no obvious analogies to humans. Secondary nondisjunction is the separation of the two homologous nonrecombinant X chromosomes from the partially homologous Y chromosome in an XXY female; our present understanding of this phenomenon can be appreciated by examining the discussions of secondary nondisjunction in Cooper (1948) and Grell (1976). Nondisjunction in male *Drosophila*—of the X from the Y chromosome as well as of the autosomes—has also been studied (for references and discussion, see the review by Zimmering, 1976).

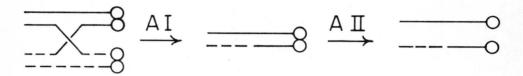

Figure 1.   The sequence of events—a normal meiosis I including crossing over followed by a failure of disjunction at anaphase II—postulated by Bridges (1916) as the cause of equational exceptions. Note that the equational-exceptional progeny are homozygous for proximal markers that were heterozygous in the parental females. (From Merriam and Frost, 1964, Exchange and nondisjunction of the X chromosomes in female *D. melanogaster, Genetics 49,* pp. 109–122.)

These studies are also not included here because male meiosis in *Drosophila* is atypical in that it is completely achiasmate; it seems, as a consequence, that *Drosophila* meiosis in males is not a likely place to find analogies useful to the elucidation of meiotic anomalies in humans.

The idea that there are two mechanically distinct modes of X chromosome nondisjunction in normal, XX, females—leading to primary and equational nondisjunction—remained current until it was noticed (by Merriam and Frost, 1964) that the sequence of events that Bridges postulated to account for equational nondisjunction (Figure 1) implies that the resulting diplo-X progeny should, in the main, be homozygous for proximally located genes while still heterozygous for more distal markers; the common observation, however, is the converse.

Merriam and Frost postulated that the observed pattern of distal homozygosis would come about if equational nondisjunction, like primary nondisjunction, was the consequence of a defective first, rather than second, meiotic division. The two modes of nondisjunction would, according to this view, differ only in that equational nondisjunction results from the abnormal segregation of an exchange, instead of a nonexchange, tetrad. This postulated sequence of events, along with that postulated to generate primary exceptions, is diagrammed in Figure 2. It can be seen from this figure that if these are the meiotic events that give rise to nondisjunction, then, among apparent primary exceptions, there should be some that carry complementary crossover X chromosomes (bottom, right in Figure 2) rather than two noncrossover Xs. Moreover, the frequency of this class should be one-half the observed frequency of equational exceptions. Merriam and Frost found both expectations realized.

It seems, therefore, most reasonable to conclude that, in *Drosophila:* 1) most nondisjunctional events occur at the first meiotic division, and 2) both recombinant and nonrecombinant tetrads can nondisjoin.

PARAMETERS OF NONDISJUNCTION

The spontaneous frequency of nondisjunction in normal *Drosophila melanogaster* females can be measured for the X chromosomes (because X chromosome "aneuploidy" changes sex rather than kills) and for the fourth chromosomes (because aneuploidy is tolerated owing to chromosome 4's small size). It has long been known

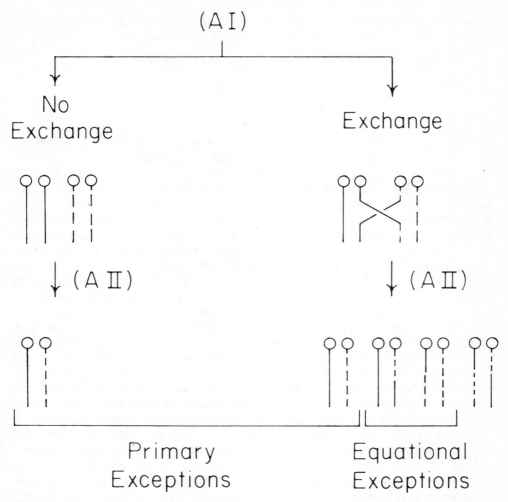

Figure 2.   The sequence of events postulated by Merriam and Frost (1964) to account for both primary and equational exceptions. They supposed a failure of disjunction of either exchange or nonexchange tetrads at anaphase I followed by normal sister-centromere disjunction at meiosis II. Note that equational exceptions are homozygous for distal markers that were heterozygous in the parental females and that a special class of nonhomozygous (apparent "primary") exceptions is expected—one that carries complementary crossover X chromosomes (bottom, right).

that the rates of nondisjunction for these two chromosomes are similar (Morgan, Bridges, and Sturtevant, 1925), implying that because the X chromosome is some 20 times larger than chromosome 4, chromosome size is not an important factor in determining the rate of nondisjunction. This rate is generally between 0.05% and 0.10% for the X chromosome (for references, see the review by Zimmering, 1976).

As a control for a series of studies on mutants affecting meiosis, Sandler et al. (1968) reported the rates of nondisjunction for both the X and fourth chromosomes in the same females. These data, in the form of a square indicating the constitution of the oocytes with respect to each chromosome along the axes, are:

	mono-4	diplo-4	nullo-4
mono-X	27,509	2	8
diplo-X	1	0	0
nullo-X	7	1	1

From these results, we can observe not only typical rates of nondisjunction and that the X and fourth chromosomes behave alike, but also two other important general attributes of nondisjunction. The first of these is that almost invariably nullo-exceptional progeny are three or more times more frequent than (the theoretically complementary class of) diplo exceptions (for references, see the review by Zimmering, 1976). In these data, as typical examples, there were one diplo-X to nine nullo-X exceptions and three diplo-4 to nine nullo-4 exceptions. The second general attribute—less securely established in *Drosophila* than in humans (for references, see, for example, the discussion by Sandler and Hecht, 1973, and the review by Baker et al., 1976) —is that double exceptions occur more frequently than would be expected by chance. Thus, in the results tabulated here, there were two X,4 double exceptions when, on the assumption of independence, only 0.004 instances were expected.

Two reasons for the excess of nullo-exceptional eggs have been suggested. Bridges (1916) suggested that there might be occasional "mechanical entanglements" of the homologs at synapsis, subsequently preventing proper anaphase movement and thus resulting in the exclusion of either homolog from the products of meiosis. Sandler and Braver (1954) suggested that an occasional failure of synapsis followed by the random segregation of the two nonrecombinant homologs could be the origin of primary exceptions and, because asynapsis leads to chromosome loss, should result in an excess of nullo-exceptional eggs. Since Merriam and Frost (1964) have shown that nondisjunction can involve both exchange and nonexchange tetrads, perhaps both suggestions are correct in some instances. Whatever the precise mechanism, however, it seems clear that some form of chromosome loss is a frequent concomitant of nondisjunction.

The cause of the nonrandomly frequent occurrence of double exceptions is reasonably clear in the case of *Drosophila*—and perhaps a similar cause obtains also for humans (Grell, 1964, 1971a). In *Drosophila,* there are many conditions under which nonhomologous chromosomes will perhaps pair with, but certainly segregate from, one another (for references, see the review by Grell, 1976). Such nonhomologous segregations will, in a fraction of cases, give rise to nondisjunction involving both participating nonhomologous chromosome pairs simultaneously. The simplest illustration is to imagine that in some meiocyte each X chromosome pairs with, and segregates from, each fourth chromosome. In one-half of such meiocytes, diplo-X,nullo-4 or nullo-X,diplo-4 double-exceptional eggs will be produced. Moreover, subsequent chromosome loss can convert either of these egg types into single exceptions or into nullo-X,nullo-4 double exceptions. Therefore, it seems reasonable to suppose that the conditions that predispose chromosomes to nondisjoin also foster nonhomologous segregations and that these segregations cause the relatively frequent occurrence of multiple nondisjunctional exceptions.

In addition to the sex and fourth chromosomes, the *Drosophila* genome contains two large (each about twice the size of the X chromosome) metacentric autosomes—chromosomes 2 and 3. Because both trisomy or monosomy for either major autosome is invariably lethal, the rates of nondisjunction for these chromosomes cannot be determined directly. This notwithstanding, there is a class of observations that makes it overwhelmingly likely that the frequencies of nondisjunction for the major autosomes are comparable to those of the X and fourth chromosomes. There now exist stocks in which the two homologs (for chromosome 2 or 3 or both) are attached to one another such that only diplo and nullo gametes are produced. If normal females are crossed to males from such attached-autosome stocks, the only surviving progeny will be those resulting from maternal nondisjunction—diplo-exceptional eggs fertilized by nullo sperm and nullo-exceptional eggs fertilized by diplo sperm. Thus, nondisjunction of the major autosomes can be detected in such crosses, but because regular progeny do not survive, the rate of nondisjunction cannot be determined. However, the number of exceptions per mother has been measured (for references, see the review by Baker et al., 1976), and this number is comparable to that for the X and fourth chromosomes. This suggests that the frequency of nondisjunction is approximately the same for each of the four chromosomes in the *Drosophila* genome.

This frequency can, however, be influenced by a number of nongenetic, as well as genetic, factors. Among the nongenetic factors, of principal interest here are the effects on nondisjunction of maternal age, chemical mutagens, and ionizing radiations.

There has been no discernible change observed in the rate of X-chromosome nondisjunction when the experiment involves aging females and measuring nondisjunction as a function of maternal age (Kelsall, 1963; Patterson, Brewster, and Winchester, 1932; Uchida 1962). However, females aged at temperatures low enough to inhibit laying eggs—so that as the female ages, so do her oocytes—exhibit substantially increased rates of nondisjunction after they are returned to normal egg-laying temperatures (Hildreth and Ulrichs 1969; Tokunaga 1970a,b). It is possible, of course, that this result is the consequence of some effect on nondisjunction of an interaction between age and low temperature, but when examined directly, nondisjunction is increased by high (35°C), rather than low, temperatures (Grell, 1971b). On the other hand, there does exist a positive synergistic interaction between maternal age (under conditions in which there is no correlation between age itself and nondisjunction) and ionizing radiation on nondisjunction (Uchida, 1962).

There is an extensive literature on the effects of ionizing radiations on nondisjunction showing, first, that x-rays increase the frequency of both diplo-X and nullo-X eggs (i.e., nondisjunction itself) but, in addition, that the frequency of nullo-X eggs is increased much more markedly than is the frequency of diplo exceptions (implying radiation effects on chromosome movement at anaphase); for a recent examination of x-rays and nondisjunction, see Savontaus (1975). This vast literature cannot be summarized here, but an excellent recent summary exists (Parker and Williamson, 1976). The effects on nondisjunction of chemical mutagens is much less developed; Lee (1976) has critically reviewed the few data there are.

GENETIC FACTORS AFFECTING NONDISJUNCTION

It is reasonably well established in *Drosophila* (and it may also be true in humans) that the regular separation of homologs at anaphase I is mediated by either of two different disjunctional systems—*exchange segregation* for tetrads having undergone exchange and *distributive segregation* for nonexchange tetrads. With respect to disjunction, the most immediate consequence of this dual system of controls is that segregation is much more regular than it would be if tetrads lacking an exchange came apart at diplotene-diakinesis and, as a consequence, frequently nondisjoined, as occurs in many forms. Thus, for example, the typical frequency of nonexchange X-chromosome tetrads is about 5% (Weinstein, 1936), whereas chromosomes 4 virtually never recombine (for references, see the review by Hochman, 1976). Nevertheless, as illustrated earlier, nondisjunction rates are no higher for the achiasmate chromosome 4 than for the X and, even in the case of the X chromosome, only a very small fraction of nonrecombinant tetrads nondisjoin. Further demonstrating this generality is that, although heterozygous X-chromosome inversions can reduce exchange and increase nondisjunction, the increase in nondisjunction is very small compared to the decrease in recombination (Sturtevant and Beadle, 1936).

This regular segregation of the vast majority of nonexchange tetrads is almost surely explained by those tetrads segregating distributively. This is most convincingly demonstrated by the patterns of segregation observed in the presence of a meiotic mutant, *nod* (no distributive disjunction), that almost completely eliminates the distributive system (Carpenter, 1973). In homozygous *nod* females, the two chromosomes 4 segregate randomly and the X chromosomes exhibit a frequency of primary nondisjunction of about 2½%, which would be expected if the 5% nonexchange tetrads segregate at random. In addition, there is extensive meiotic chromosome loss.

Thus, the first category of genic effects on nondisjunction is composed of those meiotic mutants affecting any aspect of the distributive segregational system—the only proved example of which is *nod*.

A second category of genic effects on nondisjunction is composed of recombination-defective meiotic mutants, of which there are many examples. The primary effect of recombination-defective meiotic mutants is to decrease the amount of recombination; this usually results in an increase in the frequency of nonexchange tetrads for all chromosomes. These nonexchange tetrads must disjoin distributively. However, because distributive segregation does not follow the rules of normal homology, nonhomologous segregations will often occur, leading to nondisjunction. Thus, recombination-defective meiotic mutants, because they result in many nonexchange tetrads, will appear as nondisjunction-promoting mutations.

This simple relationship between the frequency of nonexchange tetrads and nondisjunction obtains in the case of meiotic-mutant-bearing females. Over a wide range of values, Baker and Hall (1976) showed that X-chromosome nondisjunction increases as the frequency of nonexchange X tetrads cubed. In normal females, in contrast, the relationship between exchange and nondisjunction is complex. Thus, in an experiment in which the frequencies of the different-rank X-tetrads could be determined, Merriam and Frost (1964) compared these frequencies in disjunctional and nondisjunctional tetrads. If E_i is the frequency of tetrads of rank i, then, in percentages:

	Disjunctional	Nondisjunctional
E_0	4.6	26.0
E_1	65.7	24.5
E_2	28.7	47.6
E_3	1.0	2.0

It can be seen that, for reasons that remain conjectural, tetrads that nondisjoin preferentially contain either zero or two exchanges.

The third, and final, category of genic effects on nondisjunction is composed of disjunction-defective meiotic mutants that affect some aspect of the segregational mechanism that is not dependent on exchange. In *Drosophila,* four such disjunction-defectives have been discovered that affect female meiosis. Two of these, ca^{nd} (claret-nondisjunctional; Davis, 1969) and $1(1)TW$-6^{cs} (Wright, 1973), cause high frequencies of first-division nondisjunction of both exchange and nonexchange chromosomes (although segregation is somewhat more regular following exchange) and also substantial amounts of meiotic chromosome loss. Cytologically, *ca* causes abnormal anaphase I spindles (Wald, 1936), suggesting that it, and perhaps $1(1)TW$-6^{cs} also, cause nondisjunction by disrupting the orderly formation of the spindle apparatus.

These two mutants affect only female meiosis (that is, mutant males do not exhibit meiotic anomalies) and primarily or exclusively the first meiotic division. The remaining two disjunction-defectives, *mei-S332* (Davis, 1971) and *ord* (orientation-disruptor; Mason, 1976), cause similar anomalies in both sexes and increase the frequency of equational and reductional exceptions in the case of *ord,* and increase only equational nondisjunction in the case of *mei-S332*. From the genetic results and some preliminary cytology (which is done in males), Davis (for *mei-S332*) and Mason (for ord) concluded that these mutants cause defects in the mechanism that holds sister chromatids together—a general defect in the case of *ord,* a centromere-specific defect in the case of *mei-S332*.

More recently, Lawrence Goldstein has been making a detailed cytological and genetical study of these mutants. He has confirmed the earlier work and, in addition, shown that, in the case of *ord,* at very early anaphase I, just when the bivalents separate, the chromatids of the dyad also have fallen apart. Thus segregation at both divisions in *ord* homozygotes involves not a tetrad and then two dyads but, rather, four monads. This means, for example, that a "reductional nondisjunction" is really the consequence of two noncrossover chromatids, one from each homolog, proceeding to the same pole at both meiotic divisions. In the case of *mei-S332,* monads also form precociously, but later in anaphase than under the influence of *ord*.

Thus, in summary, we see that nondisjunction-producing genes can be of at least three different major classes: 1) Recombination-defective genes cause meiocytes with several nonexchange tetrads to be formed; in these, the distributive disjunction of nonhomologs results in nondisjunction. 2) Disjunction-defective meiotic mutants that affect the distributive segregational system will result directly in the nondisjunction of nonexchange chromosomes. 3) Defects in any part of the normal disjunctional mechanism—e.g., the spindle, the centromere, or the orientation mechanism—will result in nondisjunction of exchange and nonexchange chromosomes, presumably at either meiotic division.

SUMMARY

The meiotic nondisjunction of homologous chromosomes in karyotypically normal female *Drosophila melanogaster* has the following characteristics:

Nondisjunction occurs almost exclusively at the first meiotic division.
Both exchange and nonexchange tetrads can nondisjoin.
Nondisjunction is associated with chromosome loss, resulting in an excess of nullo-exceptional eggs compared with diplo-exceptional eggs.
Nondisjunction is associated with the distributive segregation of nonhomologous chromosomes, resulting in the nonrandomly frequent occurrence of multiple nondisjunctional events.
The rate of nondisjunction is of the order of 0.10% or less for each chromosome and does not vary with chromosome size.
The rate of nondisjunction can be increased by a variety of nongenic agents, including aging oocytes, high temperatures, ionizing radiations, a synergistic interaction between radiation and maternal age, several chemical mutagens, and some chromosome aberrations.
The rate of nondisjunction can be greatly increased, sometimes to values approaching the random segregation of homologs, by any of a large (and rapidly growing) number of meiotic mutants. Some of these act directly on either of the two disjunctional mechanisms operative in meiosis (disjunction-defective meiotic mutants) and others (recombination-defective meiotic mutants) act to reduce recombination, which causes, as a secondary effect, an increase in the nondisjunction of nonexchange tetrads.

REFERENCES

Baker, B. S., Carpenter, A. T. C., Esposito, M. S., Esposito, R. E., and Sandler, L. 1976. The genetic control of meiosis. Annu. Rev. Genet. 10:53–134.

Baker, B. S., and Hall, J. C. 1976. Meiotic mutants: Genic control of meiotic recombination and chromosome segregation. In M. Ashburner and E. Novitski (eds.), The Genetics and Biology of Drosophila, Vol. 1a, pp. 351–434. Academic Press, New York.

Bridges, C. B. 1916. Non-disjunction as proof of the chromosome theory of heredity. Genetics 1:1–52, 107–163.

Carpenter, A. T. C. 1973. A meiotic mutant defective in distributive disjunction in *Drosophila melanogaster*. Genetics 73:393–428.

Cooper, K. W. 1948. A new theory of secondary non-disjunction in female *D. melanogaster*. Proc. Nat. Acad. Sci. 34:179–187.

Davis, B. K. 1971. Genetic analysis of a meiotic mutant resulting in precocious sister-centromere separation in *Drosophila melanogaster*. Mol. Gen. Genetics 113:251–272.

Davis, D. G. 1969. Chromosome behavior under the influence of claret-nondisjunctional in *Drosophila melanogaster*. Genetics 61:577–594.

Grell, R. F. 1964. Distributive pairing and aneuploidy in man. Science 145:66–67.

Grell, R. F. 1971a. Distributive pairing in man? Ann. Genet. 14:165–171.

Grell, R. F. 1971b. Induction of sex chromosome nondisjunction by elevated temperature. Mutat. Res. 11:347–349.

Grell, R. F. 1976. Distributive pairing. In M. Ashburner and E. Novitski (eds.), The Genetics and Biology of Drosophila, Vol. 1a, pp. 435–486. Academic Press, New York.

Hildreth, P. E., and Ulrichs, P. C. 1969. A temperature effect on nondisjunction of the X chromosomes among eggs from aged *Drosophila* females. Genetica 40:191–197.

Hochman, B. 1976. The fourth chromosome of *Drosophila melanogaster*. In M. Ashburner and E. Novitski (eds.), The Genetics and Biology of Drosophila, Vol. 1b, pp. 903–928. Academic Press, New York.

Kelsall, P. J. 1963. Nondisjunction and maternal age in *D. melanogaster*. Genet. Res. 4: 284–289.

Lee, W. R. 1976. Chemical mutagenesis. In M. Ashburner and E. Novitski (eds.), The Genetics and Biology of Drosophila, Vol. 1c, pp. 1299–1341. Academic Press, New York.

Mason, J. M. 1976. Orientation disruptor (*ord*): A recombination and disjunction defective meiotic mutant in *Drosophila melanogaster*. Genetics 84:545–572.

Merriam, J. R., and Frost, J. N. 1964. Exchange and nondisjunction of the X chromosomes in female *D. melanogaster*. Genetics 49:109–122.

Morgan, T. H., Bridges, C. B., and Sturtevant, A. H. 1925. The genetics of Drosophila. Bibliogr. Genet. 2:1–262.

Parker, D. R., and Williamson, J. H. 1976. Segregation in oocytes. In M. Ashburner and E. Novitski (eds.), The Genetics and Biology of Drosophila, Vol. 1c, pp. 1251–1268. Academic Press, New York.

Patterson, J. T., Brewster, W., and Winchester, A. M. 1932. Effects produced by aging and X-raying eggs of *D. melanogaster*. J. Hered. 23:325–333.

Sandler, L., and Braver, G. 1954. The meiotic loss of unpaired chromosomes in *Drosophila melanogaster*. Genetics 39:365–377.

Sandler, L., and Hecht, F. 1973. Genetic effects of aneuploidy. Am. J. Hum. Genet. 25: 332–339.

Sandler, L., Lindsley, D. L., Nicoletti, B., and Trippa, G. 1968. Mutants affecting meiosis in natural populations of *Drosophila melanogaster*. Genetics 60:525–558.

Savontaus, M. L. 1975. Relationship between effects of X-rays on nondisjunction and crossing over in *Drosophila melanogaster*. Hereditas 80:195–204.

Sturtevant, A. H., and Beadle, G. W. 1936. The relations of inversions in the X chromosome of *D. melanogaster* to crossing-over and disjunction. Genetics 21:554–604.

Tokunaga, C. 1970a. The effects of low temperature and aging on nondisjunction in *Drosophila*. Genetics 65:75–94.

Tokunaga, C. 1970b. Aspects of low-temperature-induced meiotic nondisjunction in *Drosophila* females. Genetics 66:653–661.

Uchida, I. A. 1962. The effect of maternal age and radiation on the rate of nondisjunction in *D. melanogaster*. Can. J. Genet. Cytol. 4:402–408.

Wald, H. 1936. Cytologic studies on the abnormal development of the eggs of the claret mutant type of *Drosophila simulans*. Genetics 21:264–281.

Weinstein, A. 1936. The theory of multiple-strand crossing over. Genetics 21:155–199.

Wright, T. R. F. 1973. The recovery, penetrance, and pleiotrophy of X-linked, cold sensitive mutants in Drosophila. Mol. Gen. Genet. 122:101–118.

Zimmering, S. 1976. Genetic and cytogenetic aspects of altered segregation phenomena in *Drosophila*. In M. Ashburner and E. Novitski (eds.), The Genetics and Biology of Drosophila, Vol. 1b, pp. 569–613. Academic Press, New York.

OTHER FACTORS
AFFECTING
NONDISJUNCTION

Down Syndrome and Maternal Radiation

Irene A. Uchida

The high frequency of nondisjunction found in human populations is a matter of increasing concern. This serious problem is particularly evident in the continuing large numbers of Down syndrome infants observed among live births as well as the still higher frequencies among spontaneous abortions and those identified by prenatal diagnosis. Because of this high toll in human life and the ever-increasing costs of institutional and health care, much attention is being focused upon the cause of abnormal chromosome segregation with the hope that effective preventive measures can be found without having to resort to therapeutic abortion of affected fetuses.

Attention was first drawn to an association between late maternal age and radiation in the induction of nondisjunction in *Drosophila melanogaster* by Patterson, Brewster, and Winchester (1932), who observed an increase in abnormal segregation of chromosomes in aged flies exposed to x-rays. A similar increase was not found in flies that were aged but not irradiated. These observations suggested the possibility that a comparable mechanism might be operating among humans.

Epidemiological studies of the effects of radiation on human chromosome segregation have mainly been of two kinds: retrospective and prospective. Most frequent have been retrospective studies, in which mothers of Down syndrome children have been interviewed to elicit pertinent information. The results have then been compared either with age-matched nonirradiated controls or with expected frequencies. These data are fairly easy to obtain but are not always reliable because of dependence upon a mother's memory.

There are fewer prospective studies because of the many problems inherent in the methodology. However, the results should be more reliable. Women with known radiation exposure are followed to ascertain what kind of progeny are born after x-ray exposure. To circumvent the long waiting period for children to be born after radiation exposure, prolonged in some cases by a period of induced sterility, women with documented histories of previous radiological examinations can be interviewed and their children examined for the presence of Down syndrome. Ingenuity is required to locate women who had been exposed several years earlier. This method also requires large sample sizes to reveal any changes in a population frequency of approximately 1 in 800. In addition, choice of age-matched, nonirradiated controls must rely upon the mothers' memory to rule out any previous exposure, which is similar to problems inherent in retrospective studies. The possibility that the disease requiring the radiological procedure might itself contribute to abnormal chromosome segregation must also be dealt with. The most effective method to control constitutional and genetic differences is to compare the offspring born before and after x-ray exposure and to cross-match the mothers with each other for maternal age (Uchida, Holunga, and Lawler, 1968).

The results of 11 epidemiological studies on Down syndrome have been summarized (Uchida, 1977). All but 2 showed a higher frequency of affected children born to women who had been exposed to radiation than to nonirradiated controls. Only 4 studies showed a significant increase, but the general trend of the majority was in the same positive direction. Most exposures were diagnostic examinations of the abdominal region. All were preconception exposures and the doses, in general, were low. The notable exception is the study carried out in Japan following the release of the atomic bomb (Schull and Neel, 1962). Recently, however, Awa et al. (1971) identified with karyotyping a higher frequency of sex chromosome aneuploids among the exposed population.

The 1965 study of Sigler et al. that covered a 17-year period showed a significant increase in radiation exposure of mothers of Down syndrome children. However, when their study was extended to include 7 more years (Cohen et al., 1977), the result was reversed to yield a higher frequency among controls.

A third type of human population study is an investigation of the effects of background radiation in areas known for high environmental levels. Two studies, one in New York State (Gentry, Parkhurst, and Bulin, 1959) and the other in the New England states (Segall, MacMahon, and Hannigan, 1964), produced negative results. An investigation by Schuman and Gullen (1970) in Colorado, Michigan, and Minnesota showed that only in Minnesota was there an increase in Down syndrome children born in areas with higher radiation levels. For many years great interest had centered on the coastal area of Kerala in India, known for its very high level of radioactive soil. In a study carried out by Kochupillai et al. (1976), significantly higher frequencies of Down syndrome and other types of severe mental retardation of "genetic" origin were found.

Now that the groundwork has been laid, no more benefits would appear to be derived from carrying on epidemiological studies in localized areas. Past studies indicate that sample sizes are too small to be effective. The best method for tackling this problem is to initiate a large, multicountry collaborative study, with standardized methodology to collate the results. A first attempt was made in 1973 by the Nuclear Energy Agency of the Organization for Economic Co-operation and Development in Paris, but there was a disappointing lack of interest. Perhaps with the realization of the magnitude of the problem of chromosome aberrations among humans, more interest and some progress can be made to achieve this goal.

An additional problem has become evident in recent years and must be taken into account in future studies. Proof of paternal transmission of the extra chromosome in approximately 25% of Down syndrome children indicates that attention must be shifted to include the fathers in these investigations. Lowering of maternal ages observed in certain populations of trisomy 21 may be accounted for by this apparent change in the parental origin of nondisjunction and may be indicative of an unsuspected susceptibility of the male to environmental mutagens that affect chromosome segregation.

With the advent of more sophisticated banding techniques of human chromosomes, more information can be derived from karyotyping spontaneous abortions. Identification of parental transmission not only of the extra chromosome 21 but also of other acrocentric chromosomes can provide additional information.

Studies of radiation-induced mitotic nondisjunction of human lymphocytes (Uchida, Lee, and Byrnes, 1975) showed a significantly increased susceptibility of chromosomes 21 and X to abnormal segregation. These data support the relatively high frequency of mosaicism found in subjects with trisomy 21 and X-chromosome aneuploidy.

With the observation of fewer chiasmata and more univalents in aged mice, Henderson and Edwards (1968) suggested that this mechanism may account for the maternal age effect in the frequency of Down syndrome among humans. However, there was no proof that these univalents proceeded to form abnormal gametes. Following improvements in the methodology of obtaining good preparations of oocyte chromosomes in second metaphase (Tarkowski, 1966), abnormal segregation during first meiotic division could be identified. This experimental procedure provided the means to obtain proof that nondisjunction could be induced in both young and aged mice by exposing them to low doses of whole body irradiation (Uchida and Freeman, 1977; Uchida and Lee, 1974). Further studies are underway to ascertain whether or not nondisjunction can be induced in second meiotic division by examining the chromosomes of pre-implantation embryos.

Many more problems involving nondisjunction have yet to be investigated. It is difficult to provide estimates of a safe minimum radiation dosage to the gonads. Technical procedures differ from hospital to hospital. In clinics and in physicians', chiropractors', and dentists' offices, accurate records are not kept and patients easily forget past exposures or are unable to recall the type of examinations carried out. Accurate estimates of gonadal doses are unavailable and there are wide fluctuations in background radiation.

Experimental evidence of radiation effects may be relatively easy to obtain in mice, but in humans the problems are different. There are difficulties in obtaining tissue to study human oogenesis and spermatogenesis, and the effect of in vivo radiation upon these cells is impossible to ascertain.

Reevaluation of maternal age effects may result in changes in indications for genetic amniocentesis. Since it is technically impossible as well as inadvisable to perform prenatal diagnosis on all pregnant women, it may be necessary to fix an arbitrary category for genetic amniocentesis among younger women, such as a history of exposure to teratogenic agents, one of which is radiation.

It is hoped that widespread dissemination of the information in this volume on Down syndrome will alert the public to the urgency of identifying the causes of abnormal chromosome segregation in humans and place more emphasis on prevention of mental retardation than on treatment and therapy.

REFERENCES

Awa, A. A., Honda, T., Sofuni, T., Neriishi, S., Yoshida, M. C., and Matsui, T. 1971. Chromosome aberration frequencies in cultured blood cells in relation to radiation dose of A-bomb survivors. Lancet 2:903–905.

Cohen, B. H., Lilienfeld, A. M., Kramer, S., and Hyman, L. C. 1977. Parental factors in Down's syndrome—Results of the second Baltimore case-control study. In E. B. Hook and I. H. Porter (eds.), Population Cytogenetics: Studies in Humans, pp. 301–352. Academic Press, New York.

Gentry, J. T., Parkhurst, E., and Bulin, G. V. 1959. An epidemiological study of congenital malformations in New York State. Am. J. Pub. Health 49:497–513.

Henderson, S. A., and Edwards, R. G. 1968. Chiasma frequency and maternal age in mammals. Nature 218:22–28.

Kochupillai, N., Verma, I. C., Grewal, M. S., and Ramalingaswami, V. 1976. Down's syndrome and related abnormalities in an area of high background radiation in coastal Kerala. Nature 262:60–61.

Patterson, J. T., Brewster, W., and Winchester, A. M. 1932. Effects produced by aging and x-raying eggs of *Drosophila melanogaster*. J. Hered. 23:325–333.

Schull, W. J., and Neel, J. V. 1962. Maternal radiation and mongolism. Lancet 1: 537–538.

Schuman, L. M., and Gullen, W. H. 1970. Background radiation and Down's syndrome. Ann. N.Y. Acad. Sci. 171(2):441–453.

Segall, A., MacMahon, B., and Hannigan, M. 1964. Congenital malformations and background radiation in Northern New England. J. Chron. Dis. 17:915–932.

Sigler, A. T., Lilienfeld, A. M., Cohen, B. H., and Westlake, J. E. 1965. Radiation exposure in parents of children with mongolism (Down's syndrome). Bull. Johns Hopkins Hosp. 117: 374–399.

Tarkowski, A. K. 1966. An air-drying method for chromosome preparations from mouse eggs. Cytogenetics 5:394–400.

Uchida, I. A. 1977. Maternal radiation and trisomy 21. In E. B. Hook and I. H. Porter (eds.), Population Cytogenetics: Studies in Humans, pp. 285–299. Academic Press, New York.

Uchida, I. A., and Freeman, C. P. V. 1977. Radiation-induced nondisjunction in oocytes of aged mice. Nature 265:186–187.

Uchida, I. A., Holunga, R., and Lawler, C. 1968. Maternal radiation and chromosomal aberrations. Lancet 2:1045–1049.

Uchida, I. A., and Lee, C. P. V. 1974. Radiation-induced nondisjunction in mouse oocytes. Nature 250:601–602.

Uchida, I. A., Lee, C. P. V., and Byrnes, E. M. 1975. Chromosome aberrations induced *in vitro* by low doses of radiation: Nondisjunction in lymphocytes of young adults. Am. J. Human Genet. 27:419–429.

The Current Status of Alpha$_1$-Antitrypsin and Other Factors in Down Syndrome

W. Roy Breg, Robert M. Fineman,
A. Myron Johnson, and Kenneth K. Kidd

Numerous genetic marker studies have been done in Down syndrome either for the purpose of learning something about the etiology of this condition or for gene mapping following the discovery that Down syndrome patients have an extra chromosome 21. The ABO blood group system was the first locus to be studied; more recently HLA antigens, various serum proteins, and red and white blood cell enzymes showing variant forms or polymorphisms have been investigated. In most of these studies, either the results have failed to show significant differences between the observed and expected frequencies of the various phenotypes or, when differences have been found, they have not been confirmed, either because of the lack of further studies of the same system or because of the failure of other investigators to find similar differences. In many instances apparent differences could well be explained by chance fluctuations resulting from the study of relatively small samples and/or by not having appropriate controls.

However, even when apparently significant differences in the frequency of certain phenotypes have been found on studying relatively large numbers of Down syndrome and control subjects, the results often could not be confirmed by others. For instance, Brackenridge, Pitt, and Sheehy (1974) studied the erythrocyte acid phosphatase types of 171 patients and 200 controls. The frequency of the AB phenotype was reduced in Down syndrome persons, especially in females. The AB phenotype was present in 27% of Down syndrome females but in 42% of female controls ($p \approx 0.014$). When data from males and females were combined, there was still a reduction in the frequency of the AB type in Down syndrome persons ($p \approx 0.021$). However, Rundle and Sudell (1973), in studying 253 Down syndrome persons and

The studies described in this chapter were supported in part by grants from the National Institutes of Health (HD 11624 and AI 11280).

402 controls, were unable to find any deviation from the expected frequency of the erythrocyte acid phosphotase types in the Down syndrome group.

Discrepant results from various laboratories have been noted in studies of haptoglobin types. Ball et al. (1972), in studying haptoglobin types of 123 Down syndrome subjects and 117 controls, found a reduction in 2-1 types (and a concomitant increase in 1-1 and 2-2 types), which did not quite reach the 5% level of significance ($p \cong 0.057$). On the other hand, Rundle, Atkin, and Sudell (1974) were unable to show such a difference.

Despite the difficulties in finding significant differences in the distribution of protein polymorphisms in Down syndrome, we began studying the variant forms of α_1-antitrypsin (α_1AT) in Down syndrome patients in order to determine whether this polymorphic locus might give a clue to the etiology of trisomy 21.

α_1AT is one of at least nine inhibitors of proteolytic enzymes in human serum (Johnson, 1974). It is produced by the liver and is found in all body fluids. α_1AT inhibits such cellular proteases as collagenase and elastase, as well as serum trypsin; indeed, its more important function may be as an inhibitor of cellular proteases. At least 25 electrophoretic variants of α_1AT have been identified and all are believed to be codominant and determined by alleles at a single locus, referred to as Pi (protease inhibitor). The Pi variants are designated alphabetically in the order of their rates of migration on acid starch gel electrophoresis, with Pi B the most rapidly migrating form and Pi Z the slowest; M is the most common form. In addition to acid starch gel electrophoresis, newer methods—immunofixation electrophoresis and, most recently, isoelectric focusing—have permitted the identification of additional α_1AT variants. The latter method has been particularly useful in the detection of variants migrating in the M region and indistinguishable from M by acid starch gel electrophoresis.

Some α_1AT variants are associated with varying degrees of reduction in serum antitrypsin concentration and in antitrypsin activity. There are a number of well-established associations between the α_1AT variants with decreased antitrypsin activity and certain diseases (Johnson, 1974). The first such association to be discovered was that of chronic obstructive pulmonary disease and the α_1AT phenotype ZZ. An association between the same α_1AT phenotype and childhood cirrhosis has been found. In addition, there seems to be an increased frequency of SZ heterozygotes, and possibly MZ, among these affected infants. Also, the frequency of α_1AT variants is increased in infants with biliary atresia.

Of particular interest is the possible association of α_1AT variants and trisomy 21. Such a possibility was suggested by a report in 1970 by Aarskog and Fagerhol, in which they noted an apparent increased frequency of such variants in persons with various chromosomal abnormalities, especially those with sex chromosomal mosaicism. In a very small series of seven cases with sex chromosome mosaicism (none with structural rearrangements), four persons were heterozygous for an α_1AT variant; only three were homozygous for the most common type, MM. This high frequency (57%) of persons heterozygous for a variant was compared to the frequency of 10% of such persons in the general population in Norway, where their studies were conducted. Another series in that study consisted of seven 45,X (nonmosaic) patients, one of whom was an MZ heterozygote, a phenotype found in only 3% of the general population. Also, of 13 cases with trisomy 21, 2 (15%) were MS heterozygotes; the expected frequency was 4%. These results were inconclusive since the numbers studied were small; however, they were suggestive enough of an increased frequency of α_1AT variants in persons with chromosome abnormalities, particularly those with a sex chromosome mosaicism, to warrant further study.

In 1975, in an attempt to confirm the findings of Aarskog and Fagerhol, we began a study of the α_1AT phenotypes of persons with sex chromosome mosaicism. In our initial report in 1976, it was noted that of 19 cases with a sex chromosome mosaicism, some with and others without structural rearrangements, three (16%) had a variant form of α_1AT. Although this frequency was not as impressive as that Aarskog and Fagerhol had found, we felt our results were at least consistent with theirs since two of our cases appeared to be heterozygotes for an unusual variant of M known as Lamb (MM$_{Lamb}$). However, recent re-testing of these two persons by the new assay, isoelectric focusing, has shown that both have a much more common M variant, M$_2$. Since that report we have studied an additional nine cases, and four of them are heterozygous for non-M variants. Thus, of all the sex chromosome mosaics in our study, 5 of 28 (18%) have non-M variants.

After we began our study, the results of a study by Kueppers et al. (1975), which were consistent with those found by Aarskog and Fagerhol (1970), were published. Kueppers et al. studied 21 patients with a variety of sex chromosome mosaicisms, some with and others without structural abnormalities of the X chromosome. Of these 21 patients, 5 were heterozygotes, SZ or FM. This frequency (24%) was compared to a 5% frequency of heterozygotes in the general population of northern Germany, the area from which their patients had come. The combined results from the three series (Aarskog and Fagerhol, Kueppers et al., and ours) show that 13 (23%) of 56 cases studied had non-M variants detectable by acid starch gel electrophoresis. Although not as impressive as the 57% of cases heterozygous for a Pi variant found by Aarskog and Fagerhol, this frequency of 23% is greater than that found in the populations from which the subjects in these various studies had come. These results are still suggestive of an association between sex chromosome mosaicism and variants of α_1AT in the heterozygous state.

Furthermore, both Aarskog and Fagerhol (1970) and Kueppers et al. (1975) found an apparent increased frequency of cases of sex chromosome mosaicism in which one or both parents were heterozygous for α_1AT variants (demonstrated by testing of parent, or parent was an obligate heterozygote since offspring was heterozygous). There were 12 cases (63%) in which a parent was heterozygous from among 19 informative cases. Of all 43 parents on which information was available, 13 (30%) were heterozygotes.

When we began the study of patients with sex chromosome mosaicism, we decided to study Down syndrome cases as well. It seemed reasonable to consider the possibility that if α_1AT variants had played a role in the mitotic nondisjunction leading to mosaicism, Pi variants might also be associated with meiotic nondisjunction. The study by Aarskog and Fagerhol of a limited number (13) of Down syndrome patients, of whom 2 (15%) were Pi heterozygotes, did not rule out this possibility. Our study of Down syndrome patients is divided into three phases: 1) results reported in 1976 (Fineman et al., 1976), 60 patients and no controls, 2) results, presented at the Fifth International Congress of Human Genetics in October, 1976, from an additional 150 Down syndrome patients and 214 controls, and 3) Down syndrome patients (245) and control subjects (296) studied subsequently.

As reported in 1976 by Fineman et al., in our first 60 patients, 27% had a Pi variant (Table 1). More significantly, of 31 patients born to mothers 35 years old or over, 45% had a variant, but only 7% of 29 cases born when their mothers were under 30 years of age had variants. The study had been designed before data were collected to include equal numbers of Down syndrome infants born to mothers over 35 and to mothers under 30. Thus, the heterogeneity found between young and older mothers was highly significant. Since no controls had been studied, these results were also compared with an assumed 10% frequency of heterozygotes in the general population. Only the increased frequency in the older mother group was significantly different from that expected frequency. However, we could not be certain that these patients had indeed come from a population in which persons with Pi variants occur with a frequency of 10%, although some surveys in the United States had shown such a rate. It should be noted that the frequency of variants may differ significantly in a particular subpopulation with a preponderance of people whose ancestors had come from a country or area with a different rate of variants. For instance, the heterozygote frequency in blacks in the United States is only 4% and in Finland only 1%–2%, but in Spain it is 25%. A considerable difference within the same country is noted in France, where the frequency of persons with Pi variants is 16% in the south but in the north is 5%.

As noted previously, the two assays, acid starch gel electrophoresis and immunofixation, led to the detection of some M variants, which earlier were thought to be unusual. Some of these variants, which can be more reliably characterized by isoelectric focusing, have proved to be relatively common MM variants (M_2 and M_3). On reexamination of the sera of this group of patients with the isoelectric focusing technique, an increase in the frequency of patients with non-M variants in the group born to older mothers is still apparent (Table 2). Eleven of 31 patients (35%) born to mothers 35 years or older had such a variant.

Since the data from this limited study suggested an increased frequency of α_1AT variants in cases of Down syndrome with advanced maternal age, an association with possible etiological implications, it became important to see if these results could be confirmed. For this we studied an additional 150 Down syndrome persons at the

Table 1.   Frequencies of Down syndrome patients with variant Pi alleles[a]

	Maternal age			
No. of variants	< 30 ($N=29$)	35 + ($N=31$)	Total	($N=60$)
None	0.93	0.55	0.73	
One	0.07	0.39	0.23	
Two		0.06	0.03	

After Fineman et al., (1976).

[a]Frequency of persons with variants in general population assumed to be about 0.10.

Table 2.   Frequencies of Down syndrome patients with variant Pi alleles other than M$_2$ and M$_3$

| No. of variants | Maternal age | | Total | $(N=60)$ |
	$<30\ (N=29)$	$35+(N=31)$		
None	0.97	0.65	0.80	
One	0.03	0.35	0.20	
Two				

Results of reexamination of sera reported by Fineman et al. (1976) by isoelectric focusing, which reliably identifies M variants. The M variants are not considered "variants" in this tabulation.

Southbury Training School, bringing the total number studied to 210: all of those at that institution who had trisomy 21.

Each of the Down syndrome patients from the Southbury Training School has been karyotyped and shown to have trisomy 21; those patients with known trisomy 21 mosaicism or translocation have been excluded from this study. The karyotypes of Down syndrome patients from other locations, noted later, are not known to us, if in fact they have been studied. However, the heterogeneity that might result from including cases with mosaicism or translocation is unlikely to be great enough to affect significantly the results of the α_1AT studies. In addition, 214 mentally retarded persons (also at Southbury) without chromosomal abnormalities were studied for comparison.

The results from these studies using acid starch gel electrophoresis and immunofixation for Pi typing were presented at the Fifth International Congress of Human Genetics in October, 1976, and are summarized in Table 3 (Fineman et al., 1976b). This table shows the results of α_1AT typing of the sera from these persons using isoelectric focusing as well as acid starch gel electrophoresis and immunofixation methods. These results indicate that Pi variants are found more frequently in Down syndrome persons born to older mothers than in those born to younger mothers, the difference being of borderline significance. However, when compared with the frequency in control subjects, the variants are not significantly more frequent in the Down syndrome population. In fact, there is some suggestion of a decreased frequency of Pi variants in the Down syndrome patients born to mothers less than 35 years of age. Additional results concerning this point are noted later.

In an attempt to clarify the apparent discrepant results of these two phases of our study, we continued to collect data from persons with Down syndrome and from

Table 3.   Frequencies of persons with variant Pi alleles including M$_2$ and M$_3$

| No. of variant alleles | Down syndrome maternal age (years) | | Total $(N=207)$ | Controls $(N=214)$ |
	$<\ (N=99)$	$35+(N=108)$		
None	0.72	0.57	0.64	0.65
One	0.16	0.33	0.25	0.28
Two	0.12	0.10	0.11	0.07

Data presented by Fineman et al. (1976b) at the Fifth International Congress of Human Genetics, October, 1976.
$p=0.03$.

Table 4. Number of persons studied by Pi phenotyping

Group	N	Mean
Down syndrome		
Southbury 1	60	28.2
2	47	27.6
3	103	36.7
Virginia	109	27.6
New Haven	34	11.3
Utah	102	26.7
Total	455	27.5
Controls		
Southbury MR	214	33.9
Virginia MR	155	29.0
Connecticut non-MR	141	31.3
Total	510	31.7

control subjects. Dr. David Madden of the National Institutes of Health kindly provided us with serum samples that had been left from a study of Australia antigen in a Down syndrome and a control population of other patients at the Lynchburg Training School (Virginia). Also, samples were obtained from persons with Down syndrome in the New Haven area and from a group at the Utah State Training School (American Fork, Utah). Another control population, employees at the Southbury Training School and at Yale University, was also studied. The numbers of persons in these various groups, with the mean maternal age for each, are given in Table 4. We have now studied a total of 455 Down syndrome and 510 control subjects.

An examination of all the data (Table 5) shows that there is no significant difference in the frequency of Pi variants in Down syndrome and control subjects, nor is there a difference between Down syndrome persons born to older mothers (35 years or over) and those born to younger mothers (less than 35 years). In Table 5 the frequencies listed for 1976 are the same as those in Table 3, and those noted under 1978 are from the entire study, all subgroups combined, including those reported in October, 1976.

The differences in the results by maternal age from the various Down syndrome groups are shown in Table 6. In two groups, New Haven and Utah, the frequency of individuals with a Pi variant was higher in those born of younger mothers than in

Table 5. Frequencies of persons with variant Pi alleles

No. of variant alleles	Down syndrome maternal age (years)				Controls (N = 509) (1978)
	< 35		35 +		
	1976 (N = 99)	1978 (N = 193)	1976 (N = 108)	1978 (N = 208)	
None	0.72	0.60	0.57	0.58	0.62
One	0.16	0.29	0.33	0.34	0.30
Two	0.12	0.11	0.09	0.08	0.08

Table 6.   Frequency of Down syndrome persons with one or two variant Pi alleles by maternal age in various groups

| Series | Maternal age | | | | Total N |
	<35	(N)	35+	(N)	
Southbury (Oct., 1976)	0.28	(99)	0.43	(108)	207
Virginia	0.48	(46)	0.49	(43)	89
New Haven	0.86	(7)	0.37	(27)	34
Utah	0.54	(41)	0.37	(30)	71
Total	0.40	(193)	0.42	(208)	401
Controls			0.38		509

those born to older mothers. In the Southbury study, Down syndrome persons that had a variant were more common in the older maternal age group. In the Virginia Down syndrome population there was no difference in the frequency of Down syndrome cases with a Pi variant in the two age groups.

When the data from the study of all Down syndrome patients at the Southbury Training School were examined and it became apparent that the frequency of Pi variants in those patients born to older mothers was much less significant than was found in the first phase of our study, we considered the possibility that another variable might be important. In evaluating various characteristics of the groups studied it became apparent that, earlier, we had inadvertently selected for study generally younger patients, leaving an overrepresentation of older patients as the study at Southbury progressed. In examining the frequencies of Pi variants in the different age categories, a suggestive patient age effect became apparent (Table 7). Thus, older Down syndrome patients (35 years or older) had a lower frequency of variants when compared with other Down syndrome patients and with control subjects, while the younger Down syndrome patients had a higher frequency than that found in the control subjects. The difference was statistically significant at the $p = 0.018$ level. Examination of the data from our entire study shows the same trend, although to a somewhat lesser degree (Figure 1). In the two younger age groups, those under 20 years and those from 20 to 29 years of age, Down syndrome persons with a variant of any type occur more frequently than do persons with a variant in the control group. This

Table 7.   Frequencies of variant Pi alleles in Down syndrome by age of patient

| No. of variant alleles | Down syndrome age at testing | | | Controls (N=214) |
	<25 (N=61)	25–34 (N=70)	35+ (N=78)	
None	0.59	0.53	0.77	0.65
One	0.25	0.36	0.17	0.28
Two	0.16	0.11	0.06	0.07

Data from Fineman et al., 1976, *Nature 260*, p. 320.
$p = 0.018$.

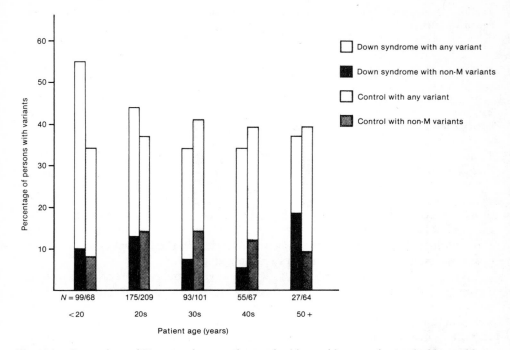

Figure 1.   Proportions of Down syndrome and control subjects with any variant and with non-M variants, whether heterozygous or homozygous, by age groups.

difference in the 20- to 29-year-old group is slight. Another analysis of the data comparing the frequencies of variants in younger and older persons is presented in Table 8. Fifty-five per cent of Down syndrome subjects less than 20 years old have one or two Pi variant alleles, whereas 39% of the older Down syndrome patients (a difference of borderline significance) and 38% of the controls have a variant. In the control groups, the frequencies of variants did not vary with the age of the test subjects. The frequencies of the various Pi alleles found in these groups are shown in Table 9. It is apparent that the increased frequency of Pi alleles in Down syndrome patients under 20 years of age is entirely accounted for by an increase in the M_2 allele.

Table 8.   Frequencies of persons with variant Pi alleles by age of patients

No. of variant alleles	Down syndrome age at testing		Control ($N = 509$)
	<20 ($N = 99$)	$20+$ ($N = 350$)	
None	0.45	0.61	0.62
One	0.45	0.29	0.30
Two	0.10	0.10	0.08

$p = 0.05$.

Table 9.   Frequencies of various Pi alleles by age of patients

Allele	Down syndrome age at testing		Control (N = 508)
	< 20 (N = 99)	20 + (N = 350)	
M	0.68	0.75	0.77
M_2	0.23	0.16	0.15
M_3	0.05	0.03	0.02
S	0.03	0.03	0.04
Z	0.01	0.02	0.01
Other	0.01	0.01	0.01

In the entire Southbury study, as reported in October, 1976, the frequency of persons who had a Pi variant was highest in the younger Down syndrome patients born to older mothers and lowest in the group of older patients born to younger mothers. However, as indicated in Table 10, the results from the complete study have failed to corroborate such a correlation. Although the younger patients (under 20 years of age) were more likely to have Pi variants (50% versus 39% for the older ones), the highest frequency was found in the group born to younger, rather than older, mothers.

Thus, from earlier phases of our study, the suggestions that there was an increased incidence of Pi variants in patients with Down syndrome born to older mothers and/or in younger patients have not been confirmed, for the most part. Suggestive evidence remains of an increased frequency of only the M_2 form of $\alpha_1 AT$ in patients under 20 years of age. We tend to think this is most likely a spurious finding without biological significance. If it is otherwise, one would have to account for: 1) the increased frequency of Down syndrome persons with the M_2 variant and then 2) a reduction of this frequency to that of the general population. The disappearance of the M_2 variant might be explained by increased mortality in persons with this variant, whereas the increased incidence of this variant in the younger patient might be related to the etiology of meiotic nondisjunction. In regard to the latter, the limited data that we have do not show an unexpectedly high frequency of M_2 variants in the parents of 61 persons with Down syndrome. However, it would be more meaningful if it were known which parents had contributed the extra chromosome 21 and if the frequency of Pi variants in these parents were compared with that in the other parents and in the general population. Perhaps the greatest reason for doubting that this is a

Table 10.   Frequencies of persons with Pi variants by patient age and maternal age

Patient age	Maternal age			Total
	< 25	25–34	35 +	
Down syndrome				
< 20	0.60	0.55	0.44	0.50
20 +	0.45	0.32	0.42	0.39
Control, all ages	0.39	0.34	0.39	0.37

real association is the near-normal activity of the M_2 molecule; the antitrypsin activity in the serum of M_2 heterozygotes (MM$_2$) is about 90%–95% of normal activity. Furthermore, there is as yet no known clinical association with any of the M variants.

REFERENCES

Aarskog, D., and Fagerhol, M. K. 1970. Protease inhibitor (Pi) phenotypes in chromosome aberrations. J. Med. Genet. 7:367.

Ball, J. R. B., Brackenridge, C. J., McKay, H., and Pitt, D. B. 1972. Haptoglobin distributions in Down's syndrome. Clin. Genet. 3:334.

Brackenridge, C. J., Pitt, D. B., and Sheehy, A. J. 1974. The distributions of seven genetic polymorphisms in patients with Down's syndrome. Clin. Genet. 5:414.

Fineman, R. M., Kidd, K. K., Johnson, A. M., and Breg, W. R. 1976a. Increased frequency of heterozygotes for α_1 antitrypsin/variants in individuals with either sex chromosome mosaicism or trisomy 21. Nature 260:320.

Fineman, R. M., Johnson, A. M., Kidd, K. K., and Breg, W. R. 1976b. Increased frequency of heterozygotes for α_1 antitrypsin (AAT) in patients with Down syndrome associated with advanced maternal age. Fifth Int. Cong. Hum. Genet., Mexico City. Excerpta Medica, Int. Cong. Series #397, Amsterdam. p. 71.

Johnson, A. M. 1974. Antiproteases and the liver. In E. F. Becker (ed.), The Liver: Normal and Abnormal Functions. M. Dekker, New York.

Kueppers, F., O'Brien, P., Passarge, E., and Rudiger, H. W. 1975. Alpha$_1$-antitrypsin phenotypes in sex chromosome mosaicism. J. Med. Genet. 12:263.

Rundle, A. T., Atkin, J., and Sudell, B. 1974. Serum polymorphisms in Down's syndrome. Humangenetik 24:105.

Rundle, A. T., and Sudell, B. 1973. Red cell polymorphisms in Down's syndrome: Gene frequencies and phenotype associations. Clin. Genet. 4:536.

THE TRISOMY STATE

Therapeutic
Approaches in Down Syndrome

Siegfried M. Pueschel

During his presentation at the 10th anniversary of the Child Development Center, Rhode Island Hospital, Dr. Park Gerald stated, "I reject categorically the concept that there is nothing we can do after a child with Down syndrome is born." I share this philosophy, although realize that genetic influences due to the supernumerary chromosome 21 are operative in utero and there is evidence of both physical and neurological deficits at the time of birth of a child with Down syndrome. Yet genetically controlled developmental and maturational processes continue into adulthood, and in many disease entities genetically induced pathological processes become apparent only in later life. Analogously, it has been suggested that some of the disabilities observed in the older child with Down syndrome are the results of such continuing genetic action upon the growing organism.

The question then arises: How can we interfere with such pathological influences and what kind of therapeutic modalities are at our disposal to counteract the evolving handicap?

This chapter does not review previous attempted treatment modalities, such as the administration of thyroid hormone, pituitary extract, vitamin E, glutamic acid, and a variety of other medications that have been discussed in recent publications (de la Cruz, 1977; Share, 1976). It focuses on a few therapeutic approaches only, and our own experience with 5-hydroxytryptophan is analyzed in detail.

PAST THERAPEUTIC ATTEMPTS

In the 1930s Niehans introduced sicca cell therapy, which has been used widely in certain parts of Europe since then. This form of treatment consists of injecting lyophilized material prepared from embryonic animal organs. It has been hypothesized that this will stimulate the growth and function of the corresponding tissues in the human body. Black, Kato, and Walker conducted a double-blind study in 1966 in order to evaluate the effects of sicca cell therapy. They injected sicca cells at 9-month intervals into 59 mentally retarded children, including 36 with Down syndrome. There was no evidence that such treatment was beneficial to the children's development. In another

217

study, Bardon (1964) found no difference between the experimental and control groups and thus concluded that sicca cell therapy is completely ineffective in the treatment of children with Down syndrome. In spite of anecdotal reports of favorable results of sicca cell therapy, recent comments in the German medical literature concur with these authors' assessments of the ineffectiveness of sicca cell treatment (Bierich, 1975; Bremer, 1975; Hitzig, 1975; Schulte, 1975).

Another approach to treatment using a conglomerate of various compounds, including vitamins, enzymes, hormones, and minerals, has been advocated in certain parts of Europe, Japan, and the United States. Although enthusiastic claims of success of such "treatment" have been made, there has not been any scientific proof that this therapeutic modality improves the ability of the child with Down syndrome. In Germany, Haubold (1963) recommended a mixture of vitamins, hormones, and minerals, which he called "basis" therapy. White and Kaplitz (1964), who attempted to treat children with Down syndrome according to Haubold's instructions, did not find any changes in the treated children. Also, other investigators did not detect improvements in mental development in the patients (Bremer, 1975; Hitzig, 1975; Tanino, 1961). In the United States, Turkel (1975) claimed that his U-series, which contains nearly 50 different substances, including vitamins, minerals, and enzymes, eliminates waste products and stimulates the child's metabolism. Based on anecdotal information, Turkel reported that there was marked improvement in treated children with Down syndrome. In order to evaluate the effectiveness of the U-series, Bumbalo et al. (1964) carried out a double-blind study following Turkel's treatment protocol. After a 12-month study period, the analysis of the data did not show a significant difference between the treatment and the placebo groups.

Dimethylsulfoxide (DMSO) also has been used in the treatment of children with Down syndrome. In particular, Chilean investigators have claimed marked improvement of Down syndrome children's overall functioning following the administration of DMSO (Aspillaga, Morizon, and Avendano, 1975). However, the poor design of the study, with its many methodological inadequacies, renders the results useless. In 1973, a short-term study was carried out in Oregon to assess the effects of DMSO on behavior and academic achievement in retarded children, including Down syndrome persons. This study revealed no significant improvement of the observed variables in the children (Gabourie, Becker, and Bateman, 1975).

Since Tu and Zellweger (1965) reported low blood serotonin concentrations in children with Down syndrome, several investigators have employed the precursor of serotonin, 5-hydroxytryptophan (5-HTP) in the treatment of children with Down syndrome. Bazelon et al. (1967) reported improvement in muscle tone, tongue protrusion, and activity level in infants with Down syndrome who had been given 5-HTP. In a follow-up study using a double-blind design and comparing Down syndrome children who received 5-HTP with a placebo group, Coleman (1973) did not find a significant difference in the study children's developmental parameters. In 1971, Partington and coworkers reported that a short-controlled trial of 5-HTP did not show any motor, behavior, or neurological improvement in children with Down syndrome. Likewise, Weise et al. (1974) administered 5-HTP to 19 children with Down syndrome. They also concluded that 5-HTP was not effective in accelerating the rate of development in children with Down syndrome, and there was no discernible clinical behavioral difference between treated and nontreated children. The designs of many of these studies leave much to be desired, and their results often do not allow definite conclusions.

CHILDREN'S HOSPITAL MEDICAL CENTER STUDY

The primary objective of the study conducted at Children's Hospital (Boston) was to evaluate the effects of 5-HTP and/or pyridoxin administration upon motor, social, language, and intellectual development in young children with Down syndrome. The underlying rationale of this study was:

1. There was ample documentation that 5-hydroxytryptamine (5-HT or serotonin) was significantly decreased in the blood of Down syndrome children when compared with 5-HT levels in the normal child.
2. There was experimental evidence that the serotonin blood level could be raised by administration of 5-HTP.
3. It had also been shown that 5-HTP improved the children's muscle tone and their motor activity. It was then postulated that increased motor activity will lead to augmented explorations of the environment at an earlier age, which in turn would affect positively their sensory input and, hence, might be beneficial to the overall development of children with Down syndrome.
4. In this context the neurophysiological role of serotonin as a neurotransmitter within the central nervous system appeared to be of particular importance (see Figure 1).

Newborn children with Down syndrome were recruited from maternity hospitals and obstetric services of general hospitals in the Greater Boston area. No specific selection process could be identified and it was assumed that the study population was representative of all children born with Down syndrome in this geographical region. Only newborn children with cytogenetically confirmed trisomy 21 who did not have additional serious handicapping conditions were enrolled. Before each child entered

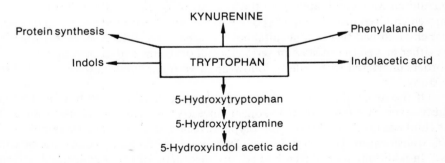

Figure 1.   Tryptophan metabolism (abbreviated).

the program the parents were informed of the study's basic principle and the double-blind design. Parents were made aware that 5-HTP was not considered to be a true treatment and we did not promise any improvement to be derived from 5-HTP administration. We emphasized the experimental nature of the study, explained the known risks and possible side effects, and an approved informed consent form was signed by the parents before enrollment of the child.

The children accepted into the study were then randomly assigned to one of four groups: 1) placebo, 2) pyridoxin, 3) 5-hydroxytryptophan, and 4) pyridoxin and 5-HTP.

The study period for an individual child commenced soon after birth. Since it was hypothesized that there are certain analogies between some of the inborn errors of metabolism with central nervous system involvement and the altered serotonin metabolism in Down syndrome, early treatment seemed to be indicated. The third birthday was chosen as the cutoff point since, at this developmental stage, more reliable data on cognitive and language functions were thought to be obtainable.

Members from nine disciplines of the Developmental Evaluation Clinic, Children's Hospital Medical Center, participated in this study: pediatrics, social service, anthropology, neurology, physical therapy, nursing, psychology, audiology, and speech and language.

An attempt was made to control some variables that ordinarily influence the child's development. Hence, parents were provided with relatively uniform guidelines of a balanced diet and asked to pay attention primarily to protein intake and those foods with a content of tryptophan metabolites. A motor stimulation program was introduced. Parents were given instructions in sensory stimulation, independence training, and were informed how to foster language acquisition. Written outlines of the diverse aspects of stimulation were provided according to the developmental stage of the child in the hope of minimizing the overstimulation by one parent and neglect of these issues by another.

Figure 2 provides a graphical description of the total study time in relation to the individual study period and the total patient load at any time during the study.

A total of 114 children with Down syndrome were admitted to the study during a 3-year period and each child was followed over a 3-year period. Of the 114 children, 89 were felt to be appropriate for inclusion in the final study sample. The 25 remaining children were eliminated from the analysis of results for the following reasons: Thirteen children died during the course of the study; with the exception of one, all these children had severe congenital heart disease. Ten children were lost; their parents either moved out of state or serious social problems and/or parental psychiatric disorders interfered with orderly follow-up. Two other children were excluded from the study.

Of the 89 children in the final study sample, there were 50 boys and 39 girls. Eighty-seven children were of European ancestry, one child was Puerto Rican, and one child was black. Eighty-six karyotypes revealed trisomy 21 and three children had D/G translocation Down syndrome. Twenty-six children had congenital heart disease. In addition, six children had seizure disorders, one had congenital leukemia, one was born with cleft palate, one had an imperforate anus, one had a hiatus hernia, one had congenital cataracts, and another developed diabetes.

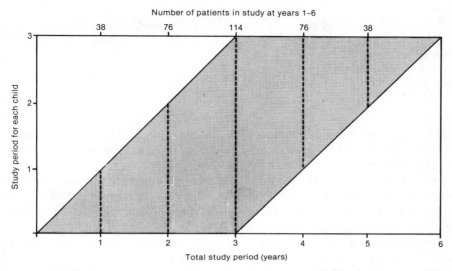

Figure 2.   Graphical description of total study period in relation to individual study period and patient load.

After breaking the drug code, we found that there were 20 children in the placebo group, 24 in the pyridoxin group, 22 in the 5-HTP group, and 23 in the pyridoxin/5-HTP group.

Investigations of factors that conceivably could have influenced the development of the young child with Down syndrome directed us to the evaluation of preconceptional, antenatal, perinatal, and neonatal historical information. Tables 1 and 2 provide a summary statement of selected variables, indicating that there was acceptable comparability among the randomized study groups.

Assessment of the initial examination of muscle tone, muscle strength, motor behavior, and blood 5-hydroxy-indol levels suggested that children in the 5-HTP group functioned slightly better at the start and had somewhat higher blood 5-hydroxy-indol levels when compared with the other groups. However, statistical analyses of these parameters did not show any significant difference.

The initial analysis was directed toward the factorial design of the study and attempted to identify 5-HTP and/or pyridoxin effects as well as interactions between those two compounds. With the exception of data from the Vineland Social Maturity Scale at 12, 24, and 36 months and on the motor scale of the Bayley at 36 months, no significant effects of drug administration were observed. There were other, nonsignificant differences that tended to be toward higher developmental values in the

Table 1.   Down syndrome-5-HTP study: analysis of antenatal histories

History	Placebo	Pyridoxin	5-HTP	Pyridoxin/5-HTP
Infections	5	4	7	4
Bleeding	4	5	10	3
Medical problems	2	3	8	6
Duration of gestation (weeks)	39.1	39.1	38.7	38.0

Table 2.   Down syndrome-5-HTP study: analysis of perinatal histories

History	Placebo	Pyridoxin	5-HTP	Pyridoxin/5-HTP
Labor difficulties	4	9	2	4
Delivery difficulties	4	3	4	5
Apgar score <8	4	2	2	3
Birth weight (kg)	3.25	3.17	2.83	3.03

5-HTP group and lower in the other three groups. These findings might suggest the possibility of some 5-hydroxytryptophan effect accompanied by a slight negative effect of pyridoxin and pyridoxin/5-HTP interaction.

As Table 3 indicates, the random assignment of children to the various treatment groups placed more children with significant heart disease in the placebo group as compared to the 5-HTP group. Once we controlled for this influencing factor, the slight 5-HTP effect tended to be removed.

In subsequent analysis, we proceeded on the assumption that there were no pyridoxin effects and no positive or negative interactions between pyridoxin and 5-HTP. We thus combined the placebo with the pyridoxin group and the 5-HTP with the 5-HTP/pyridoxin group. At the same time another nonrandomized variable was introduced into the analysis: parental follow-through. Support to parents and instructions on various aspects of care and stimulation had been provided throughout the study. For a variety of reasons parents differed in the extent to which they were able to follow through on the furnished guidance. Therefore, this factor was taken into consideration in further analysis. In regrouping, children whose parents had been less able to follow through were placed in one group, and those children whose parents had been relatively more able to follow through were placed in another group.

Two effects of the follow-through variable were hypothesized. First, it was expected that parental follow-through would likely augment development. In general, this was the case on the Bayley, Vineland, and language tests. Second, it was thought that the 5-HTP effect would be enhanced by parental follow-through because of thoroughness in giving the treatment. This did not appear to be true since the 5-HTP effects were still nonsignificant in both groups of parents.

In addition, correlational analyses were performed in order to determine whether blood levels of 5-hydroxy-indols were related to developmental progress regardless of the treatment group. For this purpose we used blood level data near the middle of the study. These 18- to 24-month blood levels of 5-hydroxy-indols were significantly different between treatment groups that received and did not receive

Table 3.   Down syndrome-5-HTP study: congenital heart defects

Defect	Placebo	Pyridoxin	5-HTP	Pyridoxin/5-HTP	Total
Mild	1	1	4	3	9
Moderate	6	4	1	1	12
Severe	1	1	0	3	5
None	12	17	17	17	63
Total	20	23	22	24	89

5-HTP. However, no significant correlation of these blood levels with any measures of developmental and growth parameters were observed.

Subsequent multiple regression analyses revealed no significant effect of 5-HTP administration, although a borderline significant effect was found with the language variable.

SUMMARY

This comprehensive longitudinal study did not show any appreciable benefit from the administration of pyridoxin, 5-HTP, or pyridoxin/5-HTP. There was no significant improvement in motor, mental, and social development with any of these treatment approaches.

In general, there is no effective medical treatment available for Down syndrome children that would improve their overall function. In recent years, increased emphasis has been placed on early intervention efforts whereby children with Down syndrome were subjected to stimulation in the sensory, motor, language, and cognitive areas. It has been suggested that many children with Down syndrome seem to have benefited from such early intervention practices.

REFERENCES

Aspillaga, M. J., Morizon, G., and Avendano, I. 1975. Dimethyl sulfoxide therapy in severe retardation in mongoloid children. In S. Jacob and R. Herschler (eds.), Biological Actions of Dimethyl Sulfoxide, pp. 421–431. New York Academy of Sciences, New York.

Bardon, L. M. 1964. Siccacell treatment in mongolism. Lancet 2:234–235.

Bazelon, M., Paine, R. S., Cowie, V. A., Hunt, P., Houck, J., and Mahanand, D. 1967. Reversal of hypotonia in infants with Down's syndrome by administration of 5-Hydroxytryptophan. Lancet 2:1130.

Bierich, J. R. 1975. Stellungnahme zur Frage der Indikation der Frisch-bzw. Sicca-Zelltherapie beim mongolismus aus padiatrisch-endokrinologischer Sicht. Mschr. Kinderheilk. 123:671–674.

Black, D. B., Kato, J. G., and Walker, G. W. H. 1966. A study of improvement in mentally retarded children accruing from siccacell therapy. Am. J. Ment. Defic. 70(4):499–508.

Bremer, H. J. 1975. Stellungnahme zur Zelltherapie bei Kindern unter besonderer Berucksichtigung padiatrisch-metaboloscher Fragen. Mschr. Kinderheilk. 123:674–675.

Bumbalo, T. S., Morelewicz, H. V., and Berens, D. L. 1964. Treatment of Down's syndrome with the "U" series of drugs. JAMA 187:125.

Coleman, M. 1973. Serotonin in Down's Syndrome. American Elsevier, New York.

de la Cruz, F. 1977. Medical management of mongolism or Down syndrome. In P. Mittler (ed.), Research to Practice in Mental Retardation: Biomedical Aspects, Vol. III. University Park Press, Baltimore.

Gabourie, J., Becker, J., and Bateman, B. 1975. Oral dimethyl sulfoxide in mental retardation, Part 1: Preliminary behavioral and psychometric data. In S. Jacob and R. Herschler (eds.), Biological Actions of Dimethyl Sulfoxide, pp. 449–459. New York Academy of Sciences, New York.

Haubold, H., Wunderlich, Ch., and Loew, W. 1963. Grundzüge der therapeutischen Beeinflussbarkeit von entwicklungsgehemmten mongoloiden Kindern im Sinne einer Nachreifungsbehandlung. Med. Klin. 58:991.

Hitzig, W. H. 1975. Stellungnahme zur Frischzellenbehandlung bei Kindern unter besonderer Berucksichtigung des Down-Syndroms und andersartiger cerebraler Schadigungen. Mschr. Kinderheilk. 123:676–678.

Partington, M. W., MacDonald, M. R. A., and Tu, J. B. 1971. 5-Hydroxytryptophan (5-HTP) in Down's syndrome. Dev. Med. Clin. Child Neurol. 13:362–372.

Schulte, F. J. 1975. Stellungnahme zur Behandlung des Down-Syndroms, speziell zur Zelltherapie aus neurophysiologisch/neuropadiatrischer Sicht. Mschr. Kinderheilk. 123:683–685.

Share, J. B. 1976. Review of drug treatment for Down's syndrome persons. Am. J. Ment. Defic. 80:388–393.

Tanino, Y. 1961. A long-term administration of multiple vitamins to mongoloid children and observation of the resultant improvement. Ann. Paediatr. Jap. 7:56.

Tu, J., and Zellweger, H. 1965. Blood serotonin deficiency in Down's syndrome. Lancet 2:715.

Turkel, H. 1975. Medical amelioration of Down's syndrome incorporating the ortho-molecular approach. J. Ortho-Mol. Psychiatry 4:102–115.

Weise, P., Koch, R., Shaw, K. N. F., and Rosenfeld, M. 1974. The use of 5-HTP in the treatment of Down's syndrome. Pediatrics 54(2):165–168.

White, D., and Kaplitz, S. E. 1964. Treatment of Down's syndrome with a vitamin-mineral-hormonal preparation. Int. Congr. Sci. Stud. Ment. Retard. 3:224.

Chromosome 21
Specific Segments That Cause
the Phenotype of Down Syndrome

Robert L. Summitt

One of the most dependable rules in biology states that, in general, any human with trisomy for all of chromosome 21 has Down syndrome and that every human who has Down syndrome has trisomy 21. Ample evidence (Gustavson, 1964; Niebuhr, 1974; Turpin and Lejeune, 1961; Zellweger and Mikamo, 1961) has made it clear that the phenotype of the person with Down syndrome due to a Robertsonian D-21 or G-21 translocation is in no way different from that in the person with simple trisomy 21.

The earliest evidence that expression of the phenotype of Down syndrome might not require the presence of an *entire* third chromosome 21 was provided by reports of patients with typical or perhaps less severe expression of the Down phenotype in which chromosome 47 was a small acrocentric, but was smaller than other chromosomes in the G group (Dent, Edwards, and Delhanty, 1963; Hall, 1963; Ilbery, Lee, and Winn, 1961).

Escobar, Sanchez, and Yunis (1974), Escobar and Yunis (1974), Noel, Quack, and Rethore (1976), Schinzel, Schmid, and Mürset (1974), and Wilroy et al. (1977) have demonstrated that specific component features of trisomy 13 and del (13q) syndromes may be attributable to trisomy and deletion of *specific segments* of the long arm of chromosome 13. This assignment was made possible by the study of translocations segregating in several families, using G- and Q-banding techniques. It is probably less difficult to study rearrangements for the purpose of making such assignments when the chromosome involved is as large as chromosome 13, in contrast to smaller chromosomes, such as 21. However, information has accumulated that allows assignment of the total Down syndrome phenotype to a specific segment of 21q.

Niebuhr summarized the data available until 1974. A number of bisatellited and other 21-G translocations had been reported that produced complete or less complete trisomy 21 (Table 1). Jernigan, Curl, and Keeler (1974), Lejeune et al. (1965), Niebuhr (1974), Sachdeva, Wodnicki, and Smith (1971), Vogel (1972), and Zellweger,

This work was supported in part by Special Project No. 900, Division of Health Services, MCHS, HSMHA, DHEW, and by a grant from the National Foundation-March of Dimes.

225

Table 1. Tandem translocations producing Down syndrome

Source	Phenotype	Karyotype
Zellweger et al. (1963)	Typical Down syndrome	tan(21;G)
Warkany and Soukup (1963)	Mild expression of Down phenotype	tan(21;G)
Lejeune et al. (1965)	Typical Down syndrome	tan(21;G)
Richards et al. (1965)	Typical Down syndrome but less severe mental defect than usual	tan(21;G)
Soudek et al. (1966)	Typical Down syndrome but with above-average intelligence	tan(21;G) arising from rob (21;G) by pericentric inversion
Cohen and Davidson (1967)	Typical Down syndrome ? less severe mental retardation	tan(21;22)
Garson et al. (1970)	Typical Down phenotype but mild mental defect	tan(21;?)
	Typical Down phenotype but ? less developmental delay than usual	tan(21;?)
Sachdeva et al. (1971)	Typical Down syndrome	tan(21;21)
Vogel (1972)	Typical Down syndrome	tan(21;21)
Bartsch-Sandhoff and Schade (1963)	Mild expression of Down phenotype	tan(21;21)
Jernigan et al. (1974)	Typical Down syndrome	tan(21;21)
Niebuhr (1974)	Typical Down syndrome	tan(21;21)

226

Mikamo, and Abbo (1963) described tandem 21-G translocations in patients with the typical Down syndrome phenotype. However, other patients with similar translocations (Table 1) presented less severe manifestations of the Down phenotype, relative particularly to mental retardation. Richards, Stewart, and Sylvester's (1965) patient was said to be typical of Down syndrome in appearance, but her IQ of 50 at age 41 years was thought to be unusually high. The abnormal chromosome was bisatellited. Warkany and Soukup (1963) reported a child with some signs of Down syndrome but whose phenotype was less severe than usual. The exact nature of the abnormal chromosome could not be determined. Soudek, Laxová, and Adámek (1966) described siblings who had inherited a tandem 21-G translocation from their mother. Both had the typical phenotype of Down syndrome but were more intelligent and had apparently normal speech. The abnormal chromosome arose from a Robertsonian translocation by pericentric inversion. Cohen and Davidson (1967) also reported affected sibs with a tandem 21-22 translocation, inherited from a carrier mother. The abnormal chromosome was not q-distal to q-distal since a centric fragment was also seen. Both had the typical Down phenotype but with higher than usual intelligence. Garson et al. (1970) described two probands with questionably less severe mental retardation than is usually seen in Down syndrome. The exact nature of the abnormal chromosome was not known. Bartsch-Sandhoff and Schade (1963) reported yet another mildly affected child with a bisatellited tandem 21-21 translocation.

Based on this information, Niebuhr (1974) postulated that "gradation of the clinical features" of Down syndrome "is due to loss of varying amounts distally at the long arm of chromosome 21" and that the very distal segment of the long arm (q22) "may be pathogenetic for" Down syndrome. It is interesting that Soudek et al.'s (1966) patients should have been mildly affected since their postulated mechanism (inversion in an inherited 21-G Robertsonian translocation chromosome) should not have involved any 21q loss.

The advent of newer techniques for chromosome banding has provided further evidence in support of Niebuhr's hypothesis. Several cases exemplify that evidence. The report by Aula, Leisti, and Von Koskull (1973) was quite interesting. It involved four relevant cases. The first patient was "slightly retarded" and manifested such features of Down syndrome as short stature, brachycephaly, microcephaly, dysmorphic ears, flat face, oblique palpebral fissures, Brushfield spots, epicanthal folds, furrowed tongue, and dermatoglyphic alterations. She was trisomic for a small acrocentric element perhaps half the size of chromosome 21. Such a deletion might involve the loss of band q22. Close scrutiny of G-banded chromosomes suggested, however, that the deletion might be interstitial, involving band q11 and part of q21, but preserving q22. Patient 2 was severely retarded, with microcephaly, brachycephaly, oblique palpebral fissures, epicanthal folds, depressed nasal bridge, and hypotonia. She was also trisomic for a small acrocentric, smaller than 21 and 22. The authors estimated preservation of 67% of the length of the accessory 21q, which would include a portion of q22. Patient 3 was similar, and was trisomic for an estimated 60% of 21q. Patient 4 (Figure 1) was clinically typical of Down syndrome and had an apparent 15-21 translocation, but the 21-derived portion of the translocation chromosome included only bands q21 and q22. These four cases indicated that

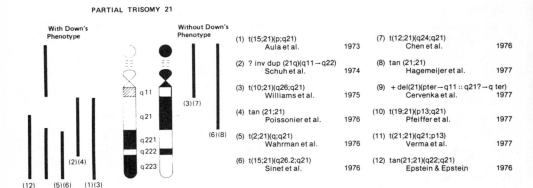

PARTIAL TRISOMY 21

With Down's Phenotype

Without Down's Phenotype

(1) t(15;21)(p;q21)
  Aula et al.   1973

(2) ? inv dup (21q)(q11→q22)
  Schuh et al.   1974

(3) t(10;21)(q26;q21)
  Williams et al.   1975

(4) tan (21;21)
  Poissonier et al.   1976

(5) t(2;21)(q;q21)
  Wahrman et al.   1976

(6) t(15;21)(q26.2;q21)
  Sinet et al.   1976

(7) t(12;21)(q24;q21)
  Chen et al.   1976

(8) tan (21;21)
  Hagemeijer et al.   1977

(9) + del(21)(pter→q11 :: q21?→q ter)
  Cervenka et al.   1977

(10) t(19;21)(p13;q21)
  Pfeiffer et al.   1977

(11) t(21;21)(q21;p13)
  Verma et al.   1977

(12) tan(21;21)(q22;q21)
  Epstein & Epstein 1976

Figure 1.   Schematic representation of chromosome 21 (R-banding on left, G-banding on right). The vertical black lines to the left of the chromosomes indicate those segments trisomic in patients exhibiting features of Down syndrome; lines to the right of the chromosomes indicate those segments trisomic in patients who do not exhibit features of Down syndrome. The numbers in parentheses below the vertical lines refer to the designations of karyotypes in cases represented, which are enumerated on the far right. (Adapted from Hagemeijer and Smit, 1977, with permission.)

trisomy involving a chromosome 21 that may lack at least a *portion* of band q22 mitigates the severity of the Down phenotype, whereas absence of band q11 and band q21 in the accessory chromosome still allows full expression of the syndrome.

  This was further supported by G- and Q-banding analysis in a family reported by Williams et al. in 1975. The proband had typical Down syndrome and in his karyotype was an elongated chromosome 10q and two normal chromosomes 21 in a total complement of 46. The phenotypically normal mother's karyotype (Figure 2) included a balanced presumptively reciprocal 10-21 translocation, with the 21 breakpoint (Figure 3) estimated to be in band q21. Her phenotypically normal sister later delivered a female infant (Figure 4) with Down syndrome and the der(10) (Figure 5) of the translocation. A brother of the mother (Figure 6), also with Down syndrome, had a similar karyotype. The proband's maternal grandmother and her sister carried the translocation (Figure 7), and the sister had a son (Figure 8) with mild mental retardation but no clinical features of Down syndrome except small, dysmorphic ears. His karyotype (Figure 9) included 47 chromosomes, the accessory chromosome being the der(21) of the translocation. This study indicated that the Down syndrome phenotype is the result of trisomy for 21q distal to band q21. While trisomy for the pter→q21 segment does not produce Down syndrome, it may produce some degree of mental retardation (Figure 1).

  Poissonier et al.'s (1976) study of a patient with a tandem 21-21 translocation and Down syndrome using R- and T-banding indicated trisomy for the segment q21→q22.2 but excluding q22.3 (Figure 1). This further narrowed the segment of 21q responsible for the Down phenotype to band q22, and specifically to q22.1 and perhaps q22.2.

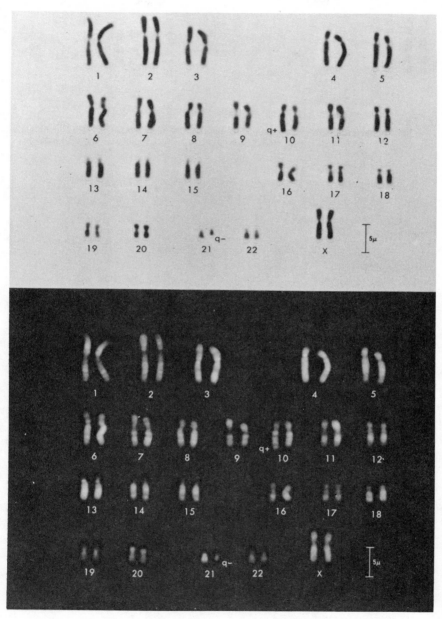

Figure 2.   Karyotype of mother of infant with Down syndrome. The mother's karyotype shows a balanced presumptively reciprocal 10-21 translocation: 46,XX,rcp(10;21)(q26;q21). (Reprinted with permission from Williams et al., 1975, Familial Down syndrome due to t(10;21) translocation: Evidence that the Down phenotype is related to trisomy of a specific segment of chromosome 21, *American Journal of Human Genetics 27,* pp. 478–485.)

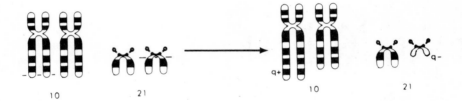

Figure 3.   Schematic representation of G-banded metaphase chromosomes involved in balanced presumptively reciprocal translocation shown in Figure 2, showing breakpoints at 10q26 and 21q21.

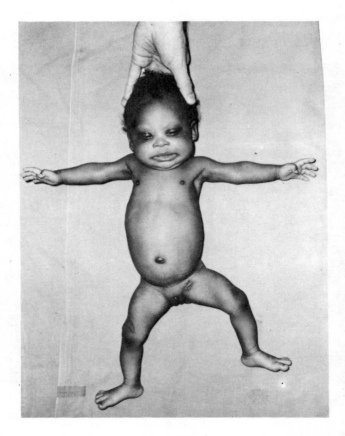

Figure 4.   Infant with typical Down syndrome and karyotype 46,XX,der(10),rcp(10;21)(q26;q21)mat.

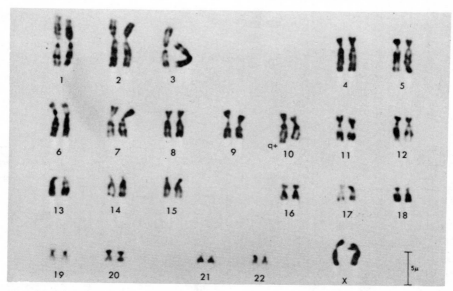

Figure 5.   G-banded karyotype of infant depicted in Figure 4, 46,XX,der(10),rcp(10;21)(q26;q21)mat.

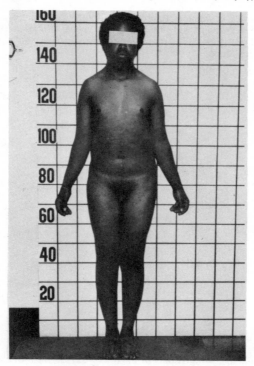

Figure 6.   Eighteen-year old boy with Down syndrome and karyotype 46,XY,der(10),rcp(10;21)(q26;21) mat. (Reprinted with permission from Williams et al., 1975, Familial Down syndrome due to t(10;21) translocation: Evidence that the Down phenotype is related to trisomy of a specific segment of chromosome 21, *American Journal of Human Genetics 27*, pp. 478–485.)

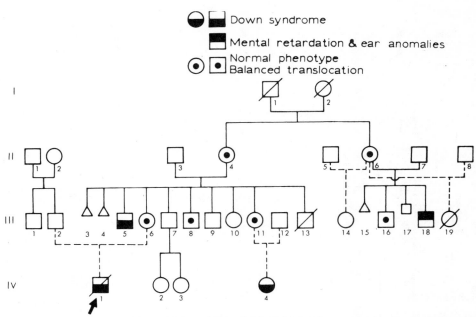

Figure 7. Pedigree of family in which a reciprocal (10;21)(q26;q21) translocation is segregating. (Reprinted with permission from Williams et al., 1975, Familial Down syndrome due to t(10;21) translocation: Evidence that the Down phenotype is related to trisomy of a specific segment of chromosome 21, *American Journal of Human Genetics 27*, pp. 478–485.)

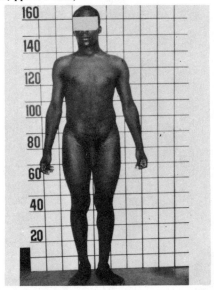

Figure 8. Twenty-year-old man with trisomy of the (pter→q21) segment of chromosome 21, who does not have Down syndrome but who is mildly mentally retarded. His karyotype is 47,XY, + der(21), rcp(10;21)(q26;q21)mat. (Reprinted with permission from Williams et al., 1975, Familial Down syndrome due to t(10;21) translocation: Evidence that the Down phenotype is related to trisomy of a specific segment of chromosome 21, *American Journal of Human Genetics 27*, pp. 478–485.)

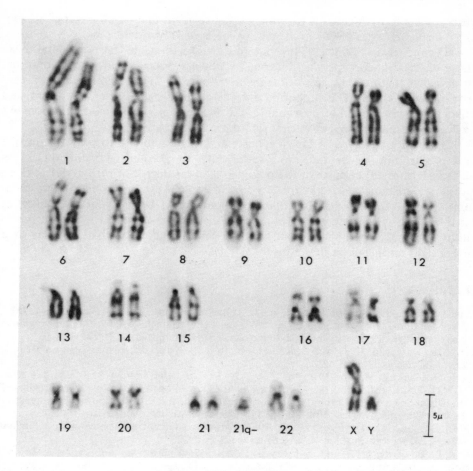

Figure 9.   Karyotype 47,XY, + der(21),rcp(10;21)(q26;q21)mat of patient depicted in Figure 8. (Reprinted with permission from Williams et al., 1975, Familial Down syndrome due to t(10;21) translocation: Evidence that the Down phenotype is related to trisomy of a specific segment of chromosome 21, *American Journal of Human Genetics 27,* pp. 478–485.)

The cases (Figure 1) reported by Cervenka, Gorlin, and Djavadi (1977) (an interstitial deletion preserving the entire q22 band), Chen, Tyrkus, and Woolley (1976), Epstein and Epstein (1976), Pfeiffer, Kessel, and Soer (1977), Schuh, Korf, and Salwen (1974), Verma et al. (1977), and Wahrman et al. (1976) all supported previous data.

Sinet et al. (1976) reported further on the patient described by Poissonier et al. (1976), who had the Down phenotype and in whom the trisomic segment was restricted to that including 21q21 → 21q22.1. The authors provided evidence for the localization of the determinant for the enzyme, superoxide dismutase (SOD), to band q22.1. The authors' report included two other cases in which a patient with typical Down syndrome had trisomy for 21q22 → 21qter and another (Figure 1) in which the phenotype was not that of Down syndrome and in whose cells SOD was not increased. This last patient was trisomic for the segment pter→q21. Sinet et al. suggested a role for excess SOD in the pathogenesis of Down syndrome.

Hagemeijer and Smit (1977) reported a child with slight developmental delay whose physical phenotype was not that of Down syndrome and whose abnormal chromosome (Figure 1) was bisatellited with trisomy for 21pter→q21, much like case 1 of Sinet et al. (1976). This supported the previous evidence of Sinet, our group, and others that trisomy for 21q proximal to q22 does not produce Down syndrome but may result in some degree of mental retardation.

Thus, the phenotype of Down syndrome *is* attributable to trisomy for the q22 band of chromosome 21 and, more specifically, to q22.1 and possibly q22.2. As might be suspected, because of the presence of some degree of mental defect in all autosomal imbalances, trisomy for 21q proximal to q22 can produce mental retardation. Although the individual component anomalies of Down syndrome cannot at this time be assigned with any certainty to a specific sequence of trisomic segments within band q22, the application of prophase and prometaphase banding may shed further light on this point in the future.

REFERENCES

Aula, P., Leisti, J., and Von Koskull, H. 1973. Partial trisomy 21. Clin. Genet. 4:241–251.

Bartsch-Sandhoff, M., and Schade, H. 1963. Zwei subterminale Heterochromatin-regionen bei einer seltenen Form einer 21/21-Translokation. Humangenetik 18:329–336.

Cervenka, J., Gorlin, R. J., and Djavadi, G. R. 1977. Down syndrome due to partial trisomy 21q. Clin. Genet. 11:119–121.

Chen, H., Tyrkus, M., and Woolley, P. V., Jr. 1976. Partial Trisomy 21 Due to Maternal t(12;21) Translocation: Further Evidence That the Down Phenotype Is Related to Trisomy of the Distal Segment of Chromosome 21. Proceedings of the Vth International Congress of Human Genetics, Mexico, Vol. 397, p. 116. Excerpta Medica, Amsterdam.

Cohen, M. M., and Davidson, R. G. 1967. Down's syndrome associated with a familial (21q−;22q+) translocation. Cytogenetics 6:321–330.

Dent, T., Edwards, J. H., and Delhanty, J. D. A. 1963. A partial mongol. Lancet 2:484–487.

Epstein, L. B., and Epstein, C. J. 1976. Localization of the gene AVG for the antiviral expression of immune and classical interferon to the distal portion of the long arm of chromosome 21. J. Infect. Dis. 133(suppl.):A56–A62.

Escobar, J. E., Sanchez, O., and Yunis, J. J. 1974. Trisomy for the distal segment of chromosome 13. A new syndrome. Am. J. Dis. Child. 128:217–220.

Escobar, J. I., and Yunis, J. J. 1974. Trisomy for the proximal segment of the long arm of chromosome 13. A new entity? Am. J. Dis. Child. 128:221–222.

Garson, O. M., Baikie, A. G., Pitt, D. B., and Newman, N. M. 1970. Down's syndrome with translocation-in-tandem. A report of two unrelated cases. Aust. Paediatr. J. 6:53–56.

Gustavson, K.-H. 1964. Down's Syndrome: A Clinical and Cytological Investigation. Almgvists and Wiksells, Uppsala, Sweden.

Hagemeijer, A., and Smit, E. M. E. 1977. Partial trisomy 21. Further evidence that trisomy of band 21q22 is essential for Down's phenotype. Hum. Genet. 38:15–23.

Hall, B. 1963. Down's syndrome (mongolism) with a morphological Philadelphia chromosome. Lancet 558.

Ilbery, P. L. T., Lee, C. W. G., and Winn, S. M. 1961. Incomplete trisomy in a mongoloid child exhibiting minimal stigmata. Med. J. Aust. 2:182–184.

Jernigan, D., Curl, N., and Keeler, C. 1974. Milledgeville Mongoloid: A rare karyotype of Down's syndrome. J. Hered. 65:254–257.

Lejeune, J., Berger, R., Vidal, O. R., and Rethore, M.-O. 1965. Un cas de translocation G-G en tandem. [A case of translocation G-G in tandem.] Ann. Genet. 8:60–62.

Niebuhr, E. 1974. Down syndrome. The possibility of a pathogenetic segment on chromosome 21. Humangenetik 21:99–101.

Noel, B., Quack, B., and Rethore, M. D. 1976. Partial deletions and trisomies of chromosome 13, mapping of bands associated with particular malformations. Clin. Genet. 9:593–602.

Pfeiffer, R. A., Kessel, E. K., and Soer, K.-H. 1977. Partial trisomies of chromosome 21 in man. Two new observations due to translocations 19;21 and 4;21. Clin. Genet. 11:207–213.

Poissonier, M., Saint-Paul, B., Dutrillaux, B., Chassaigne, M., Gruyer, P., and Blignieres-Strouk, G. de. 1976. Trisomie 21 partielle (21q.21→21q22.2). Ann. Genet. 19:69–73.

Richards, B. W., Stewart, A., and Sylvester, P. E. 1965. Reciprocal translocation and mosaicism in a mongol. J. Ment. Def. Res. 9:118–124.

Sachdeva, S., Wodnicki, J., and Smith, G. F. 1971. Fluorescent chromosomes of a tandem translocation in a mongol patient. J. Ment. Def. Res. 15:181–184.

Schinzel, A., Schmid, W., and Mürset, G. 1974. Different forms of incomplete trisomy 13. Mosaicism and partial trisomy for the proximal and distal long arm. Humangenetik 22: 287–298.

Schuh, B. E., Korf, B. R., and Salwen, M. J. 1974. A 21/21 tandem translocation with satellites on both long and short arms. J. Med. Genet. 11:297–299.

Sinet, P.-M., Couturier, J., Dutrillaux, B., Poissonier, M., Raoul, O., Rethore, M.-O., Allard, D., Lejeune, J., and Jerome, H. 1976. Trisomie 21 et superoxyde dismutase-1 (IOP-A). Tentative de localisation sur la sous bande 21q22.1. Exp. Cell Res. 97:47–55.

Soudek, D., Laxová, R., and Adámek, R. 1966. Development of translocation 21/22. Lancet 2:336–337.

Turpin, R., and Lejeune, J. 1961. Chromosome translocation in man. Lancet 1:616–617.

Verma, R. S., Peakman, D. C., Robinson, A., and Lubs, H. A. 1977. Two cases of Down syndrome with *de novo* translocation. Clin. Genet. 11:227–234.

Vogel, W. 1972. Identification of G-group chromosomes involved in a G/G tandem translocation by the Giemsa-band technique. Humangenetik 14:255–256.

Wahrman, J., Goitein, R., Richler, C., Goldman, B., Akstein, E., and Chaki, R. 1976. The mongoloid phenotype in man is due to trisomy of the distal pale G-band of chromosome 21. In P. L. Pearson and K. R. Lewis (eds.), Chromosomes Today, Vol. 5, pp. 241–248. John Wiley & Sons, New York.

Warkany, J., and Soukup, S. W. 1963. A chromosomal abnormality in a girl with some features of Down's syndrome (mongolism). J. Pediatr. 62:890–894.

Williams, J. D., Summitt, R. L., Martens, P. R., and Kimbrell, R. A. 1975. Familial Down syndrome due to t(10;21) translocation: Evidence that the Down phenotype is related to trisomy of a specific segment of chromosome 21. Am. J. Hum. Genet. 27:478–485.

Wilroy, R. S., Summitt, R. L., Martens, P., and Gooch, W. M. 1977. Partial monosomy and partial trisomy for different segments of chromosome 13 in several individuals of the same family. Ann. Genet. 20:237–242.

Zellweger, H., and Mikamo, K. 1961. Autosomal cytogenetics. Helv. Paediatr. Acta 16: 670–690.

Zellweger, H., Mikamo, K., and Abbo, G. 1963. An unusual translocation in a case of mongolism. J. Pediatr. 62:225–229.

Gene Dosage Studies in Down Syndrome
A Review

Uta Francke

The attempt to map genes to chromosomes or chromosome regions by measuring the quantitative levels of gene products in people with duplications and/or deletions of the respective chromosomes is a legitimate approach. It is based on demonstrated evidence for gene dosage effects in aneuploid plants (Carlson, 1972) and *Drosophila* (Stewart and Merriam, 1974) and on the observation of dosage compensation associated with X-chromosome inactivation in mammalian females as well as on the 50% reduction in enzyme levels found in heterozygotes for many inborn errors of metabolism.

Soon after discovery of the extra chromosome in Down syndrome, quantitative determinations of the activity of numerous enzymes were carried out on blood from these persons in an attempt to map the respective genes to chromosome 21. In red blood cells, inconsistent elevations of activity were found for more than half of the enzymes studied. Based on these results, assignments of structural genes (e.g., for phosphofructokinase) to chromosome 21 were claimed (Baikie et al., 1965) and subsequently disputed (Layzer and Epstein, 1972).

In retrospect, after gene dosage effects involving enzyme loci mapped to a number of other autosomes have been clearly demonstrated in human red blood cells, one has to conclude that trisomy 21 represents a special case. The extra chromosome 21 seems to have a more profound effect on the general cell metabolism than expected by direct action of the structural genes present on this chromosome. More recently, a "true" gene dosage effect was demonstrated for the enzyme superoxide dismutase-1 in different tissues and cell lines with monosomy and trisomy for chromosome 21 (Crosti et al., 1976; Feaster, Kwok, and Epstein, 1977; Frants et al., 1975; Gilles et al., 1976; Priscu and Sichitiu, 1975; Sichitiu et al., 1974; Sinet et al., 1974; Sinet et al., 1975a). A review of the earlier biochemical studies, although not informative for mapping of structural genes, may give some clue to specific effects of chromosome 21 aneuploidy on the cellular physiology. Table 1 summarizes the reported information on the activity of specific enzymes, the structural genes for which have now been as-

Table 1. Trisomy 21: Elevated activity of enzymes with structural loci assigned to chromosomes other than 21

Chromosome assignments[a]	Enzyme	Activity	Tissue	Reference
1	6-Phosphogluconate dehydrogenase (6PGD)	nl	E	Bartels and Kruse (1968)
		↑	E	Pantelakis et al. (1970)
1, 4	Phosphoglucomutase (PGM)	nl	E	Baikie et al. (1965), Bartels and Kruse (1968)
			E	Priscu and Sichitiu (1975)
2, 11	Acid phosphatase (ACP)	↑	L	Mellman et al. (1964), Nadler et al. (1967a), Rosner et al. (1965)
		nl	C	Nadler et al. (1967b)
3	Glutathione peroxidase (GPX)	↑	E	Sinet et al. (1975b)
		nl	C	Feaster et al. (1977)
8	Glutathione reductase (GSR)	↑	E	Bartels and Kruse (1968)
9	Galactose-1-phosphate uridyl transferase (GALT)	↑	B	Brandt et al. (1963)
			E	Ng, Bergren, and Donnell (1964)
			L	Mellman et al. (1964)
			L,E	Hsia et al. (1964), Rosner et al. (1965)
		nl	C	Nadler et al. (1967b)
10	Hexokinase (HK)	nl	E	Baikie et al. (1965), Bartels and Kruse (1968)
		↑	E	Pantelakis et al. (1970)
10	Glutamic-oxaloacetic transaminase (GOT_s)	↑	E	Bartels and Kruse (1968)
11, 12	Lactate dehydrogenase (LDH)	↑	E	Bartels and Kruse (1968)
		nl	E	Hsia et al. (1964), Pantelakis et al. (1970)
		nl	L,E	Shih et al. (1965)
17	Galactokinase (GALK)	↑	E	Donnell et al. (1965), Krone et al. (1964)
X	Glucose-6-phosphate dehydrogenase (G6PD)	↑	E	Bartels and Kruse (1968), Rosner et al. (1965)
		↑	L,E	Shih et al. (1965)
		↑	L	Mellman et al. (1964), Nadler et al. (1967b), Phillips et al. (1967)
		nl	E	Baikie et al. (1965), Hsia et al. (1964), Pantelakis et al. (1970)
		nl	C	Nadler et al. (1967a)

Key: B, whole blood; E, erythrocytes; L, leukocytes; C, cultured cells; ↑, statistically significant increase; nl, within normal range.
[a]From Human Gene Mapping 4 (1978).

signed to other chromosomes. The elevation of many enzyme activities in red cells of Down patients were statistically significant when compared to controls. These often included non-Down mentally retarded inmates of the same institutions in order to correct for possible environmental factors. If one looks more closely at these data it is clear that the mean enzyme activity in trisomic cells is rarely as high as 50% above the mean of the controls and that the distributions of activity in both populations show a large overlap (Sinet et al., 1975b). In our studies on glutathione reductase (GSR) activity, in which we assigned the structural gene for this enzyme to a region of the short arm of chromosome 8, we included 12 persons with trisomy 21 as controls (George and Francke, 1976b). Four of these had elevated GSR activity in their red blood cells comparable to the levels in patients with partial triplication of 8p, and the remaining 8 had activities in the normal range. Demonstration of a true gene dosage effect should require the consistent increase in gene product in all subjects with triplication of the respective chromosome region, unless the locus is highly polymorphic and includes alleles coding for isozymes with reduced activity. Second, elevation of activity should be consistent in different tissues for constitutive enzymes. For several red cell enzymes that were found to be elevated in erythrocytes from Down syndrome patients, normal activity in other blood cells or in cultured fibroblasts argues against a gene dosage effect.

Table 2 summarizes information on enzymes reportedly elevated in Down syndrome for which the structural gene loci have not been mapped. Catechol-O-methyl transferase (COMT) was studied because of previous indications that catecholamine metabolism in Down syndrome children is altered, e.g., dopamine β-hydroxylase in plasma is consistently decreased. COMT activity in Down syndrome patients was elevated to 40% above the mean in normal controls; however, the difference between Down and non-Down retarded persons was not significant (Gustavson et al., 1973). The author is not aware of COMT studies on other tissues, and the results on red cells probably fall into the same category as those in Table 1. These data do not constitute sufficient evidence for the assignment of the *COMT* gene to chromosome 21.

All the early studies on red cell phosphofructokinase (PFK) activity in trisomy 21 showed an increase of approximately 50% compared with controls (Baikie et al., 1965; Bartels and Kruse, 1968; Benson et al., 1968; Pantelakis et al., 1970). It was also shown, by immunological studies, that not only the activity but the respective protein was increased (Layzer and Epstein, 1972). PFK activity intermediate between normal and trisomic red cells was seen in a person with trisomy 21 mosaicism in lymphocytes (Benson et al., 1968). However, fibroblast, leukocyte, and platelet PFK levels were not increased in Down syndrome patients (Conway and Layzer, 1970; Doery et al., 1968; Layzer and Epstein, 1972). Furthermore, PFK has been shown to be composed of two nonidentical subunits with tissue-specific expression that may be coded for by different genes (Layzer and Conway, 1970). Since the red cell enzyme contains both subunits, a direct linear gene-dose relationship is made less likely unless both genes are located on chromosome 21.

Alkaline phosphatase (AP) is known to be decreased in leukemic cells from patients with chronic myelogenous leukemia (CML). The studies of alkaline phosphatase activity in cells from Down syndrome persons were based on two erroneous as-

Table 2. Trisomy 21: Elevated activity of enzymes with chromosomal gene assignment unknown

Enzyme	Activity	Tissue	Reference
Phosphofructokinase (PFK)	↑	E	Baikie et al. (1965), Bartels and Kruse (1968), Benson, Linacre, and Taylor (1968), Conway and Layzer (1970), Layzer and Epstein (1972), Pantelakis et al. (1970)
	nl	P	Doery et al. (1968)
	nl	L	Conway and Layzer (1970)
	nl	C	Layzer and Epstein (1972)
Catechol-O-methyl transferase (COMT)	↑	E	Gustavson et al. (1973)
Alkaline phosphatase (AP)	↑	L	Alter et al. (1962), King, Gillis, and Baikie (1962), Nadler et al. (1967b), O'Sullivan and Pryles (1963), Phillips et al. (1967), Trubowitz, Kirman, and Masek (1962)
	↑	L,E	Rosner et al. (1965)
	nl	C	Cox (1965), Nadler et al. (1967a)
NADPH methemoglobin reductase	↑	E	Pantelakis et al. (1970)
5' nucleotidase	↑	L	Rosner et al. (1965)

Key: E, erythrocytes; C, cultured cells; L, leukocytes; P, platelets; nl, normal range; ↑, statistically significant increase.

sumptions: first, that the Philadelphia chromosome represents a deletion of a G group chromosome rather than a translocation and, second, that the G group chromosome involved in the Philadelphia rearrangement is the same one that is trisomic in Down syndrome. Nevertheless, elevated AP activity was reported in cells from trisomy 21 subjects (Alter et al., 1962; King et al., 1962; Nadler et al., 1967b; O'Sullivan and Pryles, 1963; Phillips et al., 1967; Trubowitz et al., 1962). The complexity of the alkaline phosphatase system with tissue-specific regulation and a wide range of activity in normal controls limits its suitability for gene dosage studies.

It does not appear as if any of the as yet unassigned genes could be mapped to chromosome 21 on the basis of the reports summarized in Table 2.

Several explanations have been suggested for the apparently unspecific elevation in red cell enzymes in trisomy 21, such as macrocytosis, increased proportions of younger red cells, and shortened lifespan of leukocytes, assuming that younger red and white blood cells have increased enzyme activities (Naiman, Oski, and Mellman, 1965). When tested more specifically, none of these possible mechanisms was found to be uniformly valid (Hsia et al., 1971). In addition, normal activities have been demonstrated for a number of enzymes in cells from Down syndrome patients (Table 3). At the time of those studies, available evidence suggested that gene mapping by measuring gene dosage effects in human aneuploidy, specifically in Down syndrome, was not a feasible approach.

Due to advances in somatic cell genetics, the human gene map has been greatly expanded in the past few years (Human Gene Mapping 4, 1978). Gene dosage effects have been conclusively demonstrated in red cells and fibroblasts for enzyme loci previously assigned to the respective chromosomes by other approaches. Table 4 summarizes the results to date. Rather precise regional gene localizations have been accomplished on the basis of gene dosage effects in cases with partial chromosome triplications (gene present in three copies: *triplex*) as well as in patients with deletions having a single copy of the respective gene (designated *uniplex*).

Consequently, we should turn to the current map of chromosome 21 to look for assigned genes that might be suitable for gene dosage studies (Table 5). Superoxide

Table 3. Trisomy 21: Enzymes with normal activities

Enzyme	Tissue	Reference
Enolase	E	Bartels and Kruse (1968), Pantelarkis et al. (1970)
Phosphohexose isomerase		
Pyruvate kinase		
Triosephosphate isomerase		
Glycerate-3-phosphate dehydrogenase		
Aldolase		
Malate dehydrogenase		
Isocitrate dehydrogenase		
Catalase		
Phosphoglycerokinase		
NADPH methemoglobin reductase		
β-Glucuronidase	C	DeMars (1964)

Key: E, erythrocytes; C, cultured cells.

Table 4. Dosage effects of localized autosomal genes

Chromosome assignment	Gene product	Gene dosage	Tissue	Reference
1q2 or 3-1qter	Fumarate hydratase (FH)	Triplex	C	Braunger et al. (1977)
2p23-2pter	Acid phosphatase-1 (ACP-1)	Uniplex	E	Ferguson-Smith et al. (1973)
		Triplex	E	Magenis et al. (1975)
8p21-8p23	Glutathione reductase (GSR)	Triplex	E	George and Francke (1976b)
		Uniplex	E	de la Chapelle et al. (1976)
9q33-9qter	Adenylate kinase-1 (AK-1)	Triplex	E	Ferguson-Smith et al. (1976)
10q23.3	Glutamic oxaloacetic transaminase (GOT-1)	Triplex	C	Spritz et al. (1979)
11p12	Lactate dehydrogenase-A (LDH A)	Uniplex	E	Francke et al. (1977)
12p12.2-12pter	Glyceraldehyde-3-phosphate dehydrogenase (GAPD)	Triplex	E	Rethore et al. (1976)
12p12.2-12pter	Triose phosphate isomerase (TPI)	Triplex	E	Rethore et al. (1977)
12p11-12p13	Lactate dehydrogenase-B (LDH B)	Uniplex	E	Mayeda et al. (1974)
		Triplex	E	Rethore et al. (1975)
14q11-14q21	Nucleoside phosphorylase (NP)	Triplex	E	George and Francke (1976a)
16	Adenine phosphoribosyltransferase (APRT)	Triplex	C	Marimo and Gianelli (1975)
21q22.1	Superoxide dismutase-1 (SOD-1)	Triplex, uniplex	E	Sinet et al. (1974), Sinet et al. (1976)
21		Triplex, uniplex	C	Feaster et al. (1977)

Adapted from Krone and Wolf (1977).
Key: E, erythrocytes; C, cultured cells.

Table 5.   1978 map of chromosome 21

Locus	Gene product	Method	Region	Reference
SOD-1	Superoxide dismutase (soluble)	S		Human Gene Mapping 3 (1976)
		D	21q22.1	Sinet et al. (1976)
GARS	Glycinamide ribonucleotide synthetase	S		Moore et al. (1977)
Ag	β-lipoprotein	F		Berg, Beckman, and Beckman (1975), Jackson et al. (1974), Meera Khan et al. (1978)
AVS	Antiviral state	S		Tan, Tischfield, and Ruddle (1973)
		D		Tan et al. (1974)
		D	21q	Tan (1975), Tan and Greene (1976)
		D	21q21-qter	Epstein and Epstein (1976)

Key: S, somatic cell hybrid studies; D, dosage studies; F, family studies.

dismutase (EC 1.15.1.1) (also known as indophenol oxidase or tetrazolium oxidase) is the enzyme that eliminates the highly toxic oxygen radicals from the cell by combining them with hydrogen to form hydrogen peroxide and O_2. The gene for the dimeric soluble form of this enzyme (SOD-1) has been assigned to chromosome 21 by somatic cell hybrid studies (Human Gene Mapping 3, 1976) and the gene for the tetrameric mitochondrial form (SOD-2) to chromosome 6 (Creagan et al., 1973). The mitochondrial enzyme is not present in erythrocytes so that quantitative studies of the enzyme activity in red cells measure only the cytosol form. SOD-1 is inhibited by cyanide but the mitochondrial enzyme is not; this permits measurement of the contribution of both loci in quantitative studies carried out on fibroblasts (Feaster et al., 1977).

Dosage effects for SOD-1 were consistently demonstrated by different groups of investigators, using different methods for enzyme measurement, and in different tissues (Table 6). The relationship between gene dose and enzyme activity was linear, with a proportional increase in trisomy 21 cells and a decrease in monosomy 21 cells. SOD measurements on red cells from various persons with different partial duplications or deletions of chromosome 21 have allowed regional localization of the gene to 21q22.1 (Sinet et al., 1976).

Are there other genes assigned to chromosome 21 that could be used to study gene dosage relationships (Table 5)? The gene for glycinamide ribonucleotide synthetase (GARS) has been assigned using somatic cell hybrids between a purine requiring auxotroph Chinese hamster ovary (CHO) cell line and human lymphocytes. The human gene complementing the defect in the Chinese hamster cell line was found to co-segregate with SOD-1 and with chromosome 21 in cell hybrids (Moore et al., 1977). These studies have not established that the GARS activity present in these hybrid clones is of human origin. Actually, levels of GARS activity in hybrids were equal to those in wild-type CHO cells. The possibility that the human chromosome 21 supplies a regulatory factor has not been ruled out. If a gene dose effect for GARS could be demonstrated in human cells aneuploid for chromosome 21, the assignment of a respective gene, structural or regulatory, could be confirmed.

Table 6. Trisomy 21: Superoxide dismutase (SOD-1) gene dosage studies

Number of subjects		Method	SOD-1 levels (% of control mean)	Reference
Controls	Down syndrome			
Erythrocytes				
10	10	Activity, colorimetric NBT reduction	141	Sinet et al. (1974)
70	33	Concentration, immunological quantitative	140	Frants et al. (1975)
11	11	Densitometric analysis of electrophoretic bands	150	Sichitiu et al. (1974)
6	6	Densitometric analysis of electrophoretic bands	138	Priscu and Sichitiu (1975)
26	28	Polarographic, catalytic currents	145	Crosti et al. (1976)
9	8	Pulse radiolysis	141	Gilles et al. (1976)
Platelets				
9	11	Inhibition of chemiluminescence of luminal	156	Sinet et al. (1975a)
Fibroblasts				
6	5	Spectrophotometric NBT reduction	181	Feaster et al. (1977)
5	Monosomy 21 4	Spectrophotometric NBT reduction	60	

Linkage of *Ag,* a polymorphic β-lipoprotein in human plasma, to SOD-1 was first suggested on the basis of family studies by Jackson et al. (1974). Subsequent studies excluded close linkage of *Ag* with SOD-1 (Berg et al., 1975) and with a 21ps + (prominent satellite) variant (Meera Khan et al., 1978) and have moved this tentative gene assignment to the "in limbo" category.

A gene dosage effect, not linear but following a logarithmic scale, has been proposed for the interferon-induced antiviral state (AVS) (Tan et al., 1974). In this case the product of the purported gene on chromosome 21 is obscure, the primary action of interferon remains unknown, and the parameters measured are most likely several steps removed from the action of the gene(s) involved. These studies are of interest with respect to the long-standing, although conflicting, evidence for impairment of the immune system in Down syndrome persons. Established features are increased susceptibility to infections, increased prevalence of Australia antigen, increased incidence of leukemia, subnormal response to ϕX174 antigen, and a decreased number of circulating T cells.

Interferon is a glycoprotein of 25,000–30,000 M.W., which contains sialic acid and galactose residues. Its synthesis is induced (or de-repressed) by exposure of the cell to viruses or synthetic polynucleotides. In certain lymphocytes, interferon is also induced by mitogens or specific antigens. Interferon is excreted into the plasma or the tissue culture medium. Among its effects on other cells is the induction of the antiviral state. This process requires the presence of a cell nucleus, mRNA, and protein synthesis.

With respect to chromosomal assignments of genes involved in the interferon system, Nabholz reported in 1969 in his doctoral thesis that in mouse-human hybrids the human genes for interferon production are asyntenic with genes for interferon sensitivity. Interferon sensitivity was concordant with the expression of IPO A. Tan et al. (1973) confirmed that the sensitivity to human interferon co-segregated with the dimeric cytosol form of IPO (SOD) and with chromosome 21 in mouse-human cell hybrids. If chromosome 21 was lost from the hybrid cells, they were no longer protected by interferon against a viral infection. Simultaneously, Chany et al. (1973) reported that in monkey-mouse hybrids sensitivity to interferon co-segregated with the monkey chromosome presumably homologous to human chromosome 21.

Published data indicate that human fibroblasts with trisomy 21 are many times more sensitive to interferon than are diploid cells, but that those with monosomy 21 are less sensitive (Table 7). Results from different studies were consistent, although the methods involved in measuring the sensitivity to human interferon were variable. The effect appears to be specific for chromosome 21 imbalance since control cell lines from persons with other aneuploidies and triploidy showed a normal interferon response.

Based on interferon sensitivity of fibroblasts from persons with partial duplication of chromosome 21 due to translocations, the gene (or genes) involved in the interferon-induced antiviral state was assigned to the long arm of 21 (Tan and Greene, 1976) and, specifically, to the region distal to band 21q21 (Epstein and Epstein, 1976). Cupples and Tan (1977) reported that trisomy 21 lymphocytes are also more sensitive to human interferon as measured by a decrease in phytohemagglutinin-induced ³H-thymidine incorporation and mixed lymphocyte reaction.

Table 7.   Effect of gene dosage on the interferon-induced antiviral state (AVS)[a]

Number of cell lines		Sensitivity to human interferon[b]	Reference
(+21)	(−21)		
5		↑ 3- to 7-fold	Tan et al. (1974)
3		↑ ~4-fold logarithmic	Tan (1975)
	3	↓ ~4-fold	
11		↑ ~8-fold (range 2- to 400-fold)	Chany et al. (1975)
1		↑ 10-fold	DeClercq, Edy, and Cassiman (1976)
4		↑ 3-fold	Epstein and Epstein (1976)
	2	↓ 2-fold	

[a]Controls were human fibroblasts from skin biopsies or abortuses: diploid; triploid; trisomy 13, 18, 22.

[b]Measured as units of human interferon inhibiting 50% of viral (VSV) RNA synthesis, or reducing viral plaques by 50%, or 50% cytopathic effect inhibition, or % neutral red uptake after polyI polyC treatment.

Evidence regarding the function of the gene(s) for AVS on chromosome 21 is conflicting. Revel, Bash, and Ruddle (1976) suggested that chromosome 21 codes for the interferon receptor that is known to be host-specific. They used an antibody against chromosome 21-directed cell surface components and showed that treatment with this antibody reduced the interferon sensitivity of normal cells. DeClercq et al. (1976) found no difference in binding of interferon to cells monosomic, disomic, or trisomic for chromosome 21 and concluded that the respective gene(s) on chromosome 21 does not code for the interferon receptor.

There is also conflicting evidence regarding the non-antiviral effects of interferon. Tan (1976) reported an enhancement of the cell growth inhibitory (CGI) effect of interferon in trisomy 21 cells, and De Clercq et al. (1976) found that the non-antiviral effects of interferon were not altered in trisomy 21. The situation is further confounded by the fact that the interferon preparations used for these experiments are not pure. For instance, lymphocyte and fibroblast interferons differ chemically and immunologically. With respect to trisomy 21, all we know to date is that interferon production is normal but sensitivity to the antiviral effect of human interferon is enhanced. This may or may not be specific for genes located on chromosome 21. Late-passage fibroblasts and those from patients with cystinosis have also been reported to have increased sensitivity to interferon (Tan, Chou, and Lundh, 1975). Clearly, more detailed studies are necessary and may ultimately lead to understanding of some features of Down syndrome.

With regard to gene dosage studies in aneuploidy, the relationship between the number of structural gene copies and of gene product need not be linear when possible additional effects of the aneuploid state are considered, e.g., effects on the rates of transcription and translation, effects on secondary modification of enzyme proteins, and effects on the rate of their degradation. Furthermore, imbalance of other genes on the aneuploid chromosome segment could influence the levels of endogeneous substrates, cofactors, or inhibitors.

Table 8.   Gene dosage studies in aneuploids

Problems	Approaches
Multiple isoenzymes/subunits coded for by genes on different chromosomes, interacting (e.g., LDH) or noninteracting (e.g., PGM)	Know subunit structure and gene assignment, use electrophoretic analysis or specific inhibitors of isozymes
Enzyme polymorphism	Immunological determination of amount of protein, electrophoretic analysis, use parents and sibs as controls
Tissue-specific expression	Study enzyme activity in several tissues
Subcellular compartmentalization	Study enzyme activity in subcellular fractions
Effect of asyntenic genes on expression of enzyme locus	Use cloned cell strains from euploid/aneuploid mosaic individuals

In using the gene dosage approach for gene/chromosome assignments or regional mapping, a number of possible pitfalls have to be considered. Table 8 lists some of the presenting problems and suggestions on how to approach them.

Aside from structural gene mapping, several avenues of future research on human aneuploid cells are suggested along the following lines:

1. With more and more structural enzyme loci being mapped rather precisely on human chromosome regions, it might become possible to detect regulatory loci by gene dosage studies. Rawls and Lucchesi (1974) have shown altered activity of two enzymes in *Drosophila* hyperploid for distinct autosomal regions that were known *not* to contain the structural genes. They concluded that altered enzyme activities in segmental aneuploids can be of regulatory nature and may allow mapping of dosage-sensitive loci that regulate the activity of certain enzymes. Some of the results on elevated red cell enzyme activities reported more than 10 years ago in trisomy 21 persons may have to be reexamined in the light of these possibilities.

2. In addition to searching for dosage-sensitive loci influencing the expression of genes that are normally functioning in particular tissues, one could search for the expression of genes that are normally silent but may have been "turned on" in the aneuploid state. Chen et al. (1978) undertook such a systematic search and reported a striking increase in acetylcholinesterase (AchE) activity in cultured human fibroblasts with trisomy 2. This enzyme is normally present in nervous tissue and its activity is barely measurable in normal fibroblasts. When expressed in units of activity, fibroblasts had less than one, brain had ~1000, and trisomy 2 cells had between 12 and 28. This is a substantial increase over what would be expected in a linear gene-dose relationship and probably indicates the involvement of regulatory factors.

3. The effects of aneuploidy on the synthesis of special products could be studied directly by measuring levels of the product in the appropriate tissues, e.g., liver-

specific enzymes and other proteins in livers from Down syndrome persons compared to livers from normal controls. Fetuses aborted because of trisomy 21 could provide the necessary material.

Obviously the most elegant approach to the direct study of gene dosage involves isolation and quantitation of specific mRNAs. This has been demonstrated for deletion of single genes in the α-thalassemias and should be applicable to the study of chromosomal deletions or duplications.

REFERENCES

Alter, A. A., Lee, S. L., Pourfar, M., and Dobkin, G. 1962. Leukocyte alkaline phosphatase in mongolism: Possible chromosome marker. J. Clin. Invest. 41:1341.

Baikie, A. G., Loder, P. B., deGrouchy, G. C., and Pitt, D. B. 1965. Phosphohexokinase activity of erythrocytes in mongolism: Another possible marker for chromosome 21. Lancet 1:412.

Bartels, S., and Kruse, K. 1968. Enzymbestimmungen in Erythrozyten bei Kindern mit Down Syndrom. Humangenetik 5:305.

Benson, P. F., Linacre, B., and Taylor, A. I. 1968. Erythrocyte ATP: D-fructose-6-phosphate-1-phosphotransferase (phosphofructokinase) activity in children with normal/G trisomic mosaic Down's syndrome and in normal and Down's syndrome controls. Nature 220:1235.

Berg, K., Beckman, G., and Beckman, L. 1975. A search for linkage between the Ag and (dimeric) superoxide dismutase (SOD-1) loci. Human Gene Mapping 2. Rotterdam Conference, 1974. Birth Defects: Original Article Series 11(3):67. The National Foundation, New York.

Brandt, N. J. A., Froland, A., Mikkelsen, M., Nielsen, A., and Tolstrup, N. 1963. Galactosaemia locus and the Down's syndrome chromosome. Lancet 2:700.

Braunger, R., Kling, H., Krone, W., Schmid, M., and Olert, J. 1977. Gene dosage effect for fumarate hydratase (FH; E.C.4.2.1.2) in partial trisomy 1. Hum. Genet. 38:65.

Carlson, P. S. 1972. Locating genetic loci with aneuploids. Mol. Gen. Genet. 114:273.

Chany, C., Gregoire, A., Vignal, M., Lemaitre-Moncuit, J., Brown, P., Besancon, F., Suarez, H., and Cassaigne, R. 1973. Mechanism of interferon uptake in parental and somatic monkey-mouse hybrid cells. Proc. Nat. Acad. Sci. 70:557.

Chany, C., Vignal, M., Couillin, P., Nguyen Van Cong, Boué, J., and Boué, A. 1975. Chromosomal localization of human genes governing the interferon-induced antiviral state. Proc. Nat. Acad. Sci. 72:3129.

Chen, Y.-T., Worthy, T. E., and Krooth, R. S. 1978. Evidence for a striking increase in acetylcholinesterase activity in cultured human fibroblasts which are trisomic for chromosome two. Som. Cell Genet. 4:265.

Conway, M. M., and Layzer, R. B. 1970. Blood cell phosphofructokinase in Down's syndrome. Humangenetik 9:185.

Cox, R. P. 1965. Regulation of alkaline phosphatase in skin fibroblast cultures from patients with mongolism. Exp. Cell Res. 37:670.

Creagan, R. P., Tischfield, J. A., Ricciuti, F., and Ruddle, F. H. 1973. Chromosome assignments of genes in man using mouse-human somatic cell hybrids: Mitochondrial superoxide dismutase (indophenol oxidase-B, tetrameric) to chromosome 6. Humangenetik 20:203.

Crosti, N., Sena, A., Rigo, A., and Viglino, P. 1976. Dosage effect of SOD-A gene in 21-trisomic cells. Hum. Genet. 31:197.

Cupples, C. G., and Tan, Y. H. 1977. Effect of human interferon preparations on lymphoblastogenesis in Down's syndrome. Nature 267:165.

De Clercq, E., Edy, V. G., and Cassiman, J. J. 1976. Chromosome 21 does not code for an interferon receptor. Nature 264:249.

de la Chapelle, A., Icen, A., Aula, P., Leisti, J., Turleau, C., and deGrouchy, J. 1976. Mapping of the gene for glutathione reductase on chromosome 8. Ann. Genet. 19:253.

DeMars, R. 1964. Some studies of enzymes in cultivated human cells. Nat. Cancer Inst. Monogr. 13:181–193.

Doery, J. C. G., Hirsh, J., Garson, O. M., deGrouchy, G. C. 1968. Platelet-phosphohexokinase levels in Down's syndrome. Lancet 2:894.

Donnell, G. N., Ng, W. G., Bergren, W. R., Melnyk, J., and Koch, R. 1965. Enhancement of erythrocyte-galactokinase activity in Langdon-Down trisomy. Lancet 1:553.

Epstein, L. B., and Epstein, C. J. 1976. Localization of the gene *AVG* for the antiviral expression of immune and classical interferon to the distal portion of the long arm of chromosome 21. J. Infect. Dis. 133(suppl.):A56.

Feaster, W. W., Kwok, L. W., and Epstein, C. J. 1977. Dosage effects for superoxide dismutase-1 in nucleated cells aneuploid for chromosome 21. Am. J. Hum. Genet. 29:563.

Ferguson-Smith, M. A., Aitken, D. A., Turleau, C., and deGrouchy, J. 1976. Localization of the human ABO:Np-1:AK-1 linkage group by regional assignment of AK-1 to 9q34. Hum. Genet. 34:35.

Ferguson-Smith, M. A., Newman, B. F., Ellis, P. M., Thomson, D. M. G., and Riley, I. D. 1973. Assignment by deletion of human red cell acid phosphatase gene locus to the short arm of chromosome 2. Nature 243:271.

Francke, U., George, D. L., Brown, M. G., and Riccardi, V. M. 1977. Gene dose effect: Intraband mapping of the LDH A locus using cells from four individuals with different interstitial deletions of 11p. Cytogenet. Cell Genet. 19:197.

Frants, R. R., Eriksson, A. W., Jongbloet, P. H., and Hamers, A. J. 1975. Superoxide dismutase in Down syndrome. Lancet 2:42.

George, D. L., and Francke, U. 1976a. Gene dose effect: Regional mapping of human nucleoside phosphorylase on chromosome 14. Science 194:851.

George, D. L., and Francke, U. 1976b. Gene dose effect: Regional mapping of human glutathione reductase on chromosome 8. Cytogenet. Cell Genet. 17:282.

Gilles, L., Ferradini, C., Foos, J., and Pucheault, J. 1976. The estimation of red cell superoxide dismutase activity by pulse radiolysis in normal and trisomic 21 subjects. FEBS Letters 69:55.

Gustavson, K. H., Wetterberg, L., Bäckström, M., and Ross, S. B. 1973. Catechol-O-methyltransferase activity in erythrocytes in Down's syndrome. Clin. Genet. 4:279.

Hsia, D. Y.-Y., Inouye, T., Wong, P., and South, A. 1964. Studies on galactose oxidation in Down's syndrome. New Engl. J. Med. 270:1085.

Hsia, D. Y.-Y., Justice, P., Smith, G. F., and Dowben, R. M. 1971. Down's syndrome—A critical review of the biochemical and immunological data. Am. J. Dis. Child. 121:153.

Human Gene Mapping 3. 1976. Baltimore, Conference, 1975. Birth Defects: Original Article Series 12(7). The National Foundation, New York.

Human Gene Mapping 4. 1978. Winnipeg Conference, 1977. Birth Defects: Original Article Series 14(4). The National Foundation, New York.

Jackson, L., Falk, C. T., Allen, F. H., Jr., and Barr, M. 1974. A possible gene assignment to chromosome 21. Human Gene Mapping. New Haven Conference, 1973. Birth Defects: Original Article Series 10(3):100. The National Foundation, New York.

King, M. J., Gillis, E. M., and Baikie, A. G. 1962. Alkaline-phosphatase activity of polymorphs in mongolism. Lancet 2:1302.

Krone, W., and Wolf, U. 1977. Chromosome variation and gene action. Hereditas 86:31.

Krone, W., Wolf, U., Goedde, H. W., and Baitsch, H. 1964. Enhancement of erythrocyte-galactokinase activity in Langdon-Down trisomy. Lancet 2:590.

Layzer, R. B., and Conway, M. M. 1970. Multiple isoenzymes of human phosphofructokinase. Biochem. Biophys. Res. Comm. 40:1259.

Layzer, R. B., and Epstein, C. J. 1972. Phosphofructokinase and chromosome 21. Am. J. Hum. Genet. 24:533.

Magenis, R. E., Koler, R. D., Lovrien, E., Bigley, R. H., DuVal, M. C., and Overton, K. M. 1975. Gene dosage: Evidence for assignment of erythrocyte acid phosphatase locus to chromosome 2. Proc. Nat. Acad. Sci. 72:4526.

Marimo, B., and Gianelli, F. 1975. Gene dosage effect in human trisomy 16. Nature 256:204.

Mayeda, K., Weiss, L., Lindahl, R., and Dully, M. 1974. Localization of the human lactate dehydrogenase B gene on the short arm of chromosome 12. Am. J. Hum. Genet. 26:59.

Meera Khan, P., Szumlas-Stachowski, E., Berg, K., and Pearson, P. L. 1978. Further data on the linkage relationships between the Ag, SOD-1 and the satellite markers on chromosome 21 of man. Human Gene Mapping 4. Winnipeg Conference, 1977. Birth Defects: Original Article Series 14(4). The National Foundation, New York.

Mellman, W. J., Oski, F. A., Tedesco, T. A., Maciera-Coelho, A., and Harris, H. 1964. Leucocyte enzymes in Down's syndrome. Lancet 2:674.

Moore, E. E., Jones, C., Kao, F.-T., and Oates, D. C. 1977. Synteny between glycinamide ribonucleotide synthetase and superoxide dismutase (soluble). Am. J. Hum. Genet. 29:389.

Nabholz, M. 1969. Studies on somatic hybridization as a tool for the genetic analysis of man. Doctoral dissertation, Stanford University, Stanford, Cal.

Nadler, H. L., Inouye, T., Justice, P., and Hsia, D. Y.-Y. 1967a. Enzymes in cultivated human fibroblasts derived from patients with Down's syndrome (mongolism). Nature 213:1261.

Nadler, H. L., Monteleone, P., Inouye, T., and Hsia D. Y.-Y. 1967b. Lymphocyte and granulocyte enzyme activity in patients with Down's syndrome. Blood 30:669.

Naiman, J. L., Oski, F. A., and Mellman, W. J. 1965. Phosphokinase activity of erythrocytes in mongolism. Lancet 1:821.

Ng, W. G., Bergren, W. R., and Donnell, G. N. 1964. Galactose-1-phosphate uridyl-transferase assay by use of radioactive galactose-1-phosphate. Clin. Chim. Acta 10:337.

O'Sullivan, M. A., and Pryles, C. V. 1963. Comparison of leucocyte alkaline phosphatase determinations in 200 patients with mongolism and in 200 "familial" controls. New Engl. J. Med. 268:1168.

Pantelakis, S. N., Karaklis, A. G., Alexious, D., Vardas, E., and Valaes, T. 1970. Red cell enzymes in trisomy 21. Am. J. Hum. Genet. 22:184.

Phillips, J., Herring, R. M., Goodman, H. O., and King, J. S. 1967. Leucocyte alkaline phosphatase and erythrocyte glucose-6-phosphate dehydrogenase in Down's syndrome. J. Med. Genet. 4:268.

Priscu, R., and Sichitiu, S. 1975. Types of enzymatic overdosing in trisomy 21: Erythrocytic superoxide dismutase-AJ and phosphoglucomutase. Humangenetik 29:79.

Rawls, J. M., and Lucchesi, J. C. 1974. Regulation of enzyme activities in Drosophila. I. The detection of regulatory loci by gene dosage responses. Genet. Res. 24:59.

Rethore, M.-O., Junien, C., Malpuech, G., Baccichetti, C., Teconi, R., Kaplan, J.-C., de Romeuf, J., and Lejeune, J. 1976. Localisation du gene de la glyceraldehyde 3-phosphate deshydrogenase (G3PD) sur le segment distal du bras court du chromosome 12. Ann. Genet. 19:140.

Rethore, M.-O., Kaplan, J.-C., Junien, C., Cruveiller, J., Dutrillaux, B., Aurias, A., Carpentier, S., Lafourcade, J., and Lejeune, J. 1975. Augmentation de l'activité de la LDH-B chez un garcon trisomique 12p par malsegregation d'une translocation maternelle t(12;14) (q12;p11). Ann. Genet. 18:81.

Rethore, M.-O., Kaplan, J.-C., Junien, C., and Lejeune, J. 1977. 12pter → 12p12.2: Possible assignment of human triose phosphate isomerase. Hum. Genet. 36:235.

Revel, M., Bash, D., and Ruddle, F. H. 1976. Antibodies to a cell surface component coded by human chromosome 21 inhibit action of interferon. Nature 260:139.

Rosner, F., Ong, B. H., Paine, R. S., and Mahanand, D. 1965. Biochemical differentiation of trisomic Down's syndrome (mongolism) from that due to translocation. New Engl. J. Med. 273:1356.

Shih, L.-Y., Wong, P., Inouye, T., Makler, M., and Hsia, D. Y.-Y. 1965. Enzymes in Down's syndrome. Lancet 2:746.

Sichitiu, S., Sinet, P. M., Lejeune, J., and Frezal, J. 1974. Surdosage de la forme dimerique l'indophenoloxydase dans la trisomie 21, secondaire au surdosage genique. Humangenetik 23:65.

Sinet, P. M., Allard, D., Lejeune, J., and Jerome, H. 1974. Augmentation d'activité de la superoxide dismutase erythrocytaire dans la trisomie pour le chromosome 21. C. R. Acad. Sci. 278:3267.

Sinet, P. M., Couturier, J., Dutrillaux, B., Poissonier, M., Raoul, O., Rethore, M.-O., Allard, D., Lejeune, J., and Jerome, H. 1976. Trisomie 21 et superoxyde dismutase-1 (IPO-A). Tentative de localisation sur la sous bande 21q22.1. Exp. Cell Res. 97:47.

Sinet, P. M., LaVelle, F., Michelson, A. M., and Jerome, H. 1975a. Superoxide dismutase activities of blood platelets in trisomy 21. Biochem. Biophys. Res. Comm. 67:904.

Sinet, P. M., Michelson, A. M., Bazin, A., Lejeune, J., and Jerome, H. 1975b. Increase in glutathione peroxidase activity in erythrocytes from trisomy 21 subjects. Biochem. Biophys. Res. Comm. 67:910.

Spritz, R. A., Emanuel, B. S., Chern, C. J., and Mellman, W. J. 1979. Gene dose effect: Intraband mapping of human soluble glutamic oxaloacetic transaminase. Cytogenet. Cell Genet. 23:149.

Stewart, B. B., and Merriam, J. B. 1974. Segmental aneuploidy and enzyme activity as a method for cytogenetic localization in Drosophila melanogaster. Genetics 76:301.

Tan, Y. H. 1975. Chromosome 21 dosage effect on inducibility of antiviral gene(s). Nature 253:280.

Tan, Y. H. 1976. Chromosome 21 and the cell growth inhibitory effect of human interferon preparations. Nature 260:141.

Tan, Y. H., Chou, E. L., and Lundh, N. 1975. Regulation of chromosome 21 directed antiviral gene(s) as a consequence of age. Nature 257:310.

Tan, Y. H., and Greene, A. E. 1976. Subregional localization of the gene(s) governing the human interferon induced antiviral state in man. J. Gen. Virol. 32:152.

Tan, Y. H., Schneider, E. L., Tischfield, J., Epstein, C. J., and Ruddle, F. H. 1974. Human chromosome 21 dosage: Effect on the expression of the interferon induced antiviral state. Science 186:61.

Tan, Y. H., Tischfield, J., and Ruddle, F. H. 1973. The linkage of gene for the human interferon-induced antiviral protein and indophenol oxidase B traits to chromosome G-21. J. Exp. Med. 137:317.

Trubowitz, S., Kirman, D., and Masek, B. 1962. Leucocyte alkaline phosphatase in mongolism. Lancet 2:486.

Gene Dosage Effects in Trisomy 21

Charles J. Epstein and Lois B. Epstein

Because of the special place of trisomy 21 among the autosomal aneuploidies in the viability and frequency of affected persons, the genes on chromosome 21 have been the subject of considerable investigation by other investigators and ourselves. Four loci are now known to be on this chromosome: genes for two enzymes, superoxide dismutase-1 (*SOD-1*) (Tan, Tischfield, and Ruddle, 1973) and glycinamide ribonucleotide synthetase (*GARS*) (Moore et al., 1977), the gene for the putative interferon receptor or species-specific recognition factor (*AVG* or *AVP*)[1] (Tan et al., 1973), and one of the several genes, or sets of genes, for rRNA. In an attempt to learn something about the possible relationship of these loci to the trisomic state, several dosage studies have been carried out on two of these loci, *SOD-1* and *AVG,* and much of the reported information has been summarized elsewhere in this volume by Dr. Francke. In this chapter we review some of our own work with these two loci in cells obtained from normal persons and from subjects with Down syndrome.

SOD-1, the cupro-zinc form of superoxide dismutase, is a cytoplasmic enzyme that catalyzes the dismutation of superoxide radicals (O_2^-) to O_2 and H_2O_2 (Figure 1) (Fridovich, 1975). Superoxide is generated in a variety of cells during normal metabolic processes and in phagocytes in association with the process of phagocytosis. In addition, its generation can be enhanced by exposure of cells to radiation or drugs, and it can also be generated in vitro by enzymes like xanthine oxidase.

Since most gene dosage studies on SOD-1 had been carried out on red cells, cells that because of the frequent observation of elevated enzyme activities, are notorious for their unreliability as indicators of gene dosage in trisomy 21 (Hsia, Nadler, and Shih, 1968), we felt that studies of nucleated cells were necessary to establish a true gene dosage effect. For that reason, studies were performed of SOD-1 activities in normal and trisomic granulocytes, lymphocytes (Figure 2), and fibroblasts (Figure 3) (Feaster, Kwok, and Epstein, 1977). In both cell types, SOD-1-specific activities were

This work was supported, in part, by grants from the National Foundation-March of Dimes and the National Institutes of Health (AI-12481, GM-19527, and GM-24309). C.J.E. is an investigator of the Howard Hughes Medical Institute.

[1]*Note added in proof:* The designation *If Rec* (for interferon receptor) has now replaced *AVG* and *AVP.*

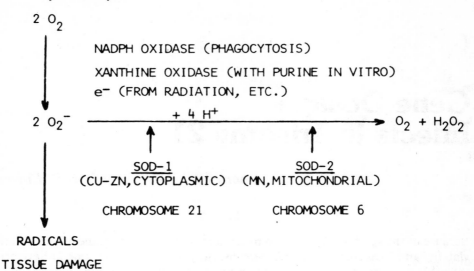

Figure 1.   The role of SOD-1 in the destruction of superoxide radicals.

significantly higher in trisomic than normal cells. The ratios of trisomic to normal activities were reasonably close to the theoretically expected value of 1.5, and these results are considered, therefore, to be indicative of a true dosage effect for SOD-1 in trisomy 21.

Although a dosage effect like that for SOD-1 is of theoretical interest, its functional implications are ultimately of considerably more importance. By itself, an alteration in the concentration of an enzyme or other gene product will not have any effect, good or bad, unless it results in a functional alteration of the cell. For this to occur with an enzyme, the enzyme would have to be functioning in a rate-limiting manner so that an alteration in enzyme concentration would be directly translated into an alteration in substrate consumed or product generated. If this were the case with SOD-1, and it is not known whether it is, it might appear that a higher specific activity would actually be *advantageous* rather than deleterious since it could result in an enhanced ability to scavenge toxic superoxide radicals induced by external agents. Such a functional alteration has not yet been demonstrated in trisomic cells, although experiments are now in progress to determine whether this might actually be the case. Furthermore, at first glance the possibility of enhanced SOD-1 activity being protective would seem to be at variance with the reports that trisomic cells are more susceptible to the induction of chromosome aberrations by radiation (Countryman, Heddle, and Crawford, 1977), an agent known to generate O_2^-. Whether these radiation effects have anything to do with superoxide remains to be determined.

One place where increased SOD-1 activity might have an effect is in phagocytosis, since superoxide has been implicated as an important component of the system responsible for killing ingested bacteria (Babior, 1978). However, bacterial killing and superoxide generation seem to occur "extracellularly" in phagocytic vacuoles (Dewald et al., 1979), and it is not clear that an altered activity of SOD-1 within the

LYMPHOCYTES

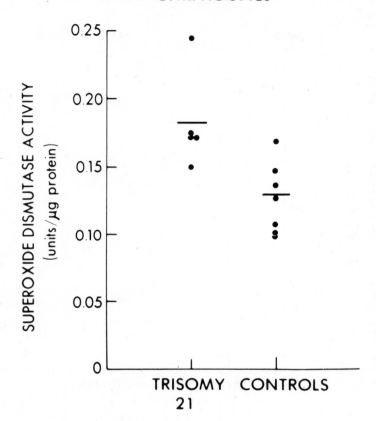

Figure 2.   SOD-1 activity in trisomy 21 and control lymphocytes.

cell will affect the concentration of superoxide on the outside. Furthermore, investigations of phagocytic function and bacterial killing by trisomic polymorphonuclear granulocytes, although suggestive of some degree of abnormality (Costello and Webber, 1976; Kretschmer et al., 1974), have not revealed a consistent defect. Therefore, at present it is not clear whether the increased activity of SOD-1 will result in any significant physiological alteration in trisomic cells and tissues.

The *A VG* locus governs the species-specific response of cells to interferons, antiviral proteins produced by many different types of cells in response to numerous stimuli, including viruses and polynucleotides (Baron and Dianzani, 1978), and by lymphocytes in response to antigens and mitogens (Epstein, 1978) (Figure 4). In hybrids between human and animal cells that segregate human chromosomes, interferon *production* has recently been shown (Meager et al., 1979) to be governed by human chromosome 9. However, human chromosome 21 is necessary to permit the hybrid cells to be able to *respond* to human interferon (Tan et al., 1973). The best data presently available suggest that *A VG* codes for the synthesis of a cell surface re-

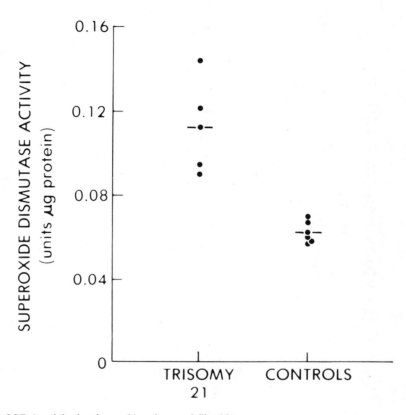

Figure 3.   SOD-1 activity in trisomy 21 and control fibroblasts.

ceptor for interferon (Revel, Bash, and Ruddle, 1976), but this still remains to be proved unequivocally.

Interferon has a multiplicity of effects on cells. Traditionally it has been identified by its ability to protect cells against viral infections, and most interferon assays are based on this antiviral effect. However, under appropriate conditions, interferon also inhibits the proliferation of a variety of cells and interferes with immune responses (Epstein, 1977).

Two major classes of interferon are recognized, the classical (type I) interferon(s), produced by leukocytes, fibroblasts, and lymphoblastoid cell lines, and immune (type II) interferon(s), produced by mitogenically and antigenically stimulated lymphocytes. The distinctions between these two classes of interferon are not sharp, and it is likely that both classes are heterogeneous in their physical, chemical, and biological properties and are actually overlapping (Epstein, 1979).

After the initial mapping of *AVG* to human chromosome 21, studies were carried out with type I interferon, which demonstrated that fibroblasts trisomic for chromosome 21 are more sensitive than normal cells to the antiviral effects of classi-

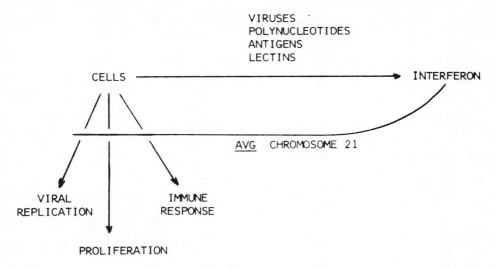

Figure 4.   The synthesis and action of interferon.

cal interferon (Tan et al., 1974). Because of our interest in the immune interferon, we repeated these studies using both type I and type II interferon (Epstein and Epstein, 1976). Again there was a significantly enhanced response to the antiviral effects of both interferons (Figure 5). When expressed in terms of the amounts of interferon necessary to reduce the number of virus plaques by half, trisomic cells were up to 10 times more sensitive than normal cells, with the mean increases in sensitivity being 3.11 and 3.05 for the type I and type II interferons, respectively. These data were taken to indicate that, despite their physical and antigenic differences, the antiviral expressions of both types of interferon are ultimately mediated by the same genetic locus.

Using the antiviral assay, it is possible to map regionally the *AVG* locus. The arrows in Figure 5 denote values obtained with a cell strain partially trisomic for the distal part of the long arm of chromosome 21 (21q21→21qter). These values are indistinguishable from those obtained with completely trisomic cells and indicate that *AVG* is located in this segment of the chromosome, the same segment responsible for the phenotype of Down syndrome itself (see Summitt, this volume). The sensitivity of this approach was borne out by the fact that a strain of fibroblasts, GM-144, originally represented as being trisomic for chromosome 21 (in a translocation), was rekaryotyped after normal responses to interferon were observed and was found to have lost the extra chromosome 21.

Perhaps the most striking feature of these data is that the increase in sensitivity to interferon in the trisomic cells is considerably greater than the 1.5-fold increase that would be expected if a simple dosage effect were operating. Although one interpretation might be that strict gene dosage is not applicable to this system, there is no real reason to believe this is the case, even though quantitation of the primary gene product has not been achieved. A more likely explanation is that the antiviral response actually being assayed is the end result of a complex series of reactions and is

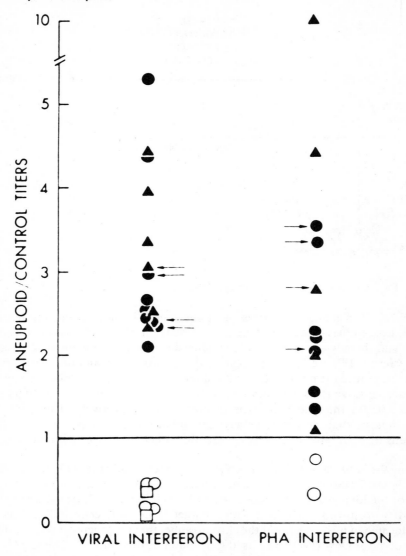

Figure 5.   The sensitivity of trisomic (closed symbols) and monosomic (open symbols) fibroblasts to the antiviral effects of type I (viral) and type II (PHA) interferon. The arrows denote values for cells partially trisomic (21q21→21qter) for chromosome 21. (Reprinted with permission from Epstein and Epstein, 1976, Localization of the gene *A VG* for the antiviral expression of immune and classical interferon to the distal portion of the long arm of chromosome 21, *Journal of Infectious Diseases 133*(suppl.), pp. A56–A62, by permission of The University of Chicago Press.)

several steps removed from the primary gene product. Assuming that the primary product is a cell surface receptor or similar molecule, then it appears that a small alteration in its concentration results, by a series of amplifications, in a proportionally much greater alteration in the measured effect.

The implications of this finding are quite significant. Since a large number of developmental and physiological processes are determined by events occurring at the cell surface, including the activities of receptors, endogenous lectins, and differentiation antigens, it is not difficult to visualize, on the basis of the *AVG* results, how a relatively small change in the concentration of a surface constituent can have a profound effect on whatever process or processes the surface constituent is involved in. Such effects could well be a principal mechanism by which aneuploidy results in abnormal development and function.

Despite increased sensitivity to the antiviral effects of interferon, which might be beneficial if interferon is administered as a therapeutic agent, there is no evidence that trisomic persons are less susceptible to viral infections. What evidence is available is to the contrary, and trisomics have been reported to be more susceptible to influenza (Siegel, 1948) and hepatitis (Hollinger et al., 1972) infections. In addition, the incidence of leukemia, which may have an underlying viral etiology, is greatly increased in persons with trisomy 21 (Rosner and Lee, 1972). These facts have led us to postulate that interferon might be having a paradoxical effect on susceptibility to viral infection in trisomic persons, an effect mediated by an increased sensitivity of the immune system of trisomics to immunosuppressive effects of interferon. Interferon does have effects on numerous systems and has been shown to inhibit lymphocyte transformation in response to mitogens, antigens, and allogeneic cells (Epstein, 1977); however, interferon is also a product of stimulated lymphocytes (Epstein, 1978). It can therefore be visualized that in trisomic persons, with their enhanced sensitivity, interferon generated in the immune response will result in a blunting or premature shutdown of the response.

As a first step in testing this hypothesis we have been examining the sensitivity of trisomic lymphocytes stimulated with mitogens and antigens to the antiproliferative effects of interferon. The data presently available indicate that the transformation (as measured by ^{3}H-thymidine incorporation) of lymphocytes stimulated by low doses of concanavalin A is inhibited to a greater extent in trisomic than in normal lymphocytes. However, the use of lectins to stimulate lymphocyte transformation has inherent difficulties, and more natural systems for investigation are now being sought.

Another cell that participates in various immune reactions is the macrophage. Recent studies have shown that the maturation of peripheral blood monocytes into macrophages in vitro is inhibited by exogenous interferon (Lee and Epstein, 1980). Again, preliminary studies indicate that monocytes from trisomic subjects are more sensitive to these effects than are monocytes from normal subjects, and concentrations of interferon that have little or no effect on the maturation of normal cells significantly inhibit the maturation of trisomic cells (Epstein, Lee, and Epstein, 1980).

The interferon system is an exceedingly complex one, and much remains to be learned about the mechanisms by which interferon acts and the numerous effects it has. Since trisomy 21 acts to perturb these responses, cells trisomic for chromosome 21 may turn out to be useful for dissecting the interferon response system. At the same time, it is hard to avoid the feeling that enhanced sensitivity to interferon may have some role in the pathogenesis of Down syndrome. However, even if its does not, the interferon system in trisomy 21 is the best model presently available for exploring how aneuploidy, by dosage effects for specific gene products, can produce significant physiological consequences.

REFERENCES

Babior, B. M. 1978. Oxygen-dependent microbial killing by phagocytes. N. Engl. J. Med. 298: 659–668.

Baron, S., and Dianzani, F. (eds.). 1978. The interferon system: A current review to 1978. Texas Rep. Biol. Med. 35:1–573.

Costello, C., and Webber, A. 1976. White cell function in Down's syndrome. Clin. Genet. 9: 603–605.

Countryman, P. I., Heddle, J. A., and Crawford, E. 1977. The repair of X-ray induced chromosomal damage in trisomy 21 and normal diploid lymphocytes. Cancer Res. 37:52–58.

Dewald, B., Baggiolini, M., Curnutte, J. T., and Babior, B. M. 1979. Subcellular localization of the superoxide-forming enzyme in human neutrophils. J. Clin. Invest. 63:21–29.

Epstein, L. B. 1977. The effects of interferons on the immune response in vitro and in vivo. In W. E. Stewart (ed.), Interferons and Their Actions, pp. 91–132. CRC Press, Cleveland.

Epstein, L. B. 1978. Mitogen and antigen induction of interferon in vitro and in vivo. Texas Rep. Biol. Med. 35:42–56.

Epstein, L. B. 1979. The comparative biology of immune and classical interferons. In S. Cohen and J. Oppenheim (eds.), Biology of the Lymphokines, pp. 443–515. Academic Press, New York.

Epstein, L. B., and Epstein, C. J. 1976. Localization of the gene *AVG* for the antiviral expression of immune and classical interferon to the distal portion of the long arm of chromosome 21. J. Inf. Dis. 133(suppl.):A56–A62.

Epstein, L. B., Lee, S. H. S., and Epstein, C. J. 1980. Enhanced sensitivity of trisomy 21 monocytes to the maturation-inhibiting effect of interferon. Cell. Immunol. 50:191–194.

Feaster, W. W., Kwok, L. W., and Epstein, C. J. 1977. Dosage effects for superoxide dismutase-1 in nucleated cells aneuploid for chromosome 21. Am. J. Hum. Genet. 29:563–570.

Fridovich, I. 1975. Superoxide dismutases. Ann. Rev. Biochem. 44:147–159.

Hollinger, F. B., Goyal, R. K., Hersh, T., Powell, H. C., Schulman, R. J., and Melnick, J. 1972. Immune response to hepatitis virus type B in Down's syndrome and other mentally retarded patients. Am. J. Epidemiol. 95:356–362.

Hsia, D. Y.-Y., Nadler, H. L., and Shih, L. 1968. Biochemical changes in chromosomal abnormalities. Ann. N.Y. Acad. Sci. 171:526–536.

Kretschmer, R. R., Lopez-Osuna, M., De La Rosa, L., and Armendares, S. 1974. Leukocyte function in Down's syndrome. Quantitative NBT reduction and bactericidal capacity. Clin. Immunol. Immunopathol. 2:449–455.

Lee, S. H. S., and Epstein, L. B. 1980. Reversible inhibition by interferon of the maturation of human peripheral blood monocytes to macrophages. Cell. Immunol. 50:177–190.

Meager, A., Graves, H., Burke, D. C., and Swallow, D. M. 1979. Involvement of a gene on human chromosome 9 in human fibroblast interferon production. Nature 280:493–495.

Moore, E. E., Jones, C., Kao, F.-T., and Oates, D. C. 1977. Synteny between glycinamide ribonucleotide synthetase and superoxide-dismutase (soluble). Am. J. Hum. Genet. 29: 389–396.

Revel, M., Bash, D., and Ruddle, F. H. 1976. Antibodies to a cell-surface component coded by human chromosome 21 inhibit action of interferon. Nature 260:139–141.

Rosner, F., and Lee, S. L. 1972. Down's syndrome and acute leukemia: Myeloblastic or lymphoblastic? Report of forty-three cases and review of the literature. Am. J. Med. 53: 203–218.

Siegel, M. 1948. Susceptibility of mongoloids to infection. I. Incidence of pneumonia, influenza A and *Shigella dysenteriae* (Sonne). Am. J. Hygiene 48:53–62.

Tan, Y. H., Schneider, E. L., Tischfield, J., Epstein, C. J., and Ruddle, F. H. 1974. Human chromosome 21 dosage: Effect on the expression of the interferon-induced antiviral state. Science 185:61–63.

Tan, Y. H., Tischfield, J., and Ruddle, F. H. 1973. The linkage of genes for the human interferon-induced antiviral protein and indophenol oxidase-B traits to chromosome G-21. J. Exp. Med. 137:317–330.

ANIMAL MODELS

Animal Models for Autosomal Trisomy

Charles J. Epstein

The causation of autosomal trisomy, and particularly trisomy 21, and the mechanisms by which it produces its deleterious effects in man have been of considerable interest. However, despite extensive investigation, much of which is documented in this volume, relatively little is known about the etiology of chromosome aberrations, and even less is known about the pathogenesis of chromosomal disorders. Insofar as the pathogenesis is concerned, the investigations of the biochemical and metabolic consequences of aneuploidy have been largely restricted to the analysis of readily obtainable cells—primarily blood cells and cultured skin fibroblasts. Although such materials have provided a fair amount of information, they have not permitted extensive studies. This is why the development of model systems for studying chromosomal aneuploidy is gaining credence.

The use of animal models for aneuploidy is based on the assumption that although the exact phenotypes may not be the same, the mechanisms of the production of abnormalities probably are. In other words, the models are viewed not so much as models of exact human disorders but as models for unraveling the mechanisms by which chromosome imbalance may produce such disorders. Several benefits of using such models can be perceived:

1. Animal models facilitate the *developmental* analysis of the pathogenesis of abnormalities, particularly during the crucial stages of organogenesis. Such studies are impossible in man because it is impossible to obtain, even with spontaneous or therapeutic abortions, material that would be appropriate for a developmental analysis. Furthermore, even if abortion material were available, it would be impossible to carry out any investigations other than static biochemical or morphological examinations.
2. The in vitro and in vivo investigations of cells and tissues other than blood elements and fibroblasts become amenable to study. This applies particularly to the central nervous system, the system most sensitive to the effects of aneuploidy in man and yet the hardest to get at.

This work was supported, in part, by grants from the USPHS (GM-24309) and from the National Foundation-March of Dimes. The author is an investigator of the Howard Hughes Medical Institute.

263

3. Aneuploid animals allow for study of the pre- and early postimplantation stages of development. This is of particular importance in the analysis of the effects of monosomy, but it applies to trisomy as well.
4. The effects of genetic and environmental factors on the phenotype of the aneuploid state can be assessed. It has been well demonstrated in human trisomy 21 that a specific genetic aberration, an extra chromosome 21, can be associated with a considerable variability of expression with regard to both physical abnormalities and intellectual impairment. This variability is presumed to reflect individual differences in genetic endowment and in exposure to undefined environmental factors, particularly in utero. A controlled analysis of these factors would not be possible in man.
5. Chromosomally unbalanced animals facilitate the performance of gene dosage studies by permitting better control of experimental conditions, by making possible the use of genetic markers, and by permitting analysis of gene products that are restricted in cellular distribution. Such dosage studies are the basis for investigating the direct molecular consequences of aneuploidy.
6. With appropriate model systems it is possible to investigate systematically all parts of the genome. This is in contrast to the situation in man in which certain types of aneuploidy are rarely or never observed and, as a result, cannot be studied even in cultured cells.
7. Aneuploid animals may ultimately provide a test system for proposed therapeutic approaches. At present no conceptual basis for therapy exists, and empirical approaches have proved unrewarding.

A limited number of models for human aneuploidy already exist. Although not an animal model, aneuploid plants have been developed and investigated (Khush, 1973). The protein patterns of trisomic strains of barley and sorghum have been analyzed (on one-dimensional polyacrylamide gels), and interesting alterations of pattern have been observed (McDaniel and Ramage, 1970; Suh et al., 1977). Perhaps somewhat closer to the human condition have been the aneuploids in *Drosophila*. Because of our great knowledge of its genetic structure and the ease with which its genome can be manipulated (Lindsley et al., 1972), this organism, which has not been very extensively investigated thus far, will undoubtedly provide considerable information about the molecular and developmental effects of aneuploidy.

Perhaps the best model for human aneuploidy is primate aneuploidy—certainly no other organism would be closer to man developmentally, biochemically, and genetically than the great apes. Trisomic primates have been recognized. One, a trisomic chimpanzee named Jama, had the chimpanzee equivalent of human trisomy 21. Of particular interest were the behavioral studies that indicated that Jama's neuromuscular development was significantly delayed (Figure 1). In general, it took Jama twice as long to acquire a skill as normal animals (McClure et al., 1969).

Unfortunately, primates are even worse to work with than humans. They are not easy to handle, do not breed readily in captivity, do not have high frequencies of aneuploid offspring, and are extremely expensive. Therefore, because of cost, rapidity of breeding, availability of genetic markers, the existence of interesting aneuploid phenotypes, and, most important, availability of methods for producing aneuploid

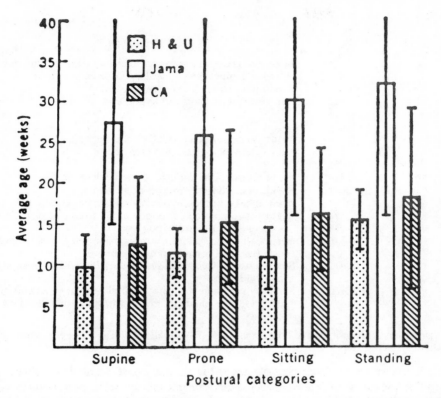

Figure 1.   A summary of the critical age norms (CA) for normal chimpanzees compared with the development of Jama, the trisomic chimpanzee, and of two control animals, Hook and Ubar (H&U). The results are given by the average ages (weeks) at which specified postural capabilities were developed. (Reprinted with permission from McClure et al., 1969, Autosomal trisomy in a chimpanzee, *Science 165,* 1010–1012.)

progeny in relatively high yields, the mouse has become the animal of choice for the development of a model system for aneuploidy.

The mouse has a total of 40 chromosomes arranged in 20 pairs: 19 pairs of autosomes and 1 pair of sex chromosomes. Therefore, a total of 19 different complete autosomal trisomies can be expected, and most of these have already been produced and investigated morphologically. The phenotypes of most of the trisomies have been studied most extensively by Gropp and his collaborators (Gropp, Giers, and Kolbus, 1974; Gropp, Kolbus, Giers, 1975) and the phenotype of trisomy 19 by White et al. (1972). Table 1 presents a summary of these phenotypes.

Except for trisomy 19, which survives to and even beyond term, all of the other trisomies result in death in utero. Some, such as trisomies 3, 5, 9, 11, 15, and 17, result in very early death by days 10 to 12, whereas others, such as trisomies 1, 12, and 13, can survive to days 14 to 16. Some produce severe hypoplasia and runting and others have relatively few generalized gross effects, suggesting that fetal death might, in some cases, result from impairment of the placenta rather than from embryonic dysfunction per se.

Table 1.   Phenotypes of mouse trisomics

Trisomy	Age at death (days)	Phenotype
1	14–15	Moderate growth retardation; facial dysplasia; brain hypoplasia; arhinencephaly and cyclopia occasionally
3	10–11	Small, unorganized, severely retarded
4	< 12	Moderate retardation and hypoplasia
	?15–16	
5	Early	
6	12–14	Moderate to severe retardation and hypoplasia
8	?12	Very severe hypoplasia and retardation
9	10–11	
10	?15	Slight retardation; slight to moderate hypoplasia
11	10–11	Small, unorganized, severely retarded
12	14–17	Exencephaly, microphthalmia; little or no retardation
13	13–15	Slight retardation and hypoplasia; no gross malformation
15	< 12	Severe retardation and hypoplasia
16	16	Very slight retardation of development and growth, myelocele (in one); congenital heart disease
17	10–12	Small, unorganized, retarded; caudal hypoplasia in survivors to 12–13 days
19	≥ term	Small reduction in size with small placentas; degenerating oocytes; cleft palate in crosses with two Rb163H metacentrics

Data from Gropp et al. (1974), Gropp et al. (1975), White et al. (1974b), and Gropp (personal communication).

A few of the trisomic phenotypes in the mouse are of particular interest. Trisomy 1 is associated with moderate growth retardation and with anomalous brain development that gives rise, in some instances, to a holoprosencephaly and even cyclopia (Gropp et al., 1975) (Figures 2, 3). Gropp (Gropp, Putz, and Zimmerman, 1976) has likened this mouse aneuploidy to human trisomy 13, which is associated with similar brain lesions. Embryos with trisomy 12, which generally develop fairly well, also have an abnormality of central nervous system morphogenesis—in this case the development of a very characteristic exencephaly, sometimes associated with microphthalmia (Gropp et al., 1975) (Figure 4). Trisomy 16 embryos have severe congenital heart disease. Trisomy 17, which is one of the early lethals, causes severe runting before death and the embryos manifest a caudal hypoplasia (Gropp et al., 1974) (Figure 5). Trisomy 19 animals do extremely well and survive to term. However, even these animals do not escape the effects of the chromosome imbalance and manifest growth retardation (Figure 6) and, to an even greater extent, placental underdevelopment throughout gestation (White et al., 1974b).

It is clear, therefore, that numerous phenotypes of interest are produced by trisomy for several of the mouse autosomes. However, before such phenotypes and the trisomic states in general become amenable to detailed investigation, it is essential to be able to obtain the necessary material with reasonable ease. Methods for doing so have recently been developed and depend upon the availability of mice with Robertsonian translocations. Although the normal laboratory mouse has 40 chromosomes,

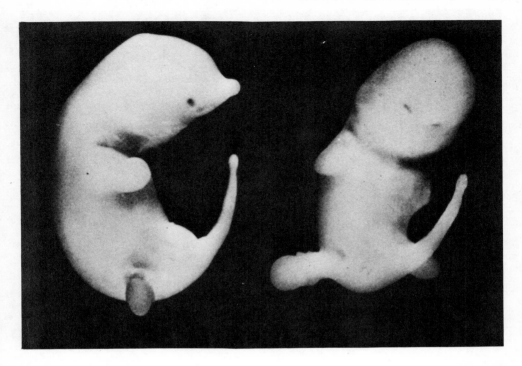

Figure 2.   Mouse embryo, 15 days, with trisomy 1. Holoprosencephaly with cyclopia is present. The scale is in millimeters. (Reprinted with permission from Gropp et al., 1976, Autosomal monosomy and trisomy causing developmental failure, *Current Topics in Pathology 62,* pp. 177–197.)

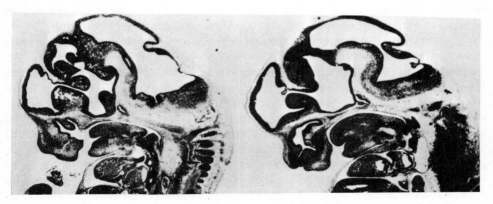

Figure 3.   Sagittal section of the head of a trisomy 1 mouse embryo at day 14 (left) compared with a normal litter mate (right). Slight retardation and orofacial hypoplasia are present. (Reprinted with permission from Gropp et al., 1975, Systematic approach to the study of trisomy in the mouse, II, *Cytogenetics and Cell Genetics 14,* pp. 42–62.)

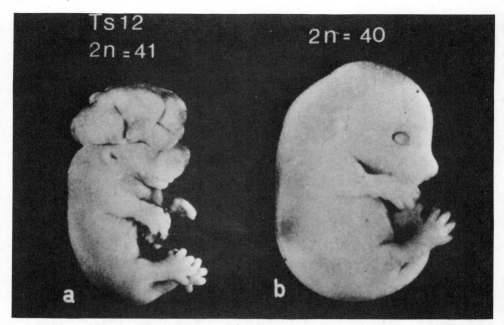

Figure 4.   Mouse embryo with trisomy 12 (a) compared with normal litter mate (b). The characteristic exencephaly is apparent. (Figure courtesy of A. Gropp.)

all of which are acrocentric or telocentric, laboratory strains and feral populations exist that carry one or more induced or spontaneous translocations. The largest numbers of each chromosome are present in mice derived from isolated valleys in Switzerland and Italy, the prototype animal being the tobacco mouse, or *Mus musculus poschiavinus* from the Valle di Poschiavo (Gropp et al., 1972). Of the over 40 such translocation chromosomes now known, over 20 have been isolated and are present singly, in a homozygous form, on a laboratory mouse background.

The essence of the breeding scheme for producing aneuploid mouse embryos is based on the observation that animals doubly heterozygous for two different translocation chromosomes that share a common arm (chromosome) tend to exhibit a high frequency of nondisjunction for the shared chromosome (Gropp et al., 1975; White et al., 1974a). Thus, as Figure 7 illustrates, trisomy for chromosome 1 can be produced by mating normal females with a male heterozygous for translocations Rb1Bnr and Rb10Bnr, which represent fusions of chromosomes 1 and 3 and chromosomes 1 and 10, respectively. In this case, the shared arm is chromosome 1. Using appropriate combinations of metacentrics, all mouse chromosomal aneuploids can, in theory, be produced, and nearly all have been. The two major problems, neither of which is insurmountable, are in isolating the necessary metacentrics and finding combinations that do not result in sterility.

The use of this breeding scheme leads to high rates of nondisjunction, and Table 2 gives values for three different trisomies. At days 12 to 13 of gestation, the proportions of trisomic embryos range from 15% to 40%, frequencies that make accumula-

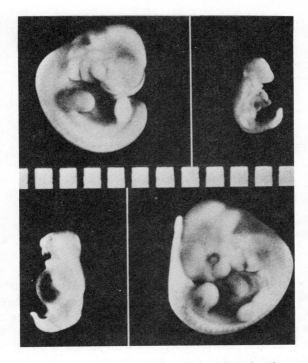

Figure 5. Mouse embryos with trisomy 17 (upper right and lower left) at day 12 compared with normal litter mates (upper left, lower right). Severe growth retardation and caudal hypoplasia are apparent. (Reprinted with permission from Gropp et al., 1974, Trisomy in the fetal backcross progeny of male and female metacentric heterozygotes of the mouse, I, *Cytogenetics and Cell Genetics 13*, pp. 511–535.)

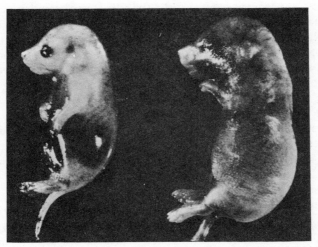

Figure 6. Mouse embryo with trisomy 19 (left) at 17.5 days of gestation. The trisomic fetus was growth retarded, weighing 520 mg in comparison with the normal litter mate (right), which weighed 965 mg. (Reprinted with permission from White et al., 1974b, Trisomy 19 in the laboratory mouse, II, *Cytogenetics and Cell Genetics 13*, pp. 232–245.)

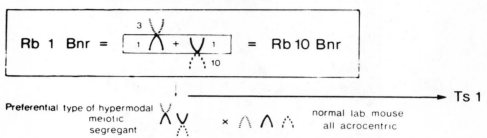

Figure 7.   Method for obtaining trisomic embryos by using mice doubly heterozygous for Robertsonian translocation chromosomes that share a common arm, in this case chromosome 1. (Figure courtesy of A. Gropp.)

tion of the necessary material readily feasible (Epstein et al., 1977). Recognition of the aneuploid embryos, which is done by chromosomal analysis of the embryonic membranes, is facilitated by the fact that trisomic embryos will have a total of 39 chromosomes with two metacentrics (Figure 8), whereas euploid embryos will have 39 chromosomes with one metacentric. Since they are so prominent, the metacentric translocation chromosomes can be observed with simple staining of the chromosomes, and detailed banding studies are not required.

In addition to the morphological studies described earlier, biochemical dosage studies have also been carried out on the mouse trisomies. Using 12- or 13-day embryos trisomic for chromosome 1, generated exactly as described earlier, gene dosage at the isocitrate dehydrogenase locus, $Id-1$ (or $Idh-1$) has been demonstrated (Table 3). The specific activity of the enzyme in trisomic embryos was 1.53 times greater than in normal embryos (Epstein et al., 1977), a ratio extremely close to the theoretical value of 1.50, which is to be expected if three $Id-1$ genes are functioning in the trisomics and two in the normals. The specificity of this result is attested to by the fact that there is no alteration in the trisomy 1 embryos of the specific activities of enzymes (G6PD, 6PGD) known to be carried on other chromosomes, or of isocitrate dehydrogenase in embryos trisomic for other chromosomes.

The only other dosage studies thus far published for aneuploid mouse embryos involve the mitochondrial malic enzyme locus, $Mod-2,$ which is carried on chromosome 7 (Table 4). Using animals either partially trisomic or monosomic for the chro-

Table 2.   Production of mouse trisomies

Mating[a]	Trisomy	Frequency at days 12–13
WS × Rbl(1.3)Bnr / Rb10(1.10)Bnr	1	14/91 (15%)
WS × Rb5(8.12)Bnr / Rb9(4.12)Bnr	12	7/23 (30%)
WS × Rbl(5.19)Wh / Rb163(9.19)H	19	11/26 (42%)

[a]WS, white Swiss; the Robertsonian translocation (Rb) chromosomes are designated by number (Rb1), series (Bnr), and arm designations (1.3 = chromosomes 1 and 3).

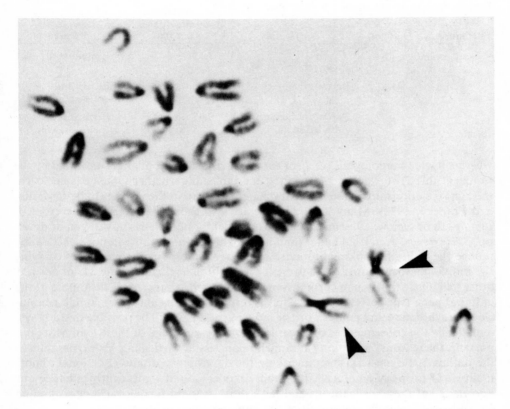

Figure 8.   Metaphase spread prepared from membranes of embryo with trisomy 19. A total of 39 chromosomes with 2 metacentrics (arrows) are present.

mosomal region carrying this locus, dosage ratios close to the expected values of 1.5 and 0.5, respectively, have been obtained (Bernstine, Russell, and Cain, 1978; Eicher and Coleman, 1977). These studies are of particular interest because they involve an enzyme that, rather than existing in soluble form, has to be integrated into an organelle. To date, dosage studies have been carried out on only relatively few such gene products, even in man.

For studying human trisomy 21, it would be useful to have a mouse model for aneuploidy of a chromosome or chromosome segment homologous to that part of the human chromosome 21 that gives rise to Down syndrome. It is not yet known

Table 3.   Enzyme activities in trisomic embryos

| Trisomy | Ratio of trisomic to normal | | |
	Id-1	G6PD	6PGD
1	1.53 ± 0.04 (6)	0.96 ± 0.05 (5)	0.94 ± 0.26 (5)
12	1.06 ± 0.05 (4)		
19	0.98 ± 0.06 (7)		

Key: Id-1, isocitrate dehydrogenase-1; G6PD, glucose-6-phosphate dehydrogenase; 6PGD, 6-phosphogluconate dehydrogenase. Mean ± S.D., numbers of samples in parentheses.

Table 4.   Gene dosage studies in the mouse

Chromosome	Locus	Aneuploidy	Ratio of activity to normal	Reference
1	*Id-1*	Trisomy (Rb1Bnr/Rb10Bnr)	1.53	Epstein et al. (1977)
7	*Mod-2*	Partial trisomy T(X;7)1Ct	1.48 (heart)	Eicher and Coleman (1977)
		Partial monosomy (deletion at *c*)	0.48 (heart) 0.55 (kidney)	Bernstine et al. (1978)

whether such a homologous segment actually exists. That it might is indicated by the results (Table 5) of experiments directed at establishing whether syntenic (same chromosome) relationships established in man also obtain in the mouse (Lalley, Minna, and Francke, 1978). Many do, but there are also those that do not. Therefore, it remains to be seen whether an exact mouse model for human trisomy 21 can be developed. However, even if it cannot (and it probably cannot), this will not significantly reduce the utility of looking at mouse embryos trisomic for chromosomes carrying the individual loci known to be present on the human chromosome 21, or for any other loci. Once the human chromosome 21 loci, such as superoxide dismutase-1, the antiviral gene (species-specific interferon response gene), and glycinamide ribonucleotide synthetase, are mapped on the mouse genome, it will be possible to study systematically the consequences of aneuploidy on the functions of these loci. More important, the reasons for looking at models relate less to particular phenotypes than to the pathogenetic mechanisms underlying the developmental and functional abnormalities. If properly employed, the mouse model should significantly enhance our knowledge of these mechanisms and, as a result, should further our understanding not only of trisomy 21, but of all of the human aneuploidies.

Table 5.   Synteny in man and mouse

Chromosome		Loci
Man	Mouse	
1p	4	*Pgm-2, Ak-2, Eno-1, Pgd*
4	5	*Pgm-1, Pep-S, Alb-1*
6p	17	*H-2, Glo-1*
7	5	*Gus, Mor-1*
10	10	*Hk-1, Pp*
11	7	*Ldh-A, Hbb*
15q	9	*Mpi-1, Pk-3*
17q	11	*Glk, Tk-1*
19	7	*Gpi-1, Pep-D*
Xq	X	*Pgk, Agal, Hprt, G6pd*

Reprinted with permission from Lalley et al. (1978), Conservation of autosomal gene synteny groups in mouse and man, *Nature 274,* pp. 160–163.

Note added in proof: The genes for SOD-1 and for the interferon receptor, now designated *If Rec,* have been shown to be located on mouse chromosome 16 (Cox, D. R., Epstein, L. B., and Epstein, C. J. 1980. Genes coding for sensitivity to interferon *(If Rec)* and superoxide dismutase (SOD-1) are linked in mouse and man and map to mouse chromosome 16. Proc. Natl. Acad. Sci. USA 77:2168–2172.).

REFERENCES

Bernstine, E. G., Russell, L. B., and Cain, C. S. 1978. Effect of gene dosage on expression of mitochondrial malic enzyme activity in the mouse. Nature 271:748–750.

Eicher, E. M., and Coleman, D. L. 1977. Influence of gene duplication and X-inactivation on mouse mitochondrial malic enzyme activity and electrophoretic patterns. Genetics 85:647–658.

Epstein, C. J., Tucker, G., Travis, B., and Gropp, A. 1977. Gene dosage for isocitrate dehydrogenase in mouse embryos trisomic for chromosome 1. Nature 267:615–616.

Gropp, A., Giers, D., and Kolbus, V. 1974. Trisomy in the fetal backcross progeny of male and female metacentric heterozygotes of the mouse. I. Cytogenet. Cell Genet. 13:511–535.

Gropp, A., Kolbus, V., and Giers, D. 1975. Systematic approach to the study of trisomy in the mouse. II. Cytogenet. Cell Genet. 14:42–62.

Gropp, A., Putz, B., and Zimmerman, U. 1976. Autosomal monosomy and trisomy causing developmental failure. Curr. Top. Pathol. 62:177–197.

Gropp, A., Winking, H., Zech, L., and Müller, H. 1972. Robertsonian chromosomal variation and identification of metacentric chromosomes in feral mice. Chromosoma 39:265–288.

Khush, G. S. 1973. Cytogenetics of Aneuploids. Academic Press, New York.

Lalley, P. A., Minna, J. D., and Francke, U. 1978. Conservation of autosomal gene synteny groups in mouse and man. Nature 274:160–163.

Lindsley, D. L., Sandler, L., Baker, B. S., Carpenter, A. T. C., Denell, R. E., Hall, J. C., Jacobs, P. A., Miklos, G. L. G., Davis, B. K., Gethmann, R. C., Hardy, R. W., Hessler, A., Miller, S. M., Nozawa, H., Parry, D. M., and Gould-Somero, M. 1972. Segmental aneuploidy and the genetic gross structure of the Drosophila genome. Genetics 71:157–184.

McClure, H. M., Belden, K. H., Pieper, W. A., and Jacobson, C. B. 1969. Autosomal trisomy in a chimpanzee: Resemblance to Down's syndrome. Science 165:1010–1012.

McDaniel, R. B., and Ramage, R. T. 1970. Genetics of a primary trisomic series in barley: Identification by protein electrophoresis. Can. J. Genet. Cytol. 12:490–495.

Suh, H. W., Goforth, D. R., Cunningham, B. A., and Liang, G. H. 1977. Biochemical characterization of six trisomics of grain sorghum. *Sorghum bicolor* (L.) Moench. Biochem. Genet. 15:611–620.

White, B. J., Tjio, J.-H., Van deWater, L., and Crandall, C. 1972. Trisomy for the smallest autosome of the mouse and identification of the T1Wh translocation chromosome. Cytogenetics 11:363–378.

White, B. J., Tjio, J.-H., Van deWater, L. C., and Crandall, C. 1974a. Trisomy 19 in the laboratory mouse. I. Frequency in different crosses at specific developmental stages and relationship of trisomy to cleft palate. Cytogenet. Cell Genet. 13:217–231.

White, B. J., Tjio, J.-H., Van deWater, L. C., and Crandall, C. 1974b. Trisomy 19 in the laboratory mouse. II. Intrauterine growth and histological studies of trisomics and their normal littermates. Cytogenet. Cell Genet. 13:232–245.

Animal Models for Studying Parental Age Effects

Edward L. Schneider and David Kram

Several epidemiological studies have demonstrated conclusively that advanced maternal age is closely related to the production of chromosomally abnormal offspring (Lilienfeld, 1969; Penrose, 1933). The term *parental age* instead of *maternal age* is used in the chapter title because the possible presence of a small paternal age effect has been suggested in Down syndrome (Stene et al., 1977). Epidemiological studies have also supported the presence of specific etiological agents for these parental age effects. These agents include x-irradiation (Cohen and Lilienfeld, 1970), infectious agents (Collman and Stoller, 1962), and autoimmunity (Dallaire and Leboeuf, 1973: Fialkow et al., 1971).

Although epidemiological studies are extremely important in detecting potential etiological agents, it is vital to complement these studies with experimental approaches. Since it is difficult to examine parental age effects in humans, a search has been made for appropriate animal model systems. In selecting animal models, there are several important considerations. First, the animal should have a relatively short lifespan. Although primates are phylogenetically closer to man, their long lifespan precludes comprehensive studies of maternal aging. Thus, rodents like the mouse or rat, with a mean lifespan of 2 to 3 years, are far more appropriate for these studies. In a similar vein, it is important that these animals have a relatively short reproductive lifespan. Mice, rats, and hamsters are suitable animals because their reproductive lifespans are less than 18 months, and often less than a year, in duration. It would also be helpful if the laboratory animals to be studied had a reproductive decline similar to that observed in man. Again, the rodent model is appropriate because, with aging, there is a significant decline in litter size. Finally, the availability of breeding colonies permits the inexpensive purchase of retired breeder mice and thus considerably shortens the time necessary to age these animals for examining maternal age effects.

UTILIZATION OF THE LABORATORY MOUSE AS A MODEL SYSTEM

We selected the laboratory mouse as our model system for several reasons. First, as outlined by others in this volume, the mouse is extremely well characterized genetically. The map of the mouse genome is the second most well defined among mammals. There are several well-established inbred strains of mice, and their reproductive capabilities have been well documented (Jackson Laboratory, 1968). In addition, there are strains that have altered reproductive capabilities. One of the best characterized is the CBA strain, which has a significantly shorter reproductive lifespan than other inbred mouse strains.

Initial attempts to use laboratory mice as models for maternal aging were discouraging. Goodlin (1965) examined the chromosome constitution of 756 neonatal mice born to mothers 15 months of age or older and could not find any chromosome aneuploidy. However, since mice are multiparous, the uterine environment may be more selective against abnormal fetuses than in man. When an earlier stage of development (10.5-day fetuses) was examined, increases in trisomy, monosomy, and mosaic aneuploidy were found as a function of maternal age (Yamamoto, Endo, and Watanabe, 1973). A maternal age-related increase in the frequency of aneuploidy was also observed, at an even earlier stage, in pre-implantation mouse embryos (Gosden, 1973). These results demonstrated that the laboratory mouse could serve as a useful model for investigating the effects of maternal age. Our own studies (Fabricant and Schneider, 1978) have confirmed the observation that fetal aneuploidy is found with increasing frequency as a function of maternal age in mice (Table 1).

The development of animal models has allowed experimental investigation of the etiological factors that have been proposed for the maternal age effect. For example, increases in fetal aneuploidy can be measured after maternal exposure to a variety of chemicals (Chrisman, 1974; Jagiello and Lin, 1973) or infectious agents (Evans, 1967).

We have utilized the mouse model to investigate etiological factors like genetic predisposition and autoimmunity. Since many inbred mouse strains were available for analysis, the relative contribution of genetic background was examined. One interesting result of these studies was the observation that the CBA strain, which has a premature reproductive decline and increased oocyte univalent frequency, demonstrated a high level of age-related fetal aneuploidy (Fabricant and Schneider, 1978).

The availability of mouse strains that feature spontaneous autoimmune diseases (A/J and NZB/J strains) has allowed investigation into this etiological factor. We found that the frequency of fetal aneuploidy in young and old females of these strains was not significantly different from that observed in immunologically normal animals (Fabricant and Schneider, 1978). In addition, induction of autoimmunity in

Table 1. Frequency of aneuploid mouse embryos as a function of maternal aging

Maternal age (months)	Aneuploid embryos
2–5	4/239 (1.7%)
7–10	17/167 (10.2%)
11 +	13/114 (11.4%)

Reprinted with permission from Fabricant and Schneider, 1978, Studies of the genetic and immunologic components of the maternal age effect, *Developmental Biology 66,* pp. 337–343.

A / J mice by thymectomy did not alter the frequency of aneuploid fetuses (Fabricant and Schneider, 1978). These observations suggest that autoimmunity does not play a major role in parental age effects.

The mouse model has probably been most extensively used to test the effect of x-irradiation on the production of genetically abnormal offspring. Exposure to x-irradiation was found to predispose female mice to the production of aneuploid fetuses (Yamamoto et al., 1973). More important, however, this effect increased with the age of the mother. Similarly, oocytes of aged mice were found to be more sensitive to radiation-induced nondisjunction than were oocytes of young mice (Uchida and Freeman, 1977). Despite these positive observations, the results of a recent study (Strausmanis et al., 1978) using over 1000 fetuses from aged mice failed to show an increased sensitivity to x-irradiation as a function of aging. Thus the relative contribution of x-irradiation to the maternal age effect is still not clear.

OTHER ANIMAL MODELS

Experimental investigation of the etiological factors of preovulatory and postovulatory oocyte aging has resulted in the development of other animal models. The alterations that occur in the hypothalamic-pituitary-ovarian axis as a woman nears menopause can result in the delayed release of oocytes, resulting in "preovulatory overripeness." Fertilization and development of such oocytes can result in reduced fertility, increased spontaneous abortions, and genetically abnormal offspring (Hertig, 1967; Jongbloet, 1975). This delay in ovulation can be artificially induced in rats by the injection of phenobarbital (Butcher, Blue, and Fugo, 1969; Freeman, Butcher, and Fugo, 1970). Administration of this drug results in ovarian retention of the mature oocytes that remain in meiotic arrest while follicular maturation continues. Such a delay in ovulation leads to decreased implantation, increased embryonic death, and genetic abnormalities like trisomies, polyploidy, and mosaicism (Butcher and Fugo, 1967).

Similarly, after ovulation, oocytes retained in the oviduct for more than the optimal period undergo degenerative changes that can result in decreased rates of fertilization and increased numbers of abnormal embryos. Because sexual activity often decreases in older couples, it has been suggested that postovulatory aging of oocytes may be a contributing factor to the production of genetically abnormal fetuses in older women (German, 1968).

The rabbit has proved to be a particularly useful animal for studying this etiological factor (Austin, 1967; Shaver and Carr, 1967, 1969). Female rabbits normally ovulate in response to coitus; this mechanism ensures that eggs are fertilized within 2 to 3 hr after ovulation. By injecting rabbits with human chorionic gonadotrophin, ovulation can be separated from coitus for controlled periods of time. Chromosome abnormalities were most frequent when ovulation and mating were separated by 8 to 9 hr.

These results indicate that several animal systems may be required to study the various etiological factors proposed for parental age effects.

WHICH DEVELOPMENTAL STAGE SHOULD BE EXAMINED

It is difficult to determine the optimal developmental stage to examine for fetal aneuploidy. For comparison and application to human parental aging, newborn studies might be the most informative. However, the results of Goodlin's (1965) study demonstrated that, at least in the laboratory mouse, aneuploidy in newborns is extremely rare. Thus, one must look earlier in development. Examination of embryos between 10 and 12 gestational days has proved to be effective for detecting maternal age-related fetal aneuploidy (Fabricant and Schneider, 1978; Yamamoto et al., 1973). However, the frequency of complete aneuploidy (2.0%–2.5%) observed at midgestation probably underestimates the frequency of chromosomally abnormal conception, since aneuploid embryos may not complete early cleavages or may fail to implant.

The chromosome constitution of pre-implantation mouse embryos was examined by Gosden (1973) as a function of aging. A 7.0% frequency of aneuploidy was observed in morulae and blastocysts collected from the oviducts 3.5 days after mating.

Many investigators have chosen to look even earlier at developmental stages before fertilization. Preparations of oocytes in the first meiotic division have been examined for frequencies of chiasmata and univalents (Henderson and Edwards, 1968; Luthardt, Palmer, and Yu, 1973; Polani and Jagiello, 1976; Speed, 1977).

Preparations of second meiotic division oocytes have also been examined for chromosome number and premature chromatid disjunction (Martin, Dill, and Miller, 1976; Rodman, 1971; Rohrborn, 1972). In the Martin et al. (1976) study, an 18.1% frequency of aneuploid oocytes was obtained. Thus the frequency of aneuploidy is clearly related to developmental stage: the earlier in development, the higher the aneuploidy. These investigations have found decreased chiasmata and increased univalents as a function of maternal age. Although the fate of univalents is unclear, abnormal segregation of these chromosomes can eventually lead to the development of aneuploid embryos.

Although examination of neonates and midgestational fetuses tends to underestimate fetal aneuploidy, examination of first meiotic oocytes may overestimate it. Polani and Jagiello (1976) showed that no correlation exists between the frequency of first meiotic division univalents and second meiotic division chromosome errors. This suggests that either oocytes with univalents divide normally or they are selected against.

We feel that the absolute rate of aneuploidy is not as important as determining why these frequencies change with maternal aging. Thus any system that is sensitive enough to detect changes in the frequency of chromosomally abnormal embryos with maternal aging will be a valuable animal model.

CORRELATION OF MORPHOLOGY AND KARYOLOGY

Ideally, karyology and morphology should correlate well. Although most chromosomal disorders in man display pleiotropic abnormalities, at least one common trisomy (triplo-X) lacks any anomalies (Hamerton, 1971). There are a number of human congenital anomalies that also feature normal karyotypes (McKusick, 1971). Thus, one should not expect perfect correlation between morphology and karyology in a mouse model. Our studies in fetuses of 10 to 14 gestational days reveal that 27% of morphologically abnormal fetuses had aneuploid karyotypes and 5% of morphologically normal fetuses had significant aneuploidy ($X^2 = 21.9$, $p < 0.05$) (Fabricant and Schneider, 1978). Thus, in the mouse model there is some degree of concordance between chromosome and morphological abnormalities.

FUTURE RESEARCH

The mouse model appears promising because it displays a maternal age-related increase in aneuploidy in oocytes as well as fetuses. While certain possible etiological factors have been tested, such as autoimmunity and x-irradiation, many other hypothesized factors need to be evaluated. Of particular interest are the effect of chemicals, hormone imbalance, and infectious agents.

One should also investigate possible paternal age effects. This may be more difficult since epidemiological evidence suggests that if a paternal age effect exists, it is small in comparison to maternal age effects (Stene et al., 1977).

REFERENCES

Austin, C. R. 1967. Chromosome deterioration in aging eggs of the rabbit. Nature 213:1018–1019.

Butcher, R. L., Blue, J. D., and Fugo, N. W. 1969. Overripeness and the mammalian ova. III. Fetal development at midgestation and at term. Fertil. Steril. 20:223–231.

Butcher, R. L., and Fugo, N. W. 1967. Overripeness and the mammalian ova. II. Delayed ovulation and chromosome anomalies. Fertil. Steril. 18:297–304.

Chrisman, C. L. 1974. Aneuploidy in mouse embryos induced by diethylstilbestrol diphosphate. Teratology 9:229–232.

Cohen, B. L., and Lilienfeld, A. M. 1970. The epidemiological study of mongolism in Baltimore. Ann. N.Y. Acad. Sci. 171:320–327.

Collman, R. D., and Stoller, A. 1962. A survey of mongoloid births in Victoria, Australia, 1942–1957. Am. J. Pub. Health 52:813–829.

Dallaire, L., and Leboeuf, G. 1973. Maternal autoimmunity and its relationship to reproductive failure. In A. Boué and C. Thibault (eds.), INSERM Symposium: Les Accidents Chromosomiques de la Reproduction, pp. 333–339. [Chromosome Accidents of Reproduction.] Institut National de la Santé et de la Recherche Medicale, Paris.

Evans, H. J. 1967. The nucleolus, virus infection, and trisomy in man. Nature 214:361–363.

Fabricant, J. D., and Schneider, E. L. 1978. Studies of the genetic and immunologic components of the maternal age effect. Dev. Biol. 66:337–343.

Fialkow, P. J., Thuline, H. C., Hecht, F., and Bryant, J. 1971. Familial predisposition to thyroid disease in Down's syndrome: Controlled immunoclinical studies. Am. J. Hum. Genet. 23:67–86.

Freeman, M. E., Butcher, R. L., and Fugo, N. W. 1970. Alteration of oocytes and follicles by delayed ovulation. Biol. Reprod. 2:209–215.

German, J. 1968. Mongolism, delayed fertilization and human sexual behavior. Nature 217:516–518.

Goodlin, R. C. 1965. Nondisjunction and maternal age in mouse. J. Reprod. Fertil. 9:355–356.

Gosden, R. G. 1973. Chromosomal anomalies of preimplantation mouse embryos in relation to maternal age. J. Reprod. Fertil. 35:351–354.

Hamerton, J. L. 1971. Human Cytogenetics. Academic Press, New York.

Henderson, S. A., and Edwards, R. G. 1968. Chiasma frequency and maternal age in mammals. Nature 218:22–28.

Hertig, A. T. 1967. The overall problem in man. In K. Benirschke (ed.), Comparative Aspects of Reproductive Failure, pp. 11–41. Springer-Verlag, Berlin.

Jackson Laboratory. 1968. Biology of the Laboratory Mouse. Dover Publications, New York.

Jagiello, G., and Lin, J. S. 1973. An assessment of the effects of mercury on the meiosis of mouse ova. Mutat. Res. 17:93–99.

Jongbloet, P. H. 1975. The effects of preovulatory overripeness of human eggs on development. In R. J. Blandau (ed.), Aging Gametes, pp. 300–329. S. Karger AG, Basel.

Lilienfeld, A. M. 1969. Epidemiology of Mongolism. Johns Hopkins Press, Baltimore.

Luthardt, F. W., Palmer, C. G., and Yu, P. L. 1973. Chiasma and univalent frequencies in aging female mice. Cytogenet. Cell Genet. 12:68–79.

McKusick, V. A. 1971. Mendelian Inheritance in Man. 3rd Ed. Johns Hopkins Press, Baltimore.

Martin, R. H., Dill, F. J., and Miller, J. R. 1976. Nondisjunction in aging female mice. Cytogenet. Cell Genet. 17:150–160.

Penrose, L. S. 1933. The relative effects of paternal and maternal age in mongolism. J. Genet. 27:219–224.

Polani, P. E., and Jagiello, G. M. 1976. Chiasmata, meiotic univalents, and age in relation to aneuploid imbalance in mice. Cytogenet. Cell Genet. 16:505–529.

Rodman, T. C. 1971. Chromatid disjunction in unfertilized ageing oocytes. Nature 223:191–193.

Rohrborn, G. 1972. Frequencies of spontaneous non-disjunction in metaphase II oocytes of mice. Humangenetik 16:123–125.

Shaver, E. L., and Carr, D. H. 1967. Chromosome abnormalities in rabbit blastocysts following delayed fertilization. J. Reprod. Fertil. 14:415–420.

Shaver, E. L., and Carr, D. H. 1969. The chromosome complement of rabbit blastocysts in relation to the time of mating and ovulation. Can. J. Genet. Cytol. 11:287–293.

Speed, R. M. 1977. The effects of aging on the meiotic chromosomes of male and female mice. Chromosoma 64:241–255.

Stene, J., Fischer, G., Stene, E., Mikkelsen, M., and Petersen, E. 1977. Paternal age effect in Down's syndrome. Ann. Hum. Genet. 40:299–306.

Strausmanis, R., Henrikson, I. B., Holmberg, M., and Ronrback, C. 1978. Lack of effect on the chromosomal non-disjunction in aged female mice after low dose x-irradiation. Mutat. Res. 49:269–274.

Uchida, I. A., and Freeman, C. P. V. 1977. Radiation-induced nondisjunction in oocytes of aged mice. Nature 265:186–187.

Yamamoto, M., Endo, A., and Watanabe, G. 1973. Maternal age dependence of chromosome anomalies. Nature 241:141–142.

Yamamoto, M., Shimada, T., Endo, A., and Watanabe, G. 1973. Effects of low dose x-irradiation on the chromosomal nondisjunction in aged mice. Nature 244:206–208.

Author Index

Subject Index